PRIMARY CARE OF THE POSTERIOR SEGMENT

PRIMARY CARE OF THE POSTERIOR SEGMENT

Larry J. Alexander, O.D.
Professor
UAB School of Optometry/The Medical Center
University of Alabama at Birmingham
Birmingham, Alabama

Appleton & Lange
East Norwalk, Connecticut/San Mateo, California

0-8385-7925-6

Notice: Our knowledge in clinical sciences is constantly changing. As new information becomes available, changes in treatment and in the use of drugs become necessary. The author   and the publisher of this volume have taken care to make certain that the doses of drugs and schedules of treatment are correct and compatible with the standards generally accepted at the time of publication. The reader is advised to consult carefully the instruction and information material included in the package insert of each drug or therapeutic agent before administration. This advice is especially important when using new or infrequently used drugs.

Copyright © 1989 by Appleton & Lange
A Publishing Division of Prentice Hall

90 91 92 93 / 10 9 8 7 6 5 4 3 2

Prentice Hall International (UK) Limited, *London*
Prentice Hall of Australia Pty. Limited, *Sydney*
Prentice Hall Canada, Inc., *Toronto*
Prentice Hall Hispanoamericana, S.A., *Mexico*
Prentice Hall of India Private Limited, *New Delhi*
Prentice Hall of Japan, Inc., *Tokyo*
Simon & Schuster Asia Pte. Ltd., *Singapore*
Editora Prentice Hall do Brasil Ltda., *Rio de Janeiro*
Prentice Hall, *Englewood Cliffs, New Jersey*

Library of Congress Cataloging-in-Publication Data
Alexander, Larry J.
    Primary care of the posterior segment / Larry J. Alexander.
       p.   cm.
    Includes index.
    ISBN 0-8385-7925-6
    1. Posterior segment (Eye)—Diseases.   I. Title.
    DNLM: 1. Eye Diseases.   WW 140 A376p
RE475.A44   1989
617.7'3—dc19
DNLM/DLC   89-136
for Library of Congress   CIP

Acquisitions Editor: R. Craig Percy
Production Editor: Eileen Lagoss Burns
Designer: Steven M. Byrum

PRINTED IN THE UNITED STATES OF AMERICA

Contents

Introduction

This text is designed for the practicing clinician and student. It is intended to be a teaching and reference text that is designed to improve patient care. It was prepared in response to questions from clinicians and students regarding the care and management of patients seen in the everyday practice of primary eye care.

There is currently no single source that outlines the diagnosis and, more importantly, the management of the retina. I have found that when a doctor asks me where to find a compilation of information covering this broad scope, no single source affords simplistic clinical answers to the problems. An atlas may present and describe a photograph of one or two patients, but as we all know the patient sitting in your office rarely matches the photograph. Many texts offer a guide to the differential diagnosis of disease processes, but rarely tell you what to do with the patient once the diagnosis is made. Several texts are available that take a histological approach to disease, but the crossover to usable clinical application is difficult for the average doctor.

I believe that to diagnose a disease, one must be able to clearly see and understand what is occurring within the structure. One must be able to understand what structures are being altered and in what way these changes present clinically. Once one diagnoses the disease, one must then be able to implement a well thought-out management plan. This text illustrates the clinicopathology of the process in schematic drawings and provides photographs of variations in clinical presentation. This text then carefully outlines management plans. In addition, a summary of each disease entity with appropriate management is provided in sections called "pearls." A clinical "pearl" index is also provided beginning on p. xv to enable quick reference on a particular topic. Numerous tables accompany the text to facilitate differential diagnosis. The text is written in a narrative fashion to facilitate pleasurable reading.

The text is comprised of five sections. These sections group diseases that are linked by a common thread. The sections include optic nerve diseases, retinal vascular diseases, macular diseases, diseases of the peripheral retina, and hereditary retinal and choroidal diseases. Each topic is addressed in a generic manner as new trends in interventive therapy seem to change on a daily basis.

I have written this text in response to the needs of clinicians. My goals were the improvement in the understanding of ocular diseases of the posterior pole and peripheral retina, the provision of a well thought-out management plan, and the improvement of patient care in the primary care setting. Remember as you read the text that to properly manage a problem, you must first be able to diagnose that problem. To properly diagnose the problem, you must first be able to see it clearly. To see the problem clearly, you must be able to understand the clinicopathology of disease and you must be a good observer.

Larry J. Alexander

Acknowledgments

I wish to acknowledge the support of Dean Henry Peters and Dean Bradford Wild in the preparation of the text. I also wish to acknowledge the excellent work of Mike Strawn at UAB Photography. Hazel Davis deserves special thanks for her excellent word processing talents.

Ken Norris served as the artist for the majority of the schematic drawings. I took my artistic renderings to Ken, who then made them look professional. He and I have signed all original works.

Dr. Rodney Nowakowski deserves recognition for his recommendations for the effective layout of the section on hereditary retinal and choroidal diseases.

Summary Tables

Clinical Pearls

PRIMARY CARE OF THE POSTERIOR SEGMENT

1

Congenital and Acquired Anomalies of the Optic Nerve Head

INTRODUCTION

To the health care practitioner looking inside the eye, the optic nerve head usually is the easiest landmark to view and one of the most important of all structures within the eye because of its intimate relationship to the neurological system. Disease of the optic nerve, however, can be the most difficult to differentially diagnose because of the subtleties associated with alteration of structure as well as the myriad of congenital variations present in the healthy population.

This discussion provides the clinician a good basis for recognition and implications of congenital variations as well as a sound background for effective differential diagnosis of acquired variations.

RELEVANT CLINICAL ANATOMY OF THE OPTIC NERVE HEAD

Gross Anatomy

The optic nerve actually is a white matter tract of the brain that is grossly divided into four portions: (1) intraocular, which is 1 mm in length and 1.60 mm in diameter and is about 4 mm superior and nasal to the fovea, (2) intraorbital, which is 25 to 30 mm in length traversing a tortuous course and about 3 to 4 mm in diameter (the diameter increases in back of the lamina because of the myelin sheathing of the nerve fibers), (3) intraosseus, which is 4 to 10 mm in length, and (4) intracranial, which is 14 to 20 mm in length. The retrobulbar optic nerve is surrounded by the same layers as the brain: the pia, the arachnoid, and the dura, and as such is subject to alterations from pressure and diseases in these areas.

The physiologic cup is apparent on most optic discs and varies considerably from person to person but is most often a mirror image of the fellow eye. Comparison of the structure of the optic nerve and comparison of the physiologic cups often will give a clue to the anomaly of the disc. There seems to be a larger physiologic cup in some races than in others. The status of the physiologic cup is not as important as the status of the neuroretinal rim in most acquired diseases of the optic nerve head. *The key to differential diagnosis of most anomalies of the optic nerve head is the side-by-side comparison of one nerve head to the other.*

The Neuroretinal Rim

The neuroretinal rim (Fig. 1–1) is classically described as the pink ring of capillary-rich tissue present on healthy optic nerve heads. In most cases, the rim is pinker or denser nasally than temporally. Just envision the neuroretinal rim as a donut and the physiologic cup as the hole in the donut. The appearance of this donut will vary from person to person, but the donut of the right eye should be a mirror image of the donut of the left eye. Optic nerve diseases, such as glaucoma or anterior ischemic optic neuropathy, cause bites to be taken out of the donut from the inside out (Figs. 1–2 to 1–4). This bite reflects compromised nerve fibers, resulting in visual field defects. Often this bite is not pasty white in color but rather a desaturation of the normally pink neuroretinal rim. Observation of bites out of the neuroretinal rim can be enhanced by using the red-free filter in the direct or binocular indirect ophthalmoscope. Again, variations in the neuroretinal rim are best seen by side-by-side comparisons of the two nerve heads.

Vascular Supply

Alteration of the larger vessels of the disc also can provide a clue to the cause of a funny-looking disc. The vascular supply to the optic nerve originates from the ophthalmic artery, which is a branch of the internal carotid system. This explains the direct relationship of internal carotid disease to retinal and nerve head emboli and infarcts. The central retinal artery enters the nerve posterior to the globe

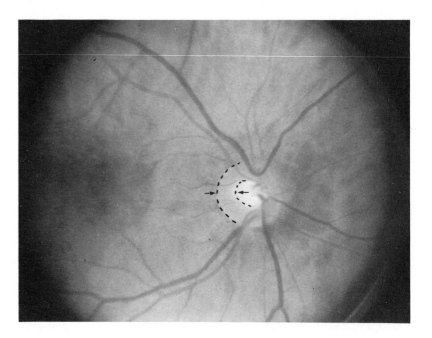

Figure 1–1. The dotted lines demarcated by the small arrows illustrate the neuroretinal rim.

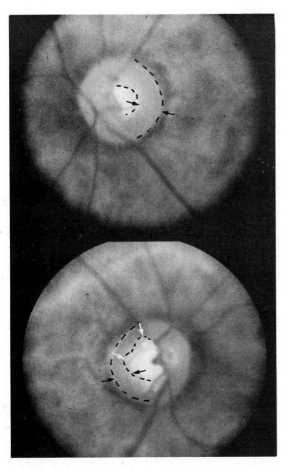

Figure 1–2. Comparison of neuroretinal rims between the two eyes is the key to diagnosis. The rim of the left disc **(top)** is intact, but the rim of the right disc **(bottom)** shows areas of notching **(white arrows)** secondary to glaucoma.

nerve head infarcts associated with such entities as anterior ischemic optic neuropathy.

Microscopic Anatomy

Nerve Fiber Layer. The optic nerve head can be separated into several regions microscopically. The surface nerve fiber layer is the most superficial of the regions. This layer consists of nonmyelinated nerve fibers entering the optic nerve from the various areas of the retina. The different areas of the retina have a specific locus on the nerve head (Fig. 1–5). The nerve fibers are separated from the overlying vitreous by a thin membrane derived from astrocytes. The nerve fibers can be envisioned as garden hoses running from a synapse at the ganglion cell to a synapse at the lateral geniculate body. The nerve impulse travels along the wall of the hose, and the center of the hose is filled with an everflowing protoplasm (axoplasm) that supplies nutrients to the fiber. Pressure on the hose, such as from increased intracranial pressure, can cause axoplasmic stasis and swelling of the nerve fibers (papilledema). Actual insult to the wall, such as that occurring with retrobulbar neuritis, can alter nerve transmission, resulting in loss or reduction in vision.

Prelaminar or Glial Region. The prelaminar or glial region is the supportive and nutritive area for the nerve fibers. This area occupies over half of the optic nerve head volume. Encircling this region is the border tissue of Elschnig, which is collagenous and acts to separate the choroid from the optic nerve.

Lamina Cribrosa Region. The lamina cribrosa region is collagenous connective and glial tissue that is continuous with and bridges the scleral canal. This sievelike tissue provides support for the exit of the nerve fibers. This can be visualized in about 35 percent of normal eyes as laminar dots at the base of the cup.

Retrolaminar Optic Nerve. The retrolaminar optic nerve is about twice the diameter of the intraocular portion because of the presence of the myeline or insulating sheath around the nerve fibers. Compromise of this myelin occurs in diseases, such as multiple sclerosis. This portion of the nerve is enclosed by the sheath of dura, arachnoid, and pia—a direct extension of the brain.

and runs forward, constricting at the lamina and entering the globe through the optic nerve head, commonly nasal to the ingress of the central retinal vein. The artery bifurcates to the superior and inferior papillary arteries to run out into the retina to supply the inner retinal layers. The central retinal vein usually forms on the disc, coursing back through the lamina, but there are occasions when this vein does not form until after passing through the lamina. The clinical example of this anomalous formation of the central retinal vein is a hemicentral retinal vein occlusion. The vein is thin-walled and very susceptible to external pressures. Most of the blood supply to the nerve head emanates from the short posterior ciliary arteries, the posterior ciliary arteries, and the pial artery. Small branches from the central retinal artery supply the most superficial layers of the optic nerve head. The blood supply to the optic nerve head is somewhat compartmentalized in nature, explaining sectoral-like

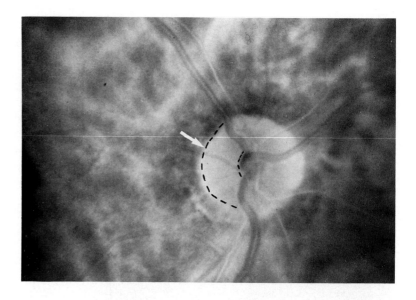

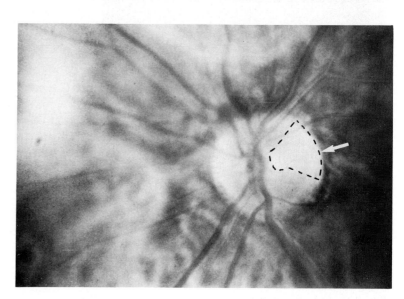

Figure 1–3. Top. The neuroretinal rim of the right disc is intact in the temporal area. **Bottom.** The neuroretinal rim of the left disc shows a bite taken at the edge of the disc. This pattern is characteristic of optic neuropathies.

DIFFERENTIAL DIAGNOSTIC TESTS FOR OPTIC NERVE HEAD ANOMALIES

Case History and Complaint

Doctors are doctors because of their deductive reasoning. They are trained to help the patient by listening to the patient and by performing tests to determine the cause of the complaint. Case history and complaint can often give a large percentage of the answer to a perplexing clinical question.

Should there be a particular complaint associated with optic nerve disease, the clinician should establish a temporal profile or a history of the complaint as it unfolds over time. The temporal profile establishes how, when, and where the symptoms first occurred. It establishes the duration of the complaint, what followed the first symptom, whether or not it recurred, circumstances surrounding the incident, and if there were associated signs or symptoms, such as headache or loss of mobility.

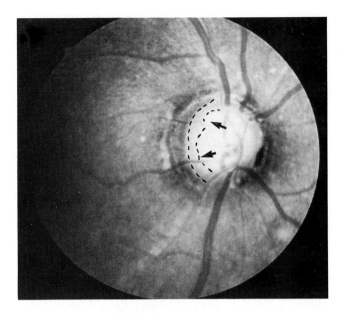

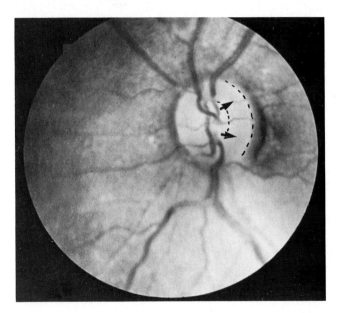

Figure 1–4. Top. The rim is compromised, especially in the area of the arrows. **Bottom.** The fellow eye is not compromised. This asymmetrical compromise of the neuroretinal rim is characteristic of glaucomatous optic atrophy. Asymmetrical visual fields usually occur as well.

In addition to the temporal profile, the clinician should consider the age and sex of the patient, the family history (pedigree), medical and medicine history, history of alcohol abuse, and history of environmental exposure. Figure 1–6 demonstrates the flow pattern of generating a good case history. Table 1–1 gives examples of symptoms that assist in diagnosis.

After determination of the complaint and case history, testing may be performed. One of the most crucial of tests is visual acuity.

Visual Acuity Testing

Certainly, visual performance analysis is the bottom line in the assessment of any eye disease. The clinician must remember that any and all tests of visual performance must be carried out through the best refractive prescription available. A significant aspect of any acuity assessment is the refraction to best visual acuity or a multiple pinhole test over the current prescription.

Visual acuity may be tested in many ways (Snellen acuities, illiterate Es) depending on the situation. In testing for diseased conditions, one also must consider assessment of functional acuities. Functional acuity can be defined as the ability to perform a vision task, such as reading. A patient with a right homonymous hemianopsia might very well be able to recognize isolated letters but would have noticeable difficulty reading a line of print. Monocular functional acuities would act as an effective means of detecting subtle ocular disease conditions.

Another consideration in visual function examination is contrast sensitivity. Tests for contrast sensitivity range from the simplest available in hand-held card form or projectable form to those generated by a computer with bracketed response curves.

Pupillary Testing

Proper pupillary testing is a crucial adjunct in testing for optic nerve disease. The swinging flashlight test or assessment for an afferent pupillary defect is the most specific test for optic nerve disease. This is also known as the Marcus-Gunn pupil test. This is a test of nerve conduction defect.

6

FIELD PROJECTION OF THE RIGHT POSTERIOR POLE

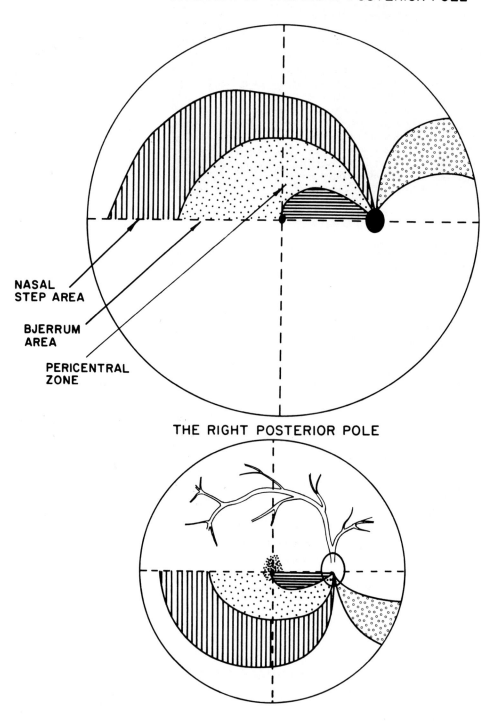

NASAL
STEP AREA

BJERRUM
AREA

PERICENTRAL
ZONE

THE RIGHT POSTERIOR POLE

Figure 1–5. Bottom. The pattern followed by the nerve fibers emanating from the right optic nerve head. **Top.** Corresponding field projection of the emanating nerve fibers.

Abbreviated Example of Case History and Complaint

Complaint: Lost vision in both eyes for 20 minutes this past weekend

Age: 35. Nurse

Sex: Female. No reported medications; no family history that would contribute to diagnosis

What time of the day? 11:00 AM

Where? A local mall. I was just walking along.

Was vision lost in both eyes or just one? Both eyes for 20 minutes

Did it come back normally? Yes

Did anything else happen during this time? Yes, I lost function of my legs.

What do you mean? I couldn't walk for about a half-hour.

Did you get a headache with this? Yes. One of my migraines.

But you told me you didn't have headaches. I forgot. ·

Did you forget to tell me anything else, like medications? Does a new experimental injectable birth control system count as medication?

Further investigation revealed a history of migraine headaches exacerbated by the injectable birth control system. Vasospasm in the vertebrobasilar area had precipitated the attacks.

Figure 1–6. Example of the generation of a case history as related to a specific complaint.

TABLE 1–1. EXAMPLES OF TEMPORAL PROFILE SYMPTOMATOLOGY

Symptom	Probable Cause
Loss of vision overnight	Common in thrombosis
5 to 15 second losses or blurs of vision	Transient obscurations of papilledema or impending central retinal vein occlusion
Abrupt loss of vision getting progressively worse	Hemorrhage
Loss of vision for a few days with a partial return	Demyelinizing disease
5 to 15 (up to 60) minute losses of vision returning to normal	Transient monocular blindness of internal carotid stenosis
Slowly progressive loss of vision	Neoplasm
Sudden bilateral contraction of fields (tubular)	Vertebrobasilar stroke sparing macular fibers
Sudden hemianopic field loss	Contralateral postchiasmal interruption of blood flow
Sudden fading of vision with postural change	Hypotensive attack; may also occur with mitral valve prolapse

HOW TO DO IT—SWINGING FLASHLIGHT TEST

This example demonstrates a case of reduced acuity secondary to optic neuropathy in the left eye.
1. Penlight on OD → OD constricts, OS constricts
2. Swing penlight to OS → OD dilates, OS dilates
3. Swing penlight to OD → OD constricts, OS constricts
4. Conclusion: OS optic nerve dysfunction or severe macular problem OS

WHEN TO DO IT—WHAT TO DO WITH THE ANSWERS

Indications	Test	Conclusion
☐ Reduced vision	☐ Swinging flashlight test	☐ Negative Marcus-Gunn test indicates reduced visual acuity, probably is caused by a macular lesion ☐ Positive Marcus-Gunn test indicates reduced visual acuity, is caused by optic nerve disease or a severe macular lesion

Should you want to enhance the view of the consensual or near response, you may darken the room and hold a Burton ultraviolet lamp about a foot from the patient to illuminate the eyes. The natural accumulation of fluorogens with age within the crystalline lens will glow without constricting the pupil. This provides an illuminated or backlit pupil on which to view the actions of the iris.

Color Vision Testing

The clinician realizes that when photoreceptors are affected in a disease process, there is a reduction or loss of function. When the cones or nerve fibers associated with the cones are involved, this will appear as some degree of color loss or desaturation. Lesions of the retina that can reduce visual acuity do not necessarily cause a proportionate reduction in color perception. Often, in-depth testing will demonstrate only mild defects. Defects in the optic nerve will, however, create faulty conduction of the nerve impulse, leading to a reduction in color perception (Table 1–2). The concept of optic nerve defects has been described as a barrier to impulse conduction within the optic nerve and to which the nerve fibers associated with cone function are preferentially sensitive. This barrier concept can be used to illustrate light comparison testing, contrast sensitivity testing, Pulfrich stereo phenomenon testing, neutral density filter testing, and evoked potential testing. In all cases, the patient presents a delayed or diminished response to stimulation. Figure 1–7 illustrates this barrier concept.

HOW TO DO IT—COLOR VISION ASSESSMENT

Must Be Performed Monocularly

---

1. The easiest and most effective method is the standard pseudoisochromatic plates from Igaku-Shoin Tokyo. These plates effectively reveal blue–yellow defects
   a. Part 1 for congenital vision defects
   b. Part 2 for acquired vision defects
2. AO HRR: Very good if you still have an old set around the office; they are no longer manufactured. AO HRR can diagnose red–green versus blue–yellow defects
3. Dvorine plates
   a. Cannot diagnose tritan defects; therefore, are of questionable value in acquired defects
   b. Designed primarily to detect congenital defects
4. D-15: Hue discrimination
   a. Mild color defectives can pass
   b. Does not distinguish between mild and moderate color deficiency
5. 100 Hue: Hue discrimination
   a. Separates normal color vision into superior, average, and low discrimination
   b. Measures zones of color confusion in congenital or acquired defects
   c. Most definitive but longest to administer

6. Desaturated D-15: Hue discrimination
   Same as D-15 but requires better hue discrimination; therefore, thought to be more sensitive

---

WHEN TO DO IT—WHAT TO DO WITH THE ANSWERS

Characteristics of Congenital Versus Acquired Color Defects

Congenital	Acquired Color Defects
☐ Usually no compromise to vision function	☐ Often altered vision function
☐ Symmetrical loss	☐ May be asymmetrical loss
☐ No change in defect over time	☐ Defect may change with status of disease
☐ Test repeatable	☐ Often poor reproducibility

Standardized color vision tests definitely have value in the assessment of diseases of the optic nerve. However, a test of color comparison provides a quick appraisal of the general status of color vision. After the patient's eyes have been equally light adapted, the clinician can present a red colored target, such as a red Mydriacyl bottle cap, to each eye alternately. The patient is asked to compare the intensity or quality of the color. The patient with a lesion of the optic nerve will report that the color is washed-out or grayish in the affected eye. This test also can be used to investigate quadrantic optic nerve defects by moving the test object

TABLE 1–2. TYPICAL DEFECTS PRODUCED BY SPECIFIC CONDITIONS

Disease	Color Defect
Optic nerve	
Glaucoma	B–Y
Dominant optic atrophy	B–Y
Alcohol optic atrophy	B–Y
Nicotine optic atrophy	R–G*
Leber's optic atrophy	R–G
Optic nerve and pathway disease	R–G
Optic neuropathy	R–G
Drusen	R–G/B–Y
Papilledema	R–G/B–Y
Macula	
Idiopathic central serous choroidopathy	B–Y
Chorioretinitis	B–Y
Diabetic maculopathy	B–Y
Hypertensive retinopathy	B–Y
Age-related maculopathy	B–Y
Stargardt's dystrophy	R–G
Vitelliform dystrophy	R–G
Central areolar dystrophy	R–G

aB, blue; G, green; R, red; Y, yellow.

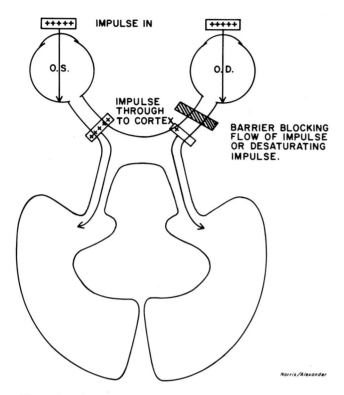

Figure 1–7. Schematic illustration of the barrier to an impulse created by an optic nerve conduction defect. *(Modified from Alexander LJ: Diseases of the optic nerve. In Bartlett JD, Jaanus SD (eds):* Clinical Ocular Pharmacology. Boston, Butterworth, 1989.)

around in the visual field. Should a field defect be present, the patient will report a color change in the cap in that part of the field.

Light Comparison Test

Another method of evaluating nerve conduction is the light comparison test. This test is a subjective evaluation of optic nerve conduction quality. It is similar to color comparison in that the patient is alternately presented a bright light and asked to compare his or her perception of the intensity or quality of the light. A patient with an optic nerve conduction defect will perceive a lower-intensity light on the affected side.

The clinician typically presents the light first to the good eye and states, "This light is worth a dollar." The light is then moved to the suspect eye, and the patient is asked, "How much is the light worth now?" I have noted, however, that patient response to this test is at best equivocal. Responses can be very misleading.

Neutral Density Filter Test

If you have a 2 log unit neutral density (2ND) filter around your office, you can use it to assist in the diagnosis of an eye with an optic nerve conduction defect. Table 1–3 illustrates the effect on visual acuity of placing a 2ND filter over a normal eye, an

eye with functional amblyopia, and an eye with an optic nerve conduction defect.

Pulfrich Stereo Phenomenon

Although I would not actively advocate this test, it is a good illustration of optic nerve conduction defects. Patients who have optic nerve disease may report that moving objects appear to look odd to them or that they are having trouble with depth perception while driving.

The Pulfrich stereo phenomenon is the binocular perception of a pendulum swinging in an elliptical path when, in fact, it is swinging in a straight path. The patient is asked to look straight ahead beyond the swinging pendulum while the pendulum bob is swung from side to side in a straight line. This illusion is created by a latency in visual signal to the cortex. This can be created artificially by placing a 2ND filter in front of one eye or by dilating one eye. It can be created also by an optic nerve conduction defect, such as that occurring in optic neuropathy or optic atrophy.

Macular Photostress Recovery Test

Macular photostress testing provides the clinician a noninvasive method of evaluation of macular physiologic function. It is important to employ tests for macular function to differentiate the cause of vision loss.

The photostress test has been defined as a dynamic test of macular performance that is based on precisely measuring the time required for an eye to recover sufficient visual function to perform a defined visual task after it has been dazzled with an intense flash of light. A prolonged photostress recovery time is thought to be secondary to altered retinal adaptation. Several studies have proven that the efficiency of retinal adaptability to stress depends not only on the photochemical mechanism of vision but also on the anatomic relationship of the photoreceptors to the retinal pigment epithelium. The photostress test serves as a sensitive discriminator between subtle maculopathy and optic neuropathy.

TABLE 1–3. NEUTRAL DENSITY FILTER TEST

Condition	Response When Filter Placed Over Eye
Normal eye	Two- to three-line reduction in acuity
Functionally-amblyopic eye	Minimal if any reduction in acuity
Eye with optic nerve conduction defect	Severe reduction in acuity

HOW TO DO IT—MACULAR PHOTOSTRESS RECOVERY TEST (MPSRT)

1. Determine the best refractive correction and place it in a trial frame
2. Use a darkened room and dark adapt one minute
3. Occlude one eye and project the line of best acuity
4. Bleach the patient's macula for 10 seconds by projecting the fixation target of the direct ophthalmoscope on the fovea
5. After bleaching, time the recovery to reading *one* line above best visual acuity
6. Repeat the procedure on the other eye after an equal time of dark adaptation
7. The average normal recovery time using this technique is 50 seconds

WHEN TO DO IT—WHAT TO DO WITH THE ANSWERS

Indications	Test	Conclusion
☐ Reduced vision		☐ If MPSRT elevated, it may indicate edema in macula
☐ Differentiating macular disease from optic nerve disease	☐ MPSRT	☐ If one eye elevated relative to the other, eye with elevated MPSRT may have edema
		☐ If no elevated MPSRT, probable optic nerve dysfunction

Amsler Grid Test

The Amsler grid test is a test of visual integrity of the macular area. The test can be sensitive if performed properly or if variations on the theme are applied effectively. Figure 1–8 illustrates the retinal area covered by Amsler grid testing. This test can be used to evaluate for retinal elevations and depressions as well as for scotomas. The Potter-Wild variation is the first significant improvement in this testing technique in years. Figure 1–9 illustrates Potter's grid (*see also* Figure 1–10).

HOW TO DO IT—STANDARD AMSLER GRID

1. Seven different charts are in the Amsler Grid Manual that test for macular integrity and metamorphopsia within a 20 degree diameter field
2. Test at 30 cm where each 5 mm square corresponds to a 1 degree visual angle

3. Use even illumination that is repeatable from time to time
4. Use the patient's correction at 30 cm
5. Ask the patient to
   a. Look at the central fixation spot
   b. Tell you if he or she sees all four corners
   c. Tell you if there are any halos or blurry spots on the chart
   d. Tell you if there are any wavy lines
   e. Draw defects on a recording grid

HOW TO DO IT—POTTER'S GRID

1. The diamond and fixation targets are red. The diamond is always temporal, that is, right side for OD testing, left side for OS testing. The diamond serves as a control of test distance
2. The patient holds the horizontal chart at arm's length with one eye closed and pulls the chart inward until the red diamond disappears in the blind spot. This is usually about 40 cm
3. The patient is asked to look for waviness or areas missing on the grid
4. The patient now repeats the test with the vertical chart

WHEN TO DO IT—WHAT TO DO WITH THE ANSWERS

Indications	Test	Conclusion
☐ Reduced vision		☐ Scotoma with no apparent macular disease indicates optic nerve dysfunction
☐ Complaints of metamorphopsia	☐ Amsler grid	☐ Metamorphopsia indicates active or resolved macular dysfunction
		☐ Scotoma with macular disease apparent indicates that the lesion is probably not active
☐ Following patients suspected of developing macular disease	☐ Home Amsler grid	

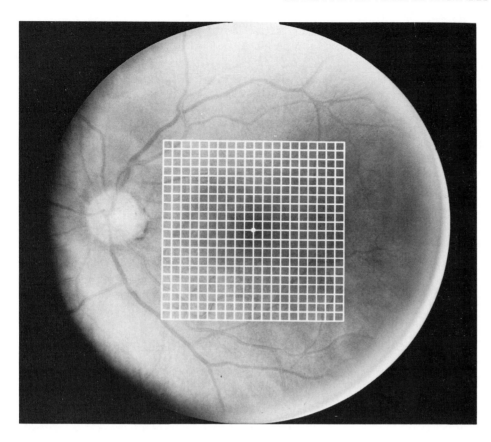

Figure 1–8. The area tested by an Amsler grid as projected onto the retinal area.

Stereoscopic Disc Viewing Techniques

The binocular indirect ophthalmoscope, the Krieger fundus lens, the Hruby lens, the center of a Goldmann three-mirror lens, and the Volk 90 and 60 diopter lens all offer an excellent view of the posterior pole. Elevations, depressions, color variations, and size differences all are key factors in diagnosing optic nerve disease. The direct ophthalmoscope just does not do it. Also remember that skill in an objective test is always better than relying on subjective patient responses.

WHEN TO DO IT—WHAT TO DO WITH THE ANSWERS—BINOCULAR INDIRECT OPHTHALMOSCOPY

Indications	Conclusion
☐ Reduced vision ☐ Flashes/floaters ☐ Aphakic and pseudophakic patients ☐ High myopes ☐ Funny-looking discs ☐ Funny-looking maculas	☐ Binocular indirect ophthalmoscopy gives information, such as elevation, depressions, better resolution, and larger field; improves ability to distinguish subtle color changes, allows a view of the peripheral retina

WHEN TO DO IT—WHAT TO DO WITH THE ANSWERS—FUNDUS LENS

Indications	Conclusion
☐ Reduced vision ☐ Altered Amsler grid ☐ Altered MPSRT ☐ Funny-looking discs	☐ Fundus lens examination gives information regarding elevations and depressions in the posterior pole when higher magnification is required

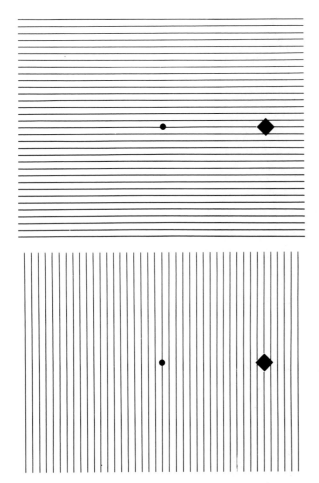

Figure 1–9. A reduced-size illustration of the macula grid test as proposed by Potter and Wild.

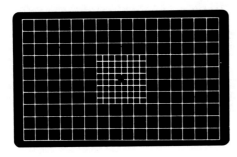

Larry J. Alexander, O.D.
Professor
UAB School of Optometry
Office: 205-934-3036 • Home: 205-822-1698
Practice: 205-934-5161

INSTRUCTIONS FOR CENTRAL VISION TEST
1. Hold Grid 14 inches away.
2. Cover left eye and look at the grid through your glasses.(Bifocal if you have one).
3. Focus on the dot and view the grid. Look for areas of the grid that are missing or wavy.
4. Repeat while covering the right eye.
5. If lines are missing or wavy call me immediately.
6. If color of dot changes when going from one eye to another, call me immediately.

Figure 1–10. A reduced-size illustration of the calling card used by the author.

Fluorescein Angiography

Fluorescein angiography is a crucial test for the differential diagnosis of retinal vascular disease and acquired serous macular disease. The technique recently has gained favor for assisting in the differential diagnosis of optic nerve disease. This is logical, since the majority of acquired optic nerve diseases would manifest delayed filling from infarcted vessels or leakage from neovascularization or inflamed discs.

Diagnostic Ultrasonography

Ultrasonography is excellent for the assessment of elevations and depressions when the crystalline lens is cloudy or the vitreous is compromised. The ultrasonographic test may be of value in suspect neoplasia or thyroid eye disease, but neurologic studies are infinitely more helpful. Figure 1–11A illustrates a normal B-scan, and Figure 1–11B illustrates a B-scan performed on a patient with buried drusen of the nerve head.

Specific Neuro-optometric Tests

Elicitation of Pain on Gross Excursion. Pain on motion of the eyes often is associated with optic neuritis. About 20 percent of patients with optic neuropathy have pain on motion of the globe, and some sources cite the percentage as being closer to 50 percent. Two important points about this symptom are (1) this is not an absolute sign of optic neuropathy, and (2) the clinician must elicit gross movements of the eyes to put enough stretch on the nerve to stimulate the pain receptors attached to the orbital wall.

Uhthoff's Symptom. Uhthoff's symptom is a loss or dimming of vision or an increase in the size of a scotoma when the body temperature is increased. This can occur while lying in the sun, while in a steam bath, or while exercising strenuously. This symptom is most often associated with loss of the myeline insulation of nerve fibers commonly occurring in demyelinizing disease.

L'Hermitte's Symptom. L'Hermitte's symptom is the sensation of electric-like shocks in the limbs and trunk when the head is flexed forward, placing the chin on the chest. This symptom is strongly suggestive of demyelinizing disease because of loss of the myelin insulation around the nerve fibers. This can, as well, be a sign of cervical injury, and, as such, the test should be performed with great care.

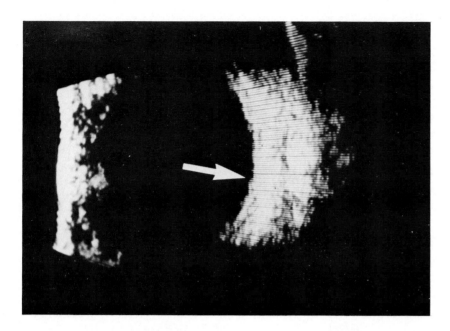

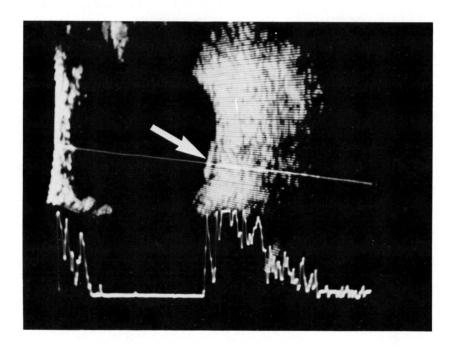

Figure 1–11. Top. A normal B-scan. **Bottom.** A B-scan with the arrow pointing to an elevated optic nerve head. The elevation in this case was secondary to buried drusen.

Tests of Cerebellar Function. Several tests of cerebellar function are available, including walking heel-to-toe down a straight line and standing with heels and toes together with eyes closed and arms outstretched (Romberg's sign). These tests usually relate to demyelinizing disease, in that coordination and balance often are compromised.

Visual Field Testing. In differentiating any disease process of the visual pathway, visual field testing is of overwhelming assistance. The subject of visual field testing is far too complicated for treatment in this discussion. The clinician should, however, remember that (1) optic nerve disease creates a hole in the visual field, (2) macular disease creates a mask over the visual field, and (3) the vertical meridians are crucial in neurologic testing (i.e., retinal disease field defects can cross the verticals, but neurologic disease field defects usually do not).

Table 1–4 summarizes diagnostic tests that may be of assistance in differentiating optic nerve diseases from macular disease.

TABLE 1–4. SUMMARY OF TESTS FOR DIFFERENTIAL DIAGNOSIS OF OPTIC NERVE VERSUS RETINAL (MACULAR) DISEASE

Test	Optic Nerve Disease	Macular Disease
Visual acuity	Reduced	Reduced
Color vision	Desaturated	May be altered depending upon severity
Light comparison test	Positive	Usually negative
Neutral density filter test	Positive	Negative
Pulfrich stereo phenomenon	Positive	Negative
Macular photostress recovery test	Negative	Positive
Pain on gross excursions	Sometimes positive	Negative
Uhthoff's symptom	Sometimes positive	Negative
L'Hermitte's symptom	Sometimes positive	Negative
Cerebellar signs	Sometimes Positive	Negative
Marcus-Gunn pupil	Positive	Negative unless gross defect
Visual fields	Hole in field	Shadow over field
Amsler grid	Scotoma	Metamorphopsia or scotoma
Fluorescein angiography	Often negative	Positive

CONGENITAL VARIATIONS OF THE OPTIC NERVE

Because of their significance in differential diagnosis, the important congenital abnormalities of the optic nerve are discussed here. Most of these anomalies are stationary rather than progressive, and many are completely benign. The majority of them is managed simply by observation alone, although a few may require surgical intervention.

Persistence of the Hyaloid System

Appearance and Layers Involved. The hyaloid artery is derived from a branch of the internal carotid artery entering the optic stalk at the 3 to 4 week embryonic stage. It typically courses forward to the lens near the end of the 4 week stage to form the tunica vasculosa lentis, the vascular supply to the developing eye. Regression of this artery usually begins at the third month and is totally regressed by the eighth month.

At the same time, the primitive epithelial papilla develops. By 7 weeks, the nerve fibers have reached the optic stalk. Bergmeister's papilla is the result of isolation of a group of primitive epithelial cells allowed to multiply to form a glial sheath around the hyaloid artery at around 4 months (Figs. 1–12 to 1–14). By the sixth month, this structure may occupy a full one third of the artery from the disc forward. During the seventh month, this structure begins to atrophy. The degree to which it atrophies and regresses determines, in part, the amount of physiologic cupping.

Incomplete regression can leave varying amounts of glial tissue on the disc or above the disc in the form of epipapillary membranes. These are usually white and almost always on the nasal side of the disc (Fig. 1–15).

A persistent hyaloid vessel (Fig. 1–16) may remain beyond full gestation. As such, it can present many pictures, from a shriveled thread trailing away from the lens (at Mittendorf's dot) to a ghost sheath coursing forward from the optic nerve head. Hyaloid artery remnants are present in 95 percent of premature infants and about 3 percent of full-term infants.

Signs and Symptoms. Signs and symptoms are usually limited to the complaint of vitreous floaters.

Prognosis and Management. Persistence of the hyaloid system usually is a benign condition except for the occasional vitreous hemorrhage that may occur should there be a patent vessel remaining in the hyaloid system.

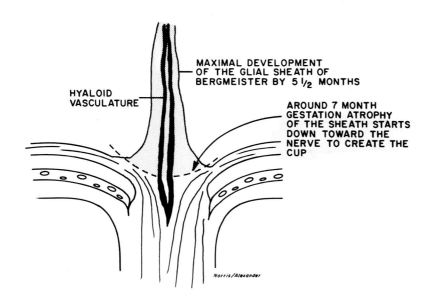

DEVELOPMENT OF
BERGMEISTER'S PAPILLA

HYALOID
VASCULATURE

MAXIMAL DEVELOPMENT
OF THE GLIAL SHEATH OF
BERGMEISTER BY 5 1/2 MONTHS

AROUND 7 MONTH
GESTATION ATROPHY
OF THE SHEATH STARTS
DOWN TOWARD THE
NERVE TO CREATE THE
CUP

Norris/Alexander

Figure 1–12. An illustration of the development of Bergmeister's papilla.

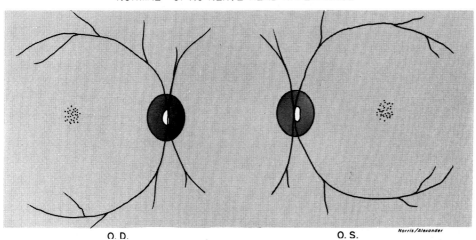

"NORMAL" OPTIC NERVE HEAD APPEARANCE

O. D.   O. S.   Norris/Alexander

Figure 1–13. A schematic of normal optic nerve head appearances. This serves to illustrate the basic concept of simultaneous comparison of optic nerve heads crucial in differential diagnosis of optic nerve head disorders.

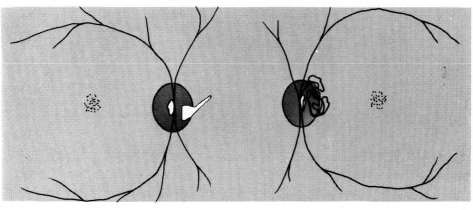

BERGMEISTER'S PAPILLA   PREPAPILLARY VASCULAR LOOP

Norris/Alexander

Figure 1–14. Illustration of the typical ophthalmoscopic presentation of Bergmeister's papilla and prepapillary vascular loops.

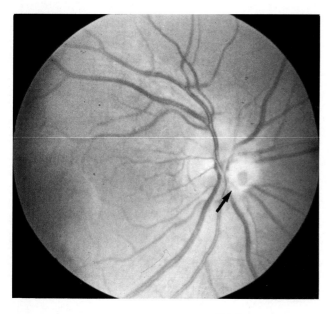

Figure 1–15. Raised area **(arrow)** on the nasal aspect of the optic nerve head, the typical location of Bergmeister's papilla.

Effective clinical management for this condition is patient education. Should a vitreous hemorrhage occur, management would consist of photocoagulation, with the possible employment of vitrectomy.

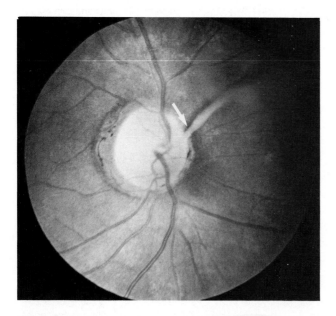

Figure 1–16. Nasal attachment of a persistent hyaloid structure **(arrow).**

PERSISTENCE OF THE HYALOID SYSTEM—PEARLS

- Regression of the hyaloid system usually complete by the eighth month
- Incomplete regression leaves varying amounts of glial tissue, usually nasal, on the disc
- Usually there are no symptoms, only a rare associated vitreous hemorrhage
- Management consists of ruling out persistent hyperplastic primary vitreous (PHPV), retinopathy of prematurity (ROP), retinoblastoma
- Routine examinations are indicated

Prepapillary Vascular Loops

Appearance and Layers Involved. Prepapillary vascular loops (Fig. 1–17) may occur on either the arterial or the venous side of the vascular system, although about 95 percent are considered arterial. These vessels appear as loops or twists extending from the optic nerve into the vitreous cavity. In 30 percent of the cases, a sheath encases the loop, indicating the embryonic nature of the vessel.

Arterial loops project varying distances into the vitreous and may move with eye movements. They usually ascend from the disc and descend back into the disc. Cilioretinal arteries also are present in about 75 percent of eyes with arterial loops emanating from the disc. There is a low incidence of bilaterality with arterial loops and no apparent association with any other ocular or systemic abnormality. These vessels most often supply the inferior retina.

Prepapillary arterial loops originate and terminate as a true branch of the central retinal artery that typically develops with but is independent of Bergmeister's papilla. Following atrophy and regression of Bergmeister's papilla, the loop remains free in the vitreous. A sheath around the loop represents incomplete regression of Bergmeister's papilla.

Prepapillary venous loops occur at about a 5 percent rate. Venous loops appear very similar to arterial loops, with the exception that the walls glisten more than arterial walls. Again, there is no apparent association of prepapillary venous loops with any systemic or ocular abnormality. Embryological development is similar to prepapillary arterial loops.

Acquired prepapillary vascular loops usually are associated with venous obstruction or a compressing optic nerve tumor. Multiple loops usually are present in the acquired variety, and the loops usually do not extend very far into the vitreous

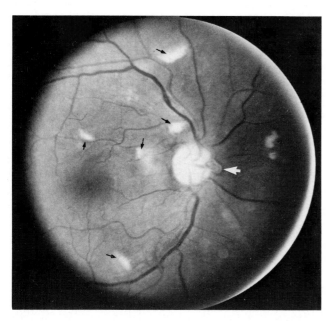

Figure 1–17. The large white arrow points to a prepapillary vascular loop, and the small black arrows point to cotton wool spots.

cavity. The acquired loops usually are referred to as "optociliary shunts."

Signs and Symptoms. Prepapillary vascular loops usually are symptomless but may be associated with transient monocular blindness, retinal artery obstruction, and vitreous hemorrhage.

Prognosis and Management. The incidence of associated retinal vascular disease is thought to be very low. In general, it can be said that prepapillary vascular loops are of no immediate threat to vision.

Management of the vascular loops consists of ruling out acquired loops, routine eye examina-

tions, and management of any complications (Table 1–5).

```
PREPAPILLARY VASCULAR LOOPS—PEARLS

• Usually unilateral, arterial, and of embryonic origin developing independent of Bergmeister's system
• Cilioretinal arteries present in 75 percent of cases
• Usually benign but may be associated with transient monocular blindness, retinal artery occlusion, and vitreous hemorrhage
• Management consists of ruling out acquired loops, patient education, and routine eye examinations
```

Miscellaneous Congenital Vascular Anomalies Associated with Optic Nerve Head

Congenital Macrovessels. An enlarged single retinal vessel can at times be seen to enter or exit the nerve head and course across the macula with branches both inferior and superior to the horizontal raphé. These are most often veins and often have arteriovenous anastomoses. There appears to be no association with systemic or ocular abnormalities. There are usually no signs or symptoms of enlarged single retinal vessels.

Management of enlarged single retinal vessels is routine eye examinations.

```
CONGENITAL MACROVESSELS—PEARLS

• Enlarged single vessel leaving the disc and crossing over the horizontal raphé
• Usually veins with possible arteriovenous anastomoses
• Management is recognition and routine examinations
```

TABLE 1–5. COMPARING PERSISTENT HYALOID ARTERIES, CONGENITAL PREPAPILLARY VASCULAR LOOPS, AND ACQUIRED PREPAPILLARY VASCULAR LOOPS

	Persistent Hyaloid Arteries	Congenital Prepapillary Vascular Loops	Acquired Prepapillary Vascular Loops
Ophthalmoscopic appearance	Single vessel, no return to disc	Vessel arising from disc and returning to disc	Often multiple loops
Extension into vitreous cavity	May run forward to lens	Usually up to one third of posterior vitreous cavity	Less than 0.5 mm
Presence of blood in vessel	Sometimes	Yes	Yes
Association with retinal vascular disease	No	No	Yes, especially venous occlusive
Complications	Vitreous hemorrhage rare	Branch arterial obstruction rare	Usually indicative of other disease processes

Racemose Angioma. Racemose angioma is an arteriovenous malformation leaving the optic nerve as an enlarged vessel, coursing through the retina, and returning to the optic nerve. This may affect vision and usually is unilateral. In more severe forms, the vessels may be so predominant as to actually obliterate vision. There is a high association with arteriovenous malformation in the central nervous system and in the skin of the face and head. These angiomas typically form at the 16th week of gestation, with the stimulus for formation being obscure.

Management of racemose angiomas includes investigation for angiomas elsewhere in the system.

RACEMOSE ANGIOMA—PEARLS

- Arteriovenous malformation leaving the optic nerve as an enlarged vessel and returning to the nerve
- Usually unilateral and, if large enough, may affect vision
- Management includes recognition and a neurological consultation to rule out angiomas in the central nervous system
- Routine eye examinations are indicated

Cilioretinal Vessels. The cilioretinal artery (Figs. 1–18 to 1–21) is not derived from the central retinal artery. It may be derived from the short posterior ciliary system or the choroidal system. Cilioretinal arteries are relatively common, occurring in at least 20 percent of eyes. Nearly 90 percent are positioned temporally and supply the inner retina in the papillomacular bundle. Cilioretinal veins occur with less frequency than do cilioretinal arteries. From an ophthalmoscopic standpoint, the cilioretinal artery appears to hook out of the temporal edge of the disc and course toward the macula. The cilioretinal artery is most easily seen in a central retinal artery occlusion because flow is maintained in the distribution area, whereas the rest of the retina becomes opaque because of oxygen starvation.

The cilioretinal vascular system is of no concern in the long-term management of the patient. It is of some benefit to patients with a central retinal artery occlusion, since a degree of vision is maintained in the distribution pattern of the cilioretinal artery. There also are instances when the cilioretinal artery may be obstructed, creating a central scotoma.

CILIORETINAL VESSELS—PEARLS

- Usually derived from the short posterior ciliary artery system or choroidal vascular system
- Occur in 20 to 25 percent of the population, 90 percent positioned temporally, hooking out of the edge of the disc and running in the papillomacular bundle
- May be patent in a central retinal artery occlusion
- Management is recognition and routine eye examinations

Myelinated Nerve Fibers

Appearance and Layers Involved. Myelinated nerve fibers (also called medulated nerve fibers) appear in many patterns and may be distributed throughout the eye. The structural changes are confined solely to the nerve fiber layer. In embry-

CILIORETINAL ARTERY   CONGENITAL MACROVESSEL

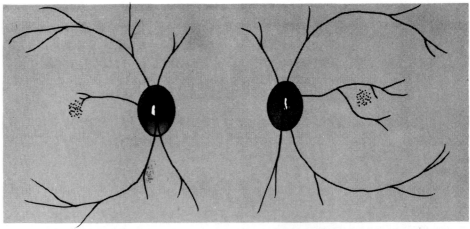

Figure 1–18. Schematic illustrating the typical appearance of a cilioretinal artery (note the hook at the edge of the disc) and a congenital macrovessel (note the crossing over the horizontal raphé and invasion into the macula).

Norris/Alexander

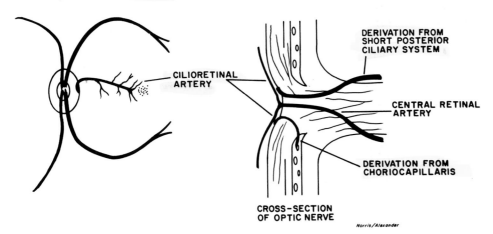

ORIGIN AND APPEARANCE OF
THE CILIORETINAL ARTERY

CILIORETINAL
ARTERY

DERIVATION FROM
SHORT POSTERIOR
CILIARY SYSTEM

CENTRAL RETINAL
ARTERY

DERIVATION FROM
CHORIOCAPILLARIS

CROSS-SECTION
OF OPTIC NERVE

Norris/Alexander

Figure 1–19. Schematic illustrating the clinical appearance and proposed origin of the cilioretinal artery.

onic development, myelination of the nerve fibers usually ceases at the level of the lamina cribrosa. If, however, the myelination persists into the eye, the characteristic appearance is that of superficial opacification with flayed edges (Fig. 1–22). This feathery pattern is very superficial and will thus block visualization of all underlying structures, such as retinal blood vessels. It may totally surround the optic nerve (Fig. 1–23).

Myelinated nerve fibers occur in about 1 percent of the population.

Signs and Symptoms. Usually, myelination of nerve fibers is of no consequence, although it has

the potential to cause visual field compromise at threshold levels. There have been some reports of association of myelinated nerve fibers with myopia, amblyopia, and strabismus. Some authors have cited examples of spontaneous appearance of myelination and of disappearance with demyelinizing disease.

Prognosis and Management. Myelinated nerve fibers typically are benign and stable, creating no long-term problems.

Management consists of definitive diagnosis and routine eye examinations.

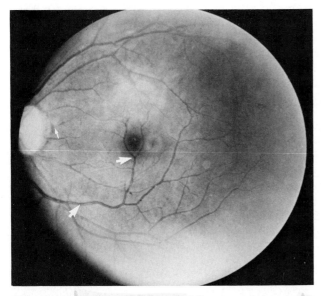

Figure 1–20. Congenital macrovessel **(large arrows)** and a cilioretinal artery **(small arrow).**

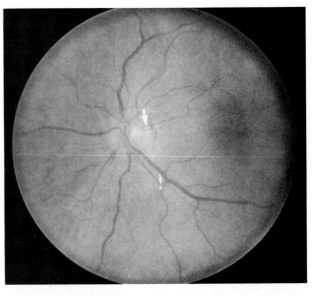

Figure 1–21. The large arrow points to the hook of a cilioretinal vessel. The small arrow points to a Hollenhorst plaque.

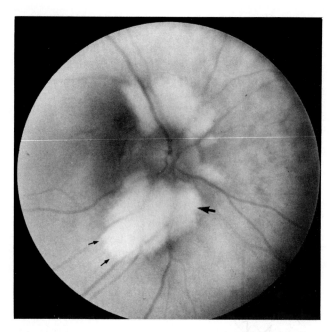

Figure 1–22. Illustration of myelinated nerve fibers. The small arrows point to the feathered or flayed edges.

MYELINATED NERVE FIBERS—PEARLS

- Superficial retinal opacification with feathered edges
- May totally surround the optic nerve
- May create visual field loss at threshold
- Management is ruling out cotton wool spots and routine examinations

---

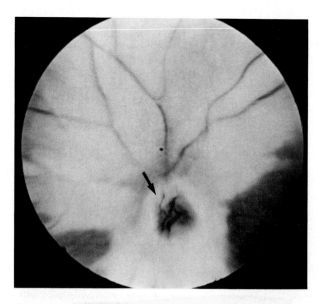

Figure 1–23. A dramatic case of myelinated nerve fibers. The arrow points to the optic disc.

Choroidal and Scleral Crescents: Circumpapillary Changes

Appearance and Layers Involved. Crescents can appear as isolated anatomic alterations or can be associated with other congenital and acquired optic nerve head anomalies. A choroidal crescent is a different color (usually darker) than the adjacent optic nerve head and retina. The choroidal crescent occurs because the retinal pigment epithelium is not abutted to the disc tissue, allowing the underlying choroid to show through (Fig. 1–24). The scleral crescent is a variation of white coloration because neither the retinal pigment epithelium nor the choroid abuts the nerve head, revealing the underlying white sclera (Fig. 1–25). The scleral crescent often is associated with high myopia because of the elongation of the eyeball. As the eye stretches, the retinal pigment epithelium and choroid are pulled away from the disc tissue. The crescents usually occur at the temporal aspect of the disc.

Signs and Symptoms. There are no particular signs or symptoms associated with crescents other than those occurring with diseases, such as progressive myopia. Physiological blind spots may be enlarged.

Prognosis and Management. Crescents in and of themselves are benign, and management consists of proper differential diagnosis. The differential diagnosis must include circumpapillary atrophy, which may occur in elderly patients. This is essentially the histopathologic equivalent of dry age-related maculopathy. Circumpapillary atrophy can be differentiated from the circumpapillary choroiditis associated with presumed ocular histoplasmosis by the presence of pigment clumping in the choroiditis (Figs. 1–26 to 1–31). **A summary of differential diagnostic features of circumpapillary changes is outlined in Table 1–6. See color plates 54 and 57.**

CHOROIDAL AND SCLERAL CRESCENTS— PEARLS

- Choroidal crescent usually is darker than the retina, occurring because the retinal pigment epithelium is not abutted to the optic nerve
- Scleral crescent is white, occurring because the retinal pigment epithelium and choroid are not abutted to the optic nerve
- Scleral crescents may be associated with ectasia of the posterior pole
- Management consists of ruling out other causes of circumpapillary changes

CRESCENT FORMATION

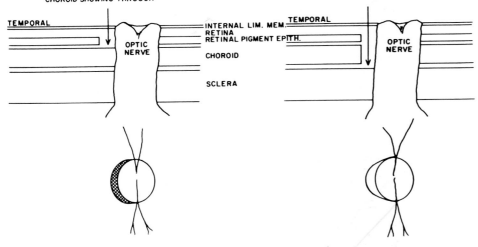

A. CHOROIDAL CRESCENT

CHOROID SHOWING THROUGH

TEMPORAL

OPTIC NERVE

B. SCLERAL CRESCENT

SCLERA SHOWING THROUGH

TEMPORAL

OPTIC NERVE

INTERNAL LIM. MEM.
RETINA
RETINAL PIGMENT EPITH.

CHOROID

SCLERA

Figure 1–24. Schematic illustrating the reason for development of a choroidal crescent **(A)** and a scleral crescent **(B)**.

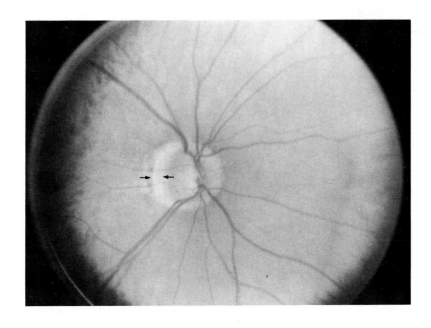

Figure 1–25. The arrows point to a scleral crescent.

CIRCUMPAPILLARY CHOROIDITIS   CIRCUMPAPILLARY ATROPHY

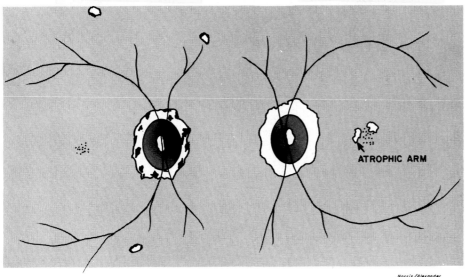

ATROPHIC ARM

Norris/Alexander

Figure 1–26. This schematic illustrates the expected patterns in circumpapillary choroiditis often associated with presumed ocular histoplasmosis and, in circumpapillary atrophy, often associated with dry age-related maculopathy.

21

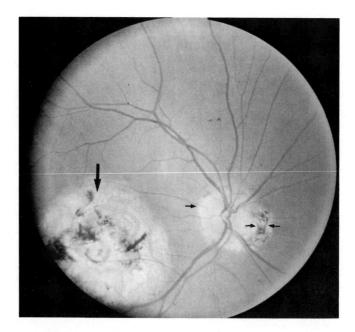

Figure 1–27. The large arrow points to a disciform macular scar, and the small arrows point to the circumpapillary choroiditis associated with this case of presumed ocular histoplasmosis syndrome.

PIGMENTED PARAVENOUS RETINOCHOROIDOPATHY

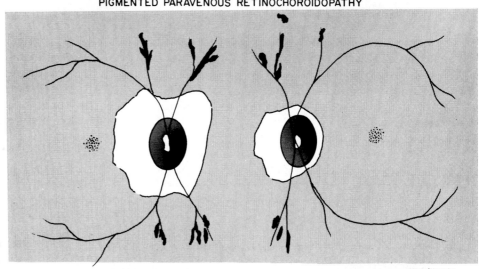

Norris/Alexander

Figure 1–28. This schematic illustrates both the circumpapillary changes and the pigmented paravenous changes in pigmented paravenous retinochoroidopathy.

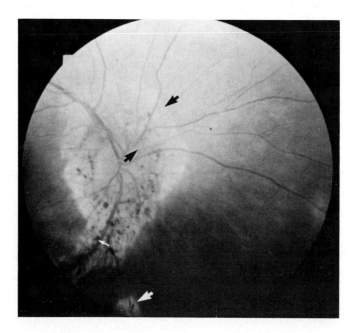

Figure 1–29. The black arrows point to the circumpapillary changes, and the white arrows point to the paravenous changes, in this case of, pigmented paravenous retinochoroidopathy.

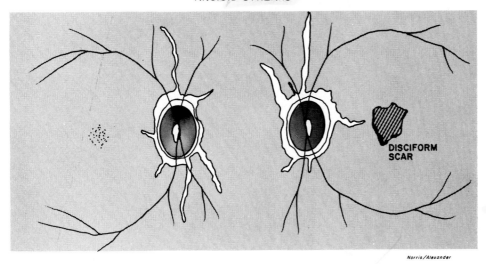

Figure 1–30. A schematic representation of angioid streaks with the circumpapillary hub from which spokes emanate. Often, a disciform scar is the result of choroidal neovascular nets.

The Tilted Disc

Appearance and Layers Involved. The optic nerve head can be tilted in any direction and usually has a crescent at the border in the direction of the downward tilt. The tilt is usually inferior nasal in the true tilted disc syndrome, whereas it usually is tilted temporally (the nasal aspect of the disc is raised) in the malinsertion syndrome. The malinsertion syndrome is very common, creating a raised nasal aspect of the disc and a depressed temporal aspect. This gives a papilledema-like appearance to the disc by direct ophthalmoscopy because the raised portion creates blurred disc margins. The malinsertion is actually an oblique insertion of the optic nerve through the scleral canal (Fig. 1–32) and is of no consequence except for confounding the differential diagnosis. Figures 1–33 to 1–37 illustrate various types of tilted discs.

The tilted disc syndrome consists of tilting of the vertical axis of the nerve head off 90 degrees, accompanied by a horizontal tilting. The tilt is usually toward the inferonasal direction, resulting in a nasal area of fundus ectasia and an accompanying crescent. If bilateral (75 percent), there also is an associated bitemporal field defect that corresponds to the area of ectatic fundus. This field defect can be made to improve by increasing the myopic correction when retesting the field. There may, however, be enough of an ectasia to physically misalign the photoreceptors, rendering them subject to the Stiles-Crawford effect. If torted enough, the receptor are desensitized, which reduces visual acuity. Oblique myopic astigmatism with slight reduction in visual acuity often is associated with the condition. Ocular situs inversus, the vessel pattern on the nerve head, is a feature of the tilted disc syndrome. In normal optic discs, the vessels leave the

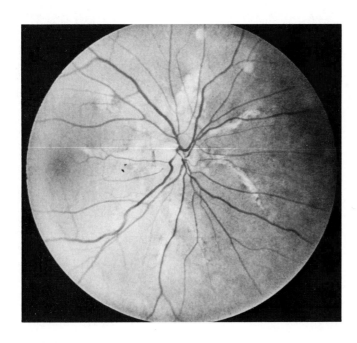

Figure 1–31. A typical case of angioid streaks.

TABLE 1–6. COMPARISON OF CIRCUMPAPILLARY CHANGES

Characteristics	Choroidal Crescent	Temporal Scleral Crescent	Circumpapillary Atrophy	Temporal Isolated Zones of Peripapillary Atrophy	Circumpapillary Choroiditis	Nasal Scleral Crescent	Angioid Streaks	Pigmented Paravenous Retinochoroidopathy
Refractive status	Not applicable	High myopia	Not applicable, possible reduced visual acuity or amblyopia	Not applicable	Not applicable	Oblique myopic astigmatism	Not applicable	Not applicable
Associated ophthalmoscopic signs	Not applicable	Thinned retina, dragged disc vessels, isolated choroidal atrophy	Possible Dry ARM[a], Peripheral drusen, CONH	Atrophy of the neuroretinal rim	Possible Peripheral chorioretinitis Disciform maculopathy	Situs inversus, nasal staphyloma	Streaks emanating from disc, possible disciform maculopathy	Pigment hyperplasia attached to veins
Associated systemic signs	Not applicable	Not applicable	AGE or in CONH, neurological and endocrine signs possible	Not applicable	Possible systemic histoplasmosis	Not applicable	Pseudoxanthoma elasticum, Paget's disease, sickle cell disease	Not applicable
Associated visual field signs	Not applicable	Possible scotomas in late stages	Enlarged blind spot	Pericentral scotomas, nasal steps	Possible Central scotoma Enlarged blind spot	Bitemporal field defects crossing verticals	Possible Central scotoma Field defects with streaks	Field defects in areas of pigment change
Associated diagnosis	Normal anatomical variant	Degenerative myopia	Age-related choroidopathy	Glaucoma	POHS	Tilted disc syndrome	Angioid streaks	Pigmented paravenous retinochoroidopathy

[a]ARM, age-related maculopathy; CONH, congenital optic nerve hypoplasia; AGE, age or age-related change. POHS, presumed ocular histoplasmosis syndrome.

MAL-INSERTION OF THE OPTIC NERVE

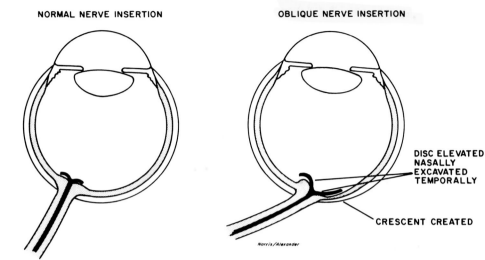

NORMAL NERVE INSERTION

OBLIQUE NERVE INSERTION

DISC ELEVATED NASALLY
EXCAVATED TEMPORALLY

CRESCENT CREATED

Norris/Alexander

Figure 1–32. Schematic illustrating the results of oblique entry of the optic nerve into the eye.

disc in a direct path toward the quadrants that they supply. In situs inversus, the temporal vessels first course toward the nasal retina before making their sharp temporal turn. Situs inversus is of no significance except for the strange appearance of the nerve head. **See color plates 2 and 3.**

Signs and Symptoms. There are no particular signs and symptoms of the tilted disc syndrome other than the bitemporal visual field defects when the condition is bilateral. The clinician must rule out chiasmal compromise in the case of bitemporal visual field defects. With tilted discs, the field defects cross over the vertical. Chiasmal compromise respects the vertical meridians of the visual field until the latter stages of chiasmal invasion.

Prognosis and Management. Tilted discs are benign, stable anatomic variations. Although they are considered by some to be variations of colobomas, there does not seem to be an increased risk

for retinal detachment as there is with other optic nerve head coloboma variations. Differential diagnosis is crucial, coupled with routine eye examination follow-up.

TILTED DISCS—PEARLS

- Malinsertion consists of elevation of the nasal aspect of the disc with temporal depression
  1. Possible scleral crescent
  2. Possible visual field alteration
  3. Rule out causes of optic disc edema and encourage routine examinations

- Tilted disc syndrome
  1. Tilting of the vertical axis of the disc with situs inversus
  2. Usually area of nasal retinal-choroidal ectasia
  3. Visual field defect corresponding to ectasia, possibly bitemporal
  4. Rule out other causes of field defects and encourage routine examinations

---

BILATERAL MALINSERTION OF THE DISCS

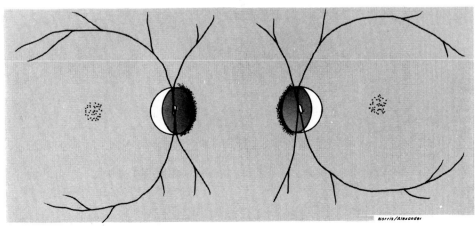

Norris/Alexander

Figure 1–33. Schematic illustrating a case of bilateral malinsertion of the discs. The nasal borders of the discs are tilted up and are blurred, and the temporal aspects of the discs are excavated with a resultant scleral crescent. This is at times referred to as "tilted discs."

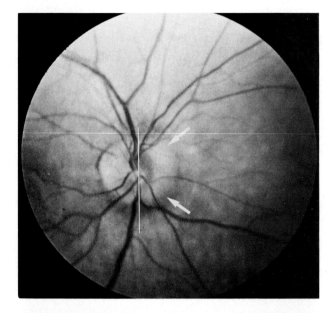

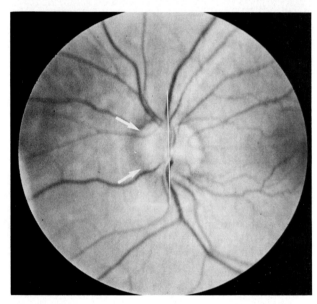

Figure 1–34. Photographs of bilaterally tilted discs (malinsertion) with the arrows pointing to elevated nasal disc margins. The tilting occurs along the vertical axis of the discs.

Circumpapillary Staphyloma

Appearance and Layers Involved. Although rare, the circumpapillary staphyloma can cause confusion from a diagnostic standpoint. This condition is characterized by an optic nerve head, usually fairly normal in appearance, lying elevated at the base of a staphyloma. Because of the stretching in the area, the surrounding retina and choroid usually show pigmentary changes (Fig. 1–38). The diagnosis is enhanced by stereoscopic viewing techniques and B-scan ultrasonography (Fig. 1–39).

The acuity usually is reduced, but instances occur with normal acuity and constricted fields.

The condition is most often unilateral and is considered to be the result of failure of development of the sclera. Tissue is not missing as it is in a coloboma, but rather the sclera is bulging or ectatic.

Signs and Symptoms. If the circumpapillary staphyloma is unilateral, the patient has reduced vision in the affected eye, with a possible squint. There is not the strong predilection toward retinal detachment as with colobomatous defects.

Prognosis and Management. Circumpapillary staphylomas must first be properly diagnosed. They are benign, self-limited conditions. The patient should wear safety glasses to protect the unaffected eye and should have routine eye examinations. **See color plate 1.**

CIRCUMPAPILLARY STAPHYLOMA—PEARLS

- Usually unilateral, with optic nerve lying elevated at the base of an area of staphyloma
- Area around disc is depigmented
- Reduced vision or constricted fields
- Diagnosis assisted by ultrasonography (B-scan)
- Management consists of patient education and provision of safety eyewear
- Routine eye examinations are indicated

Congenital Coloboma of the Optic Nerve Head

Appearance and Layers Involved. A coloboma is a hole that is the result of absence of tissue (Fig. 1–40). The varieties of colobomas of the optic nerve are many and are discussed separately. There is a fairly common thread that runs through all of these defects. In all varieties of coloboma, the affected nerve head is larger than its fellow and invariably has funny-looking vessels emanating from the disc. With stereoscopic viewing, the clinician can also expect variable excavation at some location within the nerve head.

The true congenital coloboma of the optic nerve head (Fig. 1–41) is secondary to incomplete closure of the embryonic fissure. It can be confined to the nerve head or can be present in combination with a retinochoroidal coloboma (Fig. 1–42). In either case, the site of presentation is usually the in-

UNILATERAL TILTED DISC

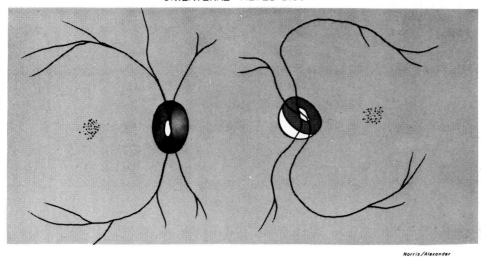

Norris/Alexander

Figure 1–35. Schematic illustrating tilting of the vertical axis of the disc.

ferior portion of the disc or retina. As stated previously, some form of unusual vessel arrangement also is present as well as enlargement of the affected nerve head. There are usually pigmentary anomalies surrounding the coloboma. Visual acuity can be reduced to light perception, and visual field changes are related to the position and extent of the colobomatous defect.

At times, glial tissue will fill the depths of the coloboma, giving an unusual appearance approaching that of the morning glory disc. Some believe that the morning glory disc and the full-blown optic nerve coloboma represent opposite limits of a continuous spectrum. There should be little difficulty in making a differential diagnosis if stereoscopic observation techniques are used. B-scan ul-

trasonography (Fig. 1–43) is also of value in differential diagnosis.

Colobomas may occur elsewhere in the ocular system, but their presence elsewhere is not necessarily the rule (Figs. 1–44 and 1–45).

Signs and Symptoms. Since the condition is congenital, the problem may appear on a routine screening for visual acuity. The patient with a coloboma of the nerve head often will report some reduction in visual acuity. There are other ocular associations with optic nerve coloboma, including myopia, hyaloid system remnants, and posterior lenticonus. Systemic associations include transphenoidal encephalocele, cardiac defects, and drug-related congenital anomalies.

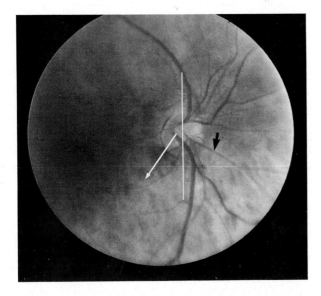
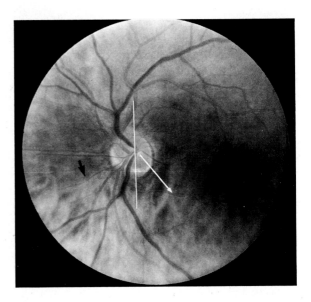

Figure 1–36. These photographs illustrate tilting of the discs off the vertical axis. The true vertical axis of the disc is illustrated by the white arrow. Often, there is a staphylomatous area of the retina in the inferior nasal zone **(black arrows)**.

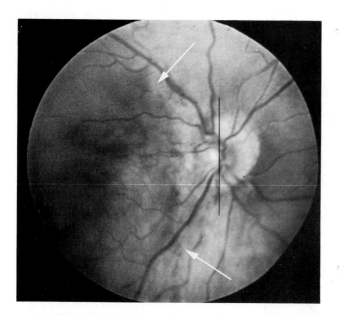 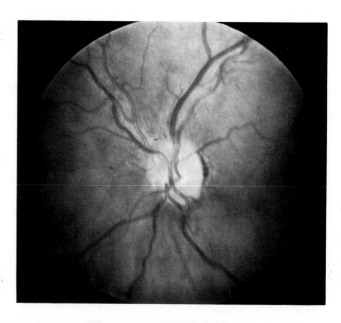

Figure 1–37. Left. The disc appears tilted in this right eye. Actually, there is a staphyloma in the macular area **(arrows)** that creates a depression temporal to the black line. **Right.** The disc in the fellow eye is normal by comparison.

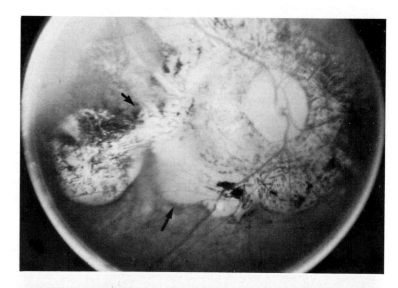

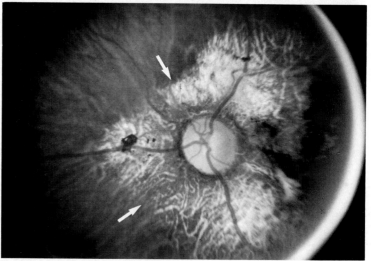

Figure 1–38. Top and Bottom. Examples of circumpapillary staphylomas.

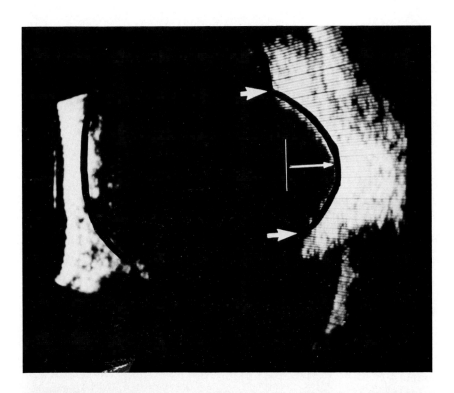

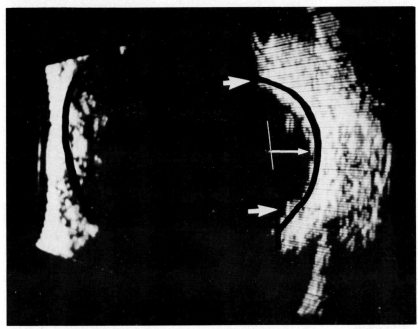

Figure 1–39. Top and Bottom. B-scan ultrasonography of posterior staphylomas. The large white arrows point to the normal retinal surface, the white lines show the expected area for the retinal surface, and the small arrows indicate the depth of the depression.

Retinochoroidal colobomas have numerous associated systemic conditions involving the cardiovascular system, the central nervous system, the musculoskeletal system, the gastrointestinal system, the genitourinary system, and the nasopharyngeal system. Chromosomal anomalies have been linked to retinochoroidal colobomas. **See color plate 4.**

Prognosis and Management. There is a strong association between optic nerve head coloboma and retinal detachment. The retina is severely stretched as it dives down into the coloboma. The physical evidence for this retinal compromise is the pigment hyperplasia that is usually present at the borders of the coloboma. The detachment often occurs in the second to third decade, involving subretinal fluid in the papillomacular area. Perhaps liquefied vitreous may leak through the areas of retinal structure compromise at the borders of the coloboma, allowing the retina to lift away. One fourth of patients with colobomas and retinal de-

CONGENITAL COLOBOMA OF THE OPTIC NERVE

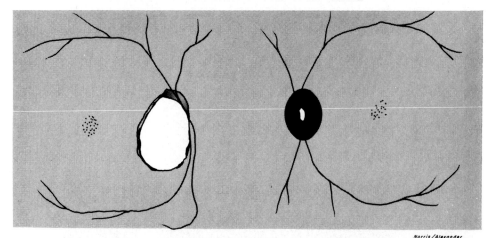

Figure 1–40. Schematic representation of a unilateral congenital coloboma of the optic nerve. The affected nerve is larger, the coloboma is surrounded by pigment, and the location is inferior.

Norris / Alexander

tachment lose vision permanently. The detachments associated with optic nerve colobomas usually are nonrhegmatogenous, whereas those in retinochoroidal colobomas usually are rhegmatogenous. There are reports of circumpapillary retinal traction associated with optic nerve colobomas.

Although the coloboma is benign and self-limited, there is concern for the development of an associated retinal detachment. The clinician must protect the eye by dissuading the patient from participation in contact sports and by the provision of maximal protective eyewear. Routine yearly eye examinations are indicated.

In patients with retinochoroidal coloboma, it is important that the clinician rule out the myriad of possibilities of associations with systemic abnormalities and chromosomal disorders.

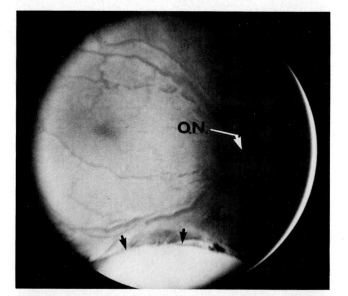

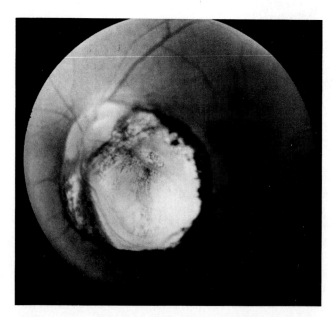

Figure 1–41. Photograph of a congenital coloboma of the left optic nerve. Note the retinal pigment epithelial hyperplasia surrounding the defect.

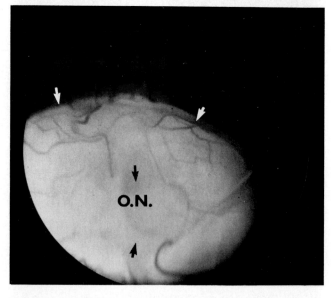

Figure 1–42. **Top.** A retinal–choroidal coloboma **(black arrows).** **Bottom.** A combined retinal–choroidal–optic nerve coloboma in the fellow eye.

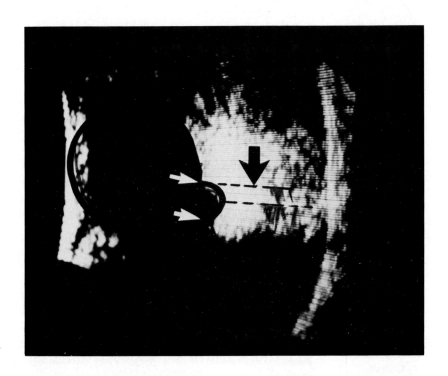

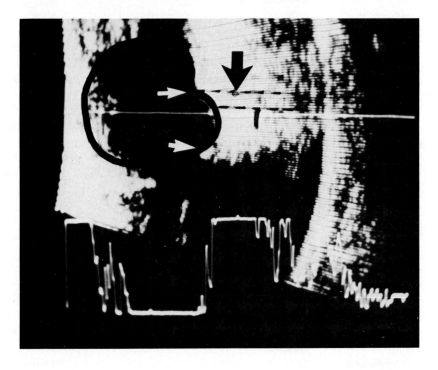

Figure 1–43. Top and Bottom. B-scan ultrasonography of the eye in Figure 1–42B taken at slightly different angles. The dotted lines demarcate the optic nerve. The white arrows point to the extent of the coloboma.

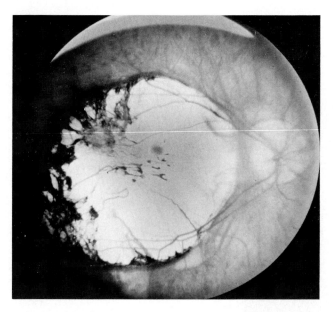

Figure 1–44. Example of a retinal–choroidal coloboma in the macular area. Note the retinal pigment epithelial hyperplasia surrounding the coloboma.

CONGENITAL COLOBOMA OF THE OPTIC NERVE HEAD—PEARLS

- Affected nerve head always is larger than its fellow, with unusual vascular pattern
- Usually inferior portion of optic nerve head with significant excavation and surround of pigment hyperplasia
- Reduced visual acuity and visual field defects are present
- Often associated with systemic abnormalities
- Strong association with nonrhegmatogenous retinal detachment in optic nerve variety and rhegmatogenous retinal detachment in retinochoriodal variety
- Management includes
  - Rule out systemic abnormalities
  - Protective eyewear
  - Patient education about signs and symptoms of retinal detachment
  - Routine yearly examinations

Morning Glory Disc

Appearance and Layers Involved. The morning glory disc (Figs. 1–46 to 1–48) is a unilaterally enlarged, funnel-shaped or scalloped area of the optic nerve head that is surrounded by an elevated ring of chorioretinal pigmentary disturbance. The condition gets its name from its resemblance to the flower. As in the optic nerve head coloboma, there is an associated enlargement of the affected disc, an abnormal vascular pattern (the vessels appear to enter and exit the disc at the margins), and an excavation when viewed using stereoscopic techniques. The vessels of the nerve head are often hidden by white central tissue. There may also be narrowing and sheathing of the arteries. Although the number of disc vessels is, in fact, normal, it appears that there are too many on the nerve head. The right eye is involved most often, and morning glory disc is seen in females twice as frequently as in males.

The embryologic origin of the morning glory disc anomaly is somewhat controversial. It is thought by some to be a variant of an optic nerve coloboma (central coloboma), and others believe it to be a variety of optic nerve dysplasia.

Signs and Symptoms. Visual acuity varies from just barely reduced to hand motion in the morning glory disc anomaly. Since it is most often unilateral, it is usually asymptomatic and may be discovered on routine vision screening. There may be an associated squint (50 percent), and there is often an association with myopia. Many ocular abnormalities have been associated with the morning glory disc anomaly, including cataracts, persistent hyaloid system and Bergmeister's papilla, persistent pupillary membrane, ciliary body cysts, microcornea and micro-ophthalmos in the contralateral eye, and Duane's retraction syndrome.

There are also related systemic abnormalities, including basal encephalocele and hypertelorism. For this reason, radiologic studies may be indicated in patients with morning glory disc anomaly should questionable neurologic signs be present. **See color plate 5.**

Prognosis and Management. The morning glory disc anomaly is a benign, nonprogressive condition, although there is a strong association with the development of nonrhegmatogenous retinal detachment confined to the posterior pole as in other forms of optic nerve head colobomas. The detachments appear to be somewhat resistent to repair.

The most important aspect of management of the morning glory disc anomaly is proper diagnosis. Because of the association with retinal detachment, contact sports should be avoided, and protective eyewear should be prescribed. Routine yearly examinations are indicated.

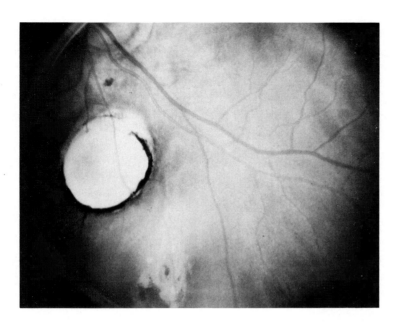

Figure 1–45. Example of a small retinal–choroidal coloboma inferior to the optic nerve.

MORNING GLORY DISC—PEARLS

- Affected nerve head is larger than its fellow, with unusual vascular pattern
- Funnel-shaped nerve head with a surround of elevated chorioretinal pigmentary disturbance
- Variable visual acuity and visual field disturbance
- Related systemic abnormalities may occur
- Strong association with nonrhegmatogenous retinal detachment
- Management includes
  - Rule out systemic abnormalities
  - Protective eyewear
  - Patient education about signs and symptoms of retinal detachment
  - Routine yearly examinations

Congenital Pits of the Optic Nerve Head

Appearance and Layers Involved. Congenital pits of the optic nerve head may vary considerably in their presentation (Figs. 1–49 to 1–51). They are a discolored area of the nerve head varying from yellowish white to olive-gray (60 percent are gray). This color variation is thought to be related to the remnants of glial retinal elements at the base of the pit. Membranous coverings over the pit also may alter the color. The shape may vary from a slitlike pit, known as the "6:45 syndrome," to round or oval. Color and shape are, however, not reliable for differential diagnosis. The 6:45 syndrome refers to the o'clock position of the pit on the right optic nerve head.

UNILATERAL MORNING GLORY DISC ANOMALY

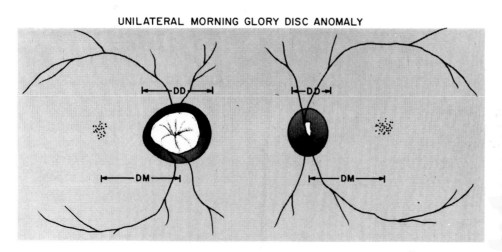

Figure 1–46. Schematic of a unilateral morning glory disc anomaly. As with all congenital optic nerve head defects, the affected disc is larger than the normal disc. Note also the reduced disc-macula/disc-disc DM/DD ratio associated with morning glory disc anomalies.

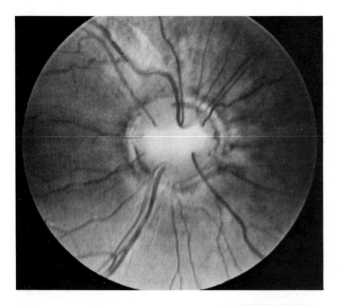

Figure 1-47. A classic presentation of a morning glory disc anomaly.

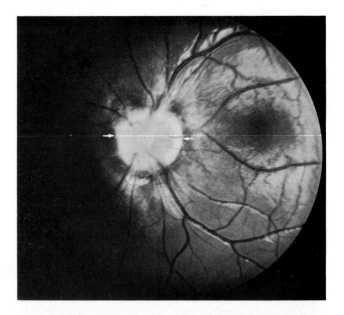

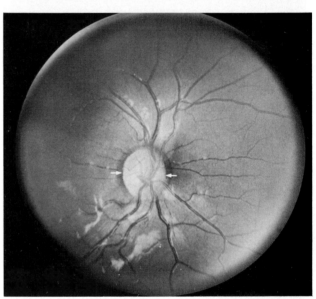

Figure 1-48. Top. The left eye with a morning glory disc. The extent of the disc is demarcated by arrows. **Bottom.** The fellow right eye has a normal-sized disc. The key to the diagnosis of congenital variations of the optic nerve is a comparison of disc sizes.

Size can be variable from 0.1 to 0.7 disc diameters, with depths from 0.5 diopters and deeper. The most common size is approximately 0.3 disc diameters. The size of the affected optic nerve head is larger than that of the unaffected eye and has an accompanying abnormal vascular pattern. Circumpapillary chorioretinal atrophy in the area of the pit is another characteristic finding, as is a cilioretinal artery (60 percent).

Pits may be located at any position on the disc, but the inferior and temporal areas are the most common. About one third of pits are located centrally. It is rare to find more than one pit per nerve head, and about 85 percent of patients have only a unilateral pit.

There is a loss of retinal ganglion cells and nerve fibers in the area of the pit that accounts for the associated visual field defect. Paradoxically, in spite of the loss of nerve fibers, there is usually no associated nerve fiber conduction defect.

The origin of the pit is controversial. Pits have been associated with incomplete closure of the fetal fissure, a coloboma-like origin. Other investigators propose that the pits result from an abnormal differentiation of the primitive epithelial papilla. Some believe that there is an associated malcommunication between the subarachnoid space surrounding the optic nerve and the optic pit. Regardless of the origin, the signs, symptoms, and prognosis are clinically well founded.

Signs and Symptoms. The patient often is unaware of the presence of an optic pit because vision usually is unaffected until the associated complica-tion of a nonrhegmatogenous retinal detachment. The pit often is discovered on a routine eye examination, especially if routine automated perimetry is performed. Approximately 60 to 70 percent of patients with pits of the nerve head have arcuate scotomas corresponding to the location of the pit. The 6:45 syndrome classically presents a pistol-grip visual field defect, which is a variation of an arcuate scotoma.

Unfortunately, a high percentage (40 to 60 percent) of patients with optic pits of the nerve head develops a nonrhegmatogenous retinal detachment

CONGENITAL PIT OF THE OPTIC NERVE

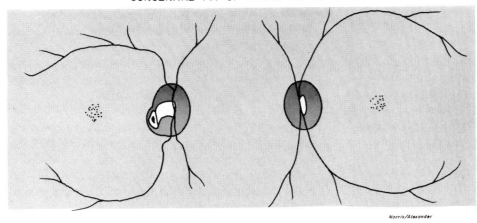

Norris/Alexander

Figure 1–49. Schematic presentation of a unilateral congenital pit of the optic nerve. As with other congenital variations, the affected optic nerve is larger. The pit is usually inferior temporal.

of the macular area extending toward the disc. The majority of these patients have temporal pits. Those with central pits rarely have detachments. The detachments associated with pits often are difficult to view because they are flat and do not undulate because of the high viscosity of the subretinal fluid. Cystic changes are seen in the elevated retina in about two thirds of the patients. These cystic changes in the inner nuclear layer may develop into lamellar macular holes. In approximately one third of the detachments, small subretinal yellow precipitates occur on the retinal surface. There appears to be a high incidence of posterior vitreous detachment associated with the serous maculopathy. The mean age of incidence of the serous mac-

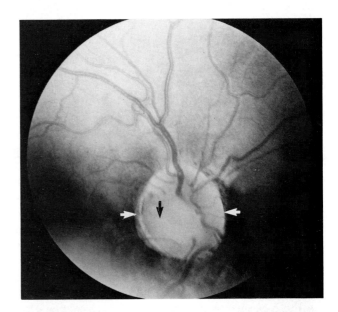

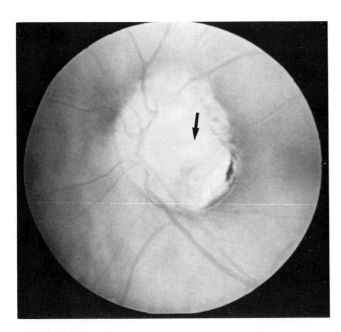

Figure 1–50. Photograph of an unusually large optic pit that borders on being classified as a coloboma. The arrow points to two very deep depressions located within the defect.

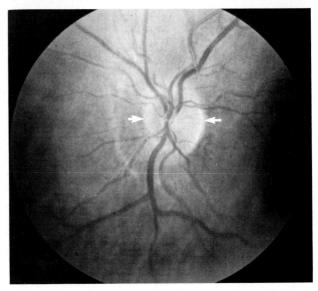

Figure 1–51. Top. Right optic nerve head with an optic pit **(black arrow).** Compare the size of the affected disc with the fellow left eye. **Bottom.**

ulopathy associated with a congenital pit of the optic nerve head is about 30 years. Symptoms of the detachment include metamorphopsia and vision reduction.

The etiology of the subretinal fluid is very controversial. Fluorescein angiography demonstrates that the serous detachment associated with a pit is distinctly different from that associated with idiopathic central serous choroidopathy and choroidal neovascularization. Virtually all pits hyperfluoresce during fluorescein angiography. With detachment, there may be a mottled macular hyperfluorescence during the venous phase. There are proponents of the theory that liquefied vitreous is responsible for the subretinal fluid. Others argue that the fluid emanates from leaking vessels within the pit. An unsubstantiated theory is the leakage of cerebrospinal fluid from the subarachnoid sheath surrounding the optic nerve. The majority of work supports the theory of a vitreous communication via the pit. **See color plate 6.**

Prognosis and Management. There is a very high incidence of serous maculopathy associated with congenital pits in the temporal aspect of the optic nerve head. Some reports state that the condition waxes and wanes, with a high percentage of spontaneous reattachment, whereas others cite the presence of subretinal fluid in up to 75 percent of cases over a 5-year follow-up. The primary prognostic indicators are size and location of the pit. There is no particular association of optic pits to any other ocular or systemic abnormality.

The controversy surrounding congenital pits of the optic nerve head continues with management. Prophylactic photocoagulation near the pits has been advocated, but results were not beneficial. In addition to photocoagulation, oral corticosteroids, optic nerve decompression, scleral buckling, and

vitrectomy have been tried in the treatment of the serous maculopathy secondary to optic pits. The only mode of therapy that may be of value is photocoagulation. Photocoagulation applied in cases of serous maculopathy results in flattening of the retina and elimination of subretinal fluid, but visual acuity does not improve significantly.

The clinician should routinely monitor the patient with a congenital pit of the optic nerve head. The patient should be given some method of monitoring the vision monocularly and should report metamorphopsia or vision loss as soon as it occurs. The longer the macula is detached, the poorer the long-term prognosis.

CONGENITAL PITS OF THE OPTIC NERVE HEAD—PEARLS

- Affected disc is larger than its fellow with unusual vascular pattern
- Most often an inferior temporal discoloration (olive-gray) that is excavated
- Usually 0.3 disc diameters in size
- Visual field defect corresponds to the pit location
- Strong association with nonrhegmatogenous retinal detachment, mean age 31 years
- Management includes
  - Patient education about signs and symptoms of retinal detachment
  - Home monitoring by Amsler Grid
  - Routine yearly examinations

Congenital Optic Nerve Hypoplasia

Appearance and Layers Involved. Congenital optic nerve hypoplasia may occur unilaterally or bilaterally (Figs. 1–52 to 1–54). The nerve head is

UNILATERAL CONGENITAL OPTIC NERVE HYPOPLASIA

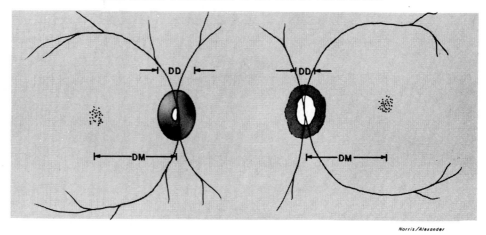

Figure 1–52. Schematic illustrating unilateral congenital optic nerve hypoplasia. The affected disc is reduced in size, which increases the DM/DD ratio. The affected disc is surrounded by a discolored area that corresponds to the size of the unaffected disc.

Norris/Alexander

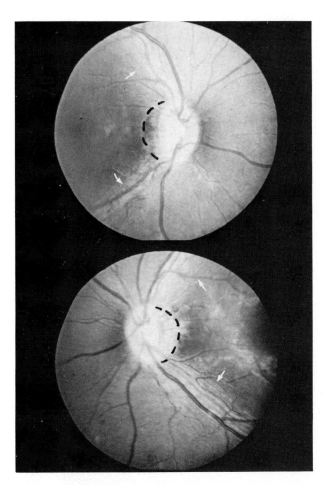

Figure 1–53. Bilateral congenital optic nerve hypoplasia. The dotted lines represent the expected disc size. The arrows point to the edges of the intact nerve fiber layer. The macular zones have a severe reduction in nerve fiber layer reflex. This patient had nystagmus.

typically one-third to one-half the size of a normally developed optic nerve. The nerve head is usually pale in comparison to the normal nerve head and usually is surrounded by a yellow zone that may be variably pigmented. This surrounding zone approximates the size of the optic nerve head if it were normal in its development. This is refered to in some reports as a "double ring sign." The reduction in size is the result of an absent or severely reduced nerve fiber layer with a corresponding absence of ganglion cells. This is all thought to be related to a failure of development of the ganglion cell layer of the retina secondary to interruption in fetal development.

The majority of patients with congenital optic nerve hypoplasia has relatively normal nerve head vasculature that exits and enters the disc centrally. The disc–macula/disc–disc (DM/DD) ratio is altered in cases of congenital optic nerve hypoplasia and may serve as a means of quantification of the condition. The normal DM/DD ratio is 2.1 to 3.2,

and values greater than 3.2 are strongly suggestive of congenital optic nerve hypoplasia.

Signs and Symptoms. Since there is a maldevelopment of the nerve fiber layer, there is a resultant variable visual acuity from normal to no light perception. The patient often may have amblyopia or strabismus (50 percent, and the majority are esotropes). The pupillary response in the affected eye is usually absent or very slowly reactive to direct light. A Marcus-Gunn pupil may then be present in cases of unilateral congenital optic nerve hypoplasia. As one would expect, nystagmus is present in a majority of bilateral cases because of poor acuity from birth. Visual fields vary considerably depending on the areas of the nerve head affected and the extent of the hypoplasia. Remember that there is a gradient regarding the degree of hypoplasia from just clinically observable to almost total absence of the nerve head.

Congenital optic nerve hypoplasia has been related to many ocular and systemic anomalies, including strabismus, nystagmus, persistent hyperplastic primary vitreous, anencephaly, hydranencephaly, septo-optic dysplasia, pituitary dysfunction (13 percent), cerebral palsy, epilepsy, porencephaly, absence of the septum pellucidum (27 percent), and facial and head abnormalities. There also has been an association with maternal ingestion of quinine to induce abortion as well as other pharmacologic implications. There is thought to be some association with maternal cytomegalovirus, syphilis, rubella and diabetes. It should be noted, however, that the majority of patients with congenital optic nerve hypoplasia has no associated systemic abnormalities. **See color plate 7.**

Prognosis and Management. Congenital optic nerve hypoplasia is a benign, self-limited condition that will not respond to intervention. The only possible concern surrounds the associated systemic anomalies.

Management of congenital optic nerve hypoplasia involves, most importantly, proper differential diagnosis to prevent unnecessary amblyopic or strabismic therapy or unnecessary extensive neurologic investigations because of a small pale optic disc and reduced vision.

Additional studies may be indicated when there is the suspicion of associated systemic anomalies. Axial tomograms, skull x-rays, CT scans, and magnetic resonance imaging may be employed to assist in the discovery of neurologic malformations and dysfunction.

Should the condition be unilateral, protective eyewear is indicated.

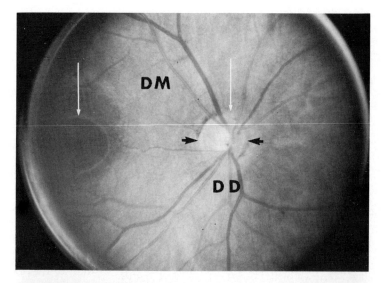

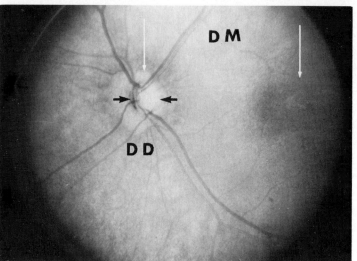

Figure 1–54. Top. The unaffected right eye with DM and DD distances indicated. **Bottom.** The fellow left eye with congenital optic nerve hypoplasia and the expected increased DM/DD. Acuity was reduced to 20/200.

CONGENITAL OPTIC NERVE HYPOPLASIA—PEARLS

- Nerve head is usually ½ to ⅓ the size of the fellow eye and pale by comparison
- Surrounded by a discolored zone the size of the normal optic nerve head
- Altered DM/DD
- Reduced vision because of maldevelopment of the nerve fiber layer
- Variable visual fields
- Association with systemic abnormalities
- Management includes
  - Proper differential diagnosis to prevent unnecessary treatment, such as amblyopia therapy
  - Rule out systemic abnormalities
  - Patient education
  - Provision of protective eyewear if unilateral
  - Routine eye examinations

■ Clinical Note on Differential Diagnosis: Optic Nerve Aplasia

Optic nerve aplasia is a rare condition in which there is total absence of the optic nerve, ganglion cells, and retinal vessels. Aplasia is considered to occur as the result of interference in the development of the optic nerve at an earlier point in gestation than that which would result in optic nerve hypoplasia.

The eye affected with aplasia often is microophthalmic with cataracts and retinal–choroidal colobomas. There is no vision at all and no pupillary response. This condition usually is unilateral. Optic nerve aplasia may or may not have related systemic anomalies.

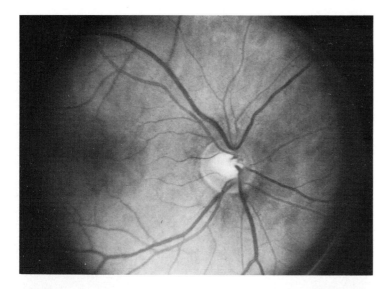

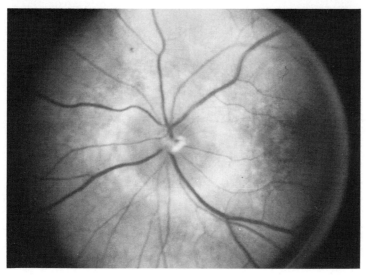

Figure 1–55. The normal-sized optic nerve head **(top)** compared to the megalopapillic left nerve head **(bottom)**. Acuity was not reduced.

Megalopapilla

Appearance and Layers Involved. Megalopapilla (Figs. 1–55 and 1–56) is a term used to describe any nerve head that is clinically larger by observation than its fellow nerve head. As discussed previously, many congenital nerve head anomalies can appear as an associated enlargement of the affected nerve. Among these variations are congenital optic nerve coloboma, congenital optic pits, the morning glory disc anomaly, and buried drusen of the nerve head. When the clinician is faced with the unilaterally enlarged optic nerve, it is important to rule out any acquired condition creating enlargement of the nerve head secondary to optic disc edema. Once congenital and acquired anomalies have been ruled out, the clinician is left with megalopapilla as a diagnosis.

The megalopapillic nerve head can have any number of appearances but usually has an unusual vascular pattern. The DM/DD will be reduced below 2.1. The condition is usually unilateral, but bilateral megalopapilla is seen occasionally. Acuity usually is unaffected, and nerve conduction defects are absent. Circumpapillary retinal pigment epithelium defects often are present.

Simultaneous comparison of the view of the nerve heads often is necessary for a differential diagnosis. This is difficult with direct ophthalmoscopy and fundus lens evaluation is enhanced with binocular indirect ophthalmoscopy and is maximized with fundus photography.

The condition is thought to evolve as the result of abnormal development of the primitive epithelial papilla.

Signs and Symptoms. Visual acuity usually is normal, and visual fields are unaffected except for

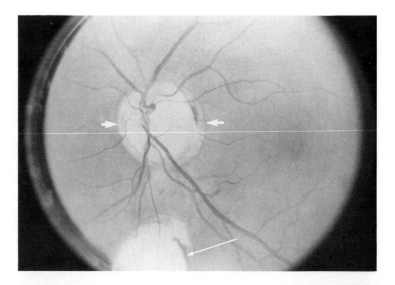

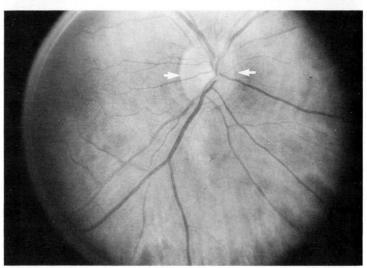

Figure 1–56. Top. The left nerve head is enlarged but flat, and acuity is normal. The long white arrow points to a retinal–choroidal coloboma. The right nerve head (**bottom**) is of normal size.

enlarged physiological blind spots. There are no associated systemic anomalies. Other congenital anomalies, such as cleft palate, may coexist.

Prognosis and Management. Megalopapilla is a benign, nonprogressive congenital anomaly that requires no management beyond proper differential diagnosis. **See color plate 8.**

MEGALOPAPILLA—PEARLS

- Unilaterally enlarged optic nerve of congenital origin, possibly secondary to abnormal development of the primitive epithelial papilla
- Reduced DM/DD
- Benign nonprogressive anomaly requiring routine eye examinations

---

Buried Drusen of the Optic Nerve Head

Appearance and Layers Involved. Buried drusen of the nerve head (Figs. 1–57 to 1–62) can create a diagnostic dilemma that certainly does not represent a benign, non-progressive condition. Buried drusen of the nerve head occur congenitally with variable clinical presentation. The drusen of the nerve head have no histopathologic correlation to retinal drusen and are as such not age-related. Optic nerve head drusen are inherited in an autosomal irregular dominant pattern, are bilateral in over 70 percent of the patients, and occur primarily in whites.

Drusen evolve slowly, often requiring decades to fully develop. In childhood, the discs appear papilledema-like, with no physiological cupping. Later, the discs become yellowish, with spherical

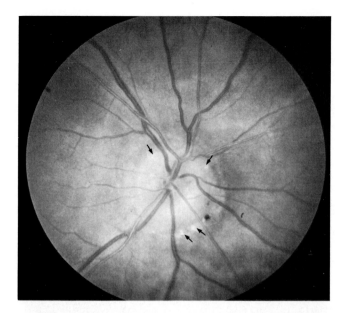

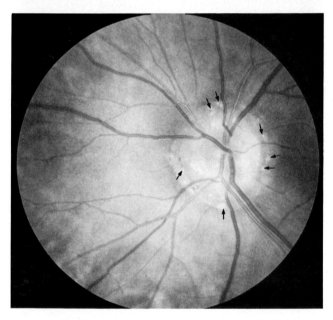

Figure 1–57. Top and Bottom. An example of bilateral optic nerve head drusen in an older patient. Both nerve heads were elevated. The arrows point to glowing buried drusen.

refractile structures surfacing. These refractile bodies transilluminate (glow) and appear more often near the nasal disc margin, although they can be seen at any location. There is often an anomalous vascular pattern on the nerve head associated with buried drusen.

The drusen of the optic nerve are confined anterior to the lamina cribrosa. The calciumlike globular deposits may be associated with alterations of axoplasmic flow and subsequent damage to the axons. It is postulated that alteration of the axons occurs before calcific deposition. The calcific deposits

can then compromise the nerve fibers and vascular supply, leading to visual field defects and circumpapillary hemorrhages.

Signs and Symptoms. Buried drusen of the nerve head give a papilledema-like appearance to the discs in younger patients and ascend within the disc to assume their refractile properties as the patient ages. Visual field defects often are present and are known to progress. The defects may be scotomas, concentric constriction, or generalized depressions.

The sharpness of the drusen can shear the blood vessels, leading to hemorrhages in, around, and over the optic nerve head.

The drusen are known to autofluoresce, which aids in differential diagnosis. Ultrasonography (see Fig. 1–62) is of tremendous assistance in the differential diagnosis from optic disc edema. The buried drusen are highly reflective with ultrasound. Even when the frequency of the ultrasound wave is reduced so that soft tissue is no longer reflective, the drusen will continue to appear. **See color plate 9.**

Prognosis and Management. Buried drusen of the optic nerve head can be visually devastating. Hemorrhages secondary to the drusen can compromise vision. The most severe complication is, however, progressive compromise of the nerve fibers and slowly progressive optic atrophy. The changes can cause a progressive visual field defect that ultimately can result in total loss of vision function.

Unfortunately, buried drusen of the optic nerve head progress unchecked. Interventive therapy is currently not available to prevent either the associated nerve fiber loss or the hemorrhages.

It is important to make the proper differential diagnosis to avoid costly and unnecessary neurological evaluations. It also is important to educate patients about the condition so that they are prepared if field loss or hemorrhages occur.

■ Clinical Note: Drusen of the Optic Nerve Head Associated with Retinitis Pigmentosa

Drusen of the nerve head can arise in patients with retinitis pigmentosa. These drusen differ somewhat from the familial drusen in that they lie just off the disc margin in the superficial retina. There certainly will be the other fundus characteristics associated with retinitis pigmentosa, but the visual field defects can confound the diagnosis. Often, it is necessary to employ electrodiagnostic testing to confirm the diagnosis.

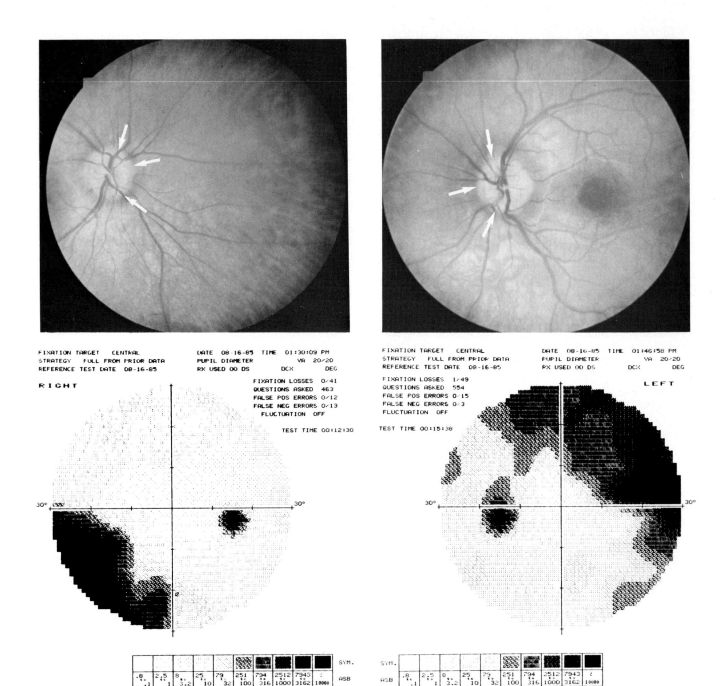

FIXATION TARGET   CENTRAL   DATE 08-16-85 TIME 01:30:09 PM
STRATEGY   FULL FROM PRIOR DATA   PUPIL DIAMETER   VA 20/20
REFERENCE TEST DATE 08-16-85   RX USED OO DS   DCX   DEG

RIGHT   FIXATION LOSSES   0/41
                                      QUESTIONS ASKED   463
                                      FALSE POS ERRORS 0/12
                                      FALSE NEG ERRORS 0/13
                                      FLUCTUATION OFF

                                              TEST TIME 00:12:30

FIXATION TARGET   CENTRAL   DATE 08-16-85 TIME 01:46:58 PM
STRATEGY   FULL FROM PRIOR DATA   PUPIL DIAMETER   VA 20/20
REFERENCE TEST DATE 08-16-85   RX USED OO DS   DCX   DEG

FIXATION LOSSES   1/49   LEFT
QUESTIONS ASKED   554
FALSE POS ERRORS 0/15
FALSE NEG ERRORS 0/3
FLUCTUATION OFF

TEST TIME 00:15:38

Figure 1–58. Top. An example of buried drusen in a younger patient. The arrows point to areas of gross optic nerve head elevation where no drusen were readily visible. **Bottom.** The field corresponding to that in top figure, demonstrating a dense defect.

Figure 1–59. Top. The fellow eye to that in Figure 58 **(top),** with the arrows again pointing to gross elevation, and **(bottom)** the corresponding field defect.

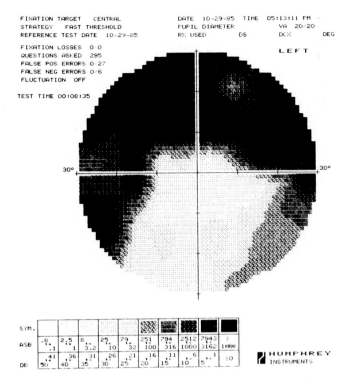

```
FIXATION TARGET   CENTRAL          DATE  10-29-85  TIME  05:13:11 PM
STRATEGY    FAST THRESHOLD         PUPIL DIAMETER            VA  20/20
REFERENCE TEST DATE  10-29-85      RX USED      DS     DCX        DEG

FIXATION LOSSES   0/0                                    LEFT
QUESTIONS ASKED   295
FALSE POS ERRORS  0/27
FALSE NEG ERRORS  0/6
FLUCTUATION  OFF

TEST TIME  00:08:35
```

30°   30°

Figure 1–60. Within 3 months, the field defect in Figure 59 **(bottom)** had progressed to this stage. This illustrates the potential for vision loss with buried drusen of the optic nerve head.

BURIED DRUSEN OF THE OPTIC NERVE HEAD—PEARLS

- Inherited in autosomal irregular pattern and are bilateral in 70 percent
- Occur primarily in whites
- Calciumlike globular deposits anterior to the lamina cribrosa that become more apparent with age. In youth, present as only a swollen disc but transilluminate as the patient ages
- The deposits can shear blood vessels, causing hemorrhage, and can alter axoplasmic flow, causing progressive field loss
- Autofluoresce to aid in differential diagnosis
- Ultrasonography is very useful in differential diagnosis
- If associated with retinitis pigmentosa, the drusen lie off the disc margin in the superficial retina
- Management includes
  - Proper diagnosis and patient education
  - Baseline fields to monitor progression
  - Patient self-monitoring of vision
  - Routine yearly examinations

INHERITED FAMILIAL OPTIC ATROPHY

The hereditary aspect of optic atrophy can be misleading when consideration is given to the facts that atrophies may be of juvenile onset and may,

in fact, progress. This discussion differentiates (1) autosomal dominant congenital optic atrophy, (2) autosomal recessive congenital optic atrophy, (3) autosomal dominant juvenile optic atrophy, (4) autosomal recessive juvenile optic atrophy, (5) Leber's hereditary optic atrophy, and (6) Behr's optic atrophy. **Differentiation of these conditions is best managed by referring to the clinical findings listed in Table 1–7.** The more common hereditary optic atrophies are discussed briefly.

Autosomal Dominant Juvenile Optic Atrophy

Appearance. Autosomal dominant juvenile optic atrophy is characterized by variable bilateral optic nerve pallor usually involving a temporal sector. (Fig. 1–63). This is, however, variable from full pallor to no clinically observable pallor and usually is the sole finding. There is a low correlation of optic nerve appearance and resultant acuity. The incidence is 1/50,000, with an autosomal dominant inheritance pattern.

Signs and Symptoms. There is a wide range in reports of visual acuity in autosomal dominant juvenile optic atrophy from near normal to 1/60. Near visual acuity may be better than distance acuity. Visual acuity may or may not be stable, but if progression occurs, it is usually mild. The onset of loss is insidious, usually occurring in a 6 to 12 year old. A blue–yellow defect often precedes the atrophy, and a wide range of field defects can occur. Most often there is a centrocecal scotoma. A Marcus-Gunn pupil is usually absent because of bilaterality. Usually, electrodiagnostic tests and dark adaptation are unaffected. Diagnosis often is made after establishment of a pedigree. **See color plate 10.**

Prognosis and Management. The condition is usually stationary, but slight progressive loss of vision may occur.

The clinician must make the correct diagnosis by ruling out potential neurological causes. Patient education and genetic counseling are certainly in order. The patient with autosomal dominant juvenile optic atrophy can expect one half of the offspring to be affected, with equal sex distribution. It is important to provide the best possible prescription and low-vision rehabilitation if necessary.

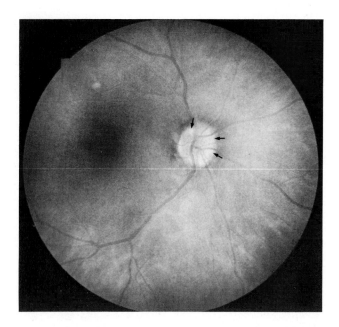
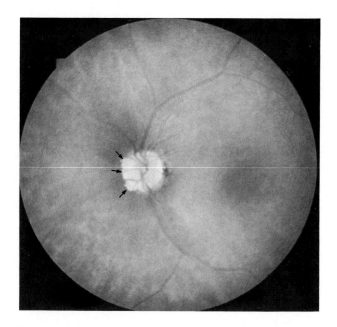

Figure 1–61. Left and Right. Optic nerve head drusen can be very asymmetrical and often will create asymmetrical field defects.

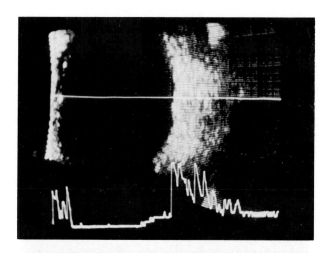
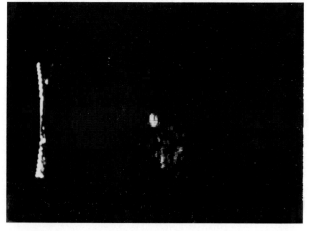

Figure 1–62. This illustrates a very valuable diagnostic tool to assist in determining the presence of buried drusen. **Top.** Elevation of the nerve head (cursor) by B-scan ultrasonography. **Bottom.** When the gain is reduced, solid structures, such as drusen and asteroid hyalosis, will continue to return signals to the transducer. The buried drusen becomes visible.

TABLE 1–7. INHERITED OPTIC ATROPHIES

Characteristic	Autosomal Dominant Juvenile Optic Atrophy	Autosomal Recessive Juvenile Optic Atrophy	Leber's Hereditary Optic Atrophy	Autosomal Dominant Congenital Optic Atrophy	Autosomal Recessive Congenital Optic Atrophy	Behr's Optic Atrophy
Inheritance pattern	Dominant	Recessive	Questionable, affects primarily males	Dominant	Recessive	Recessive
Age of onset	Insidious at 6–12 years	Insidious at 6–12 years	Acute at 10–40 years	Congenital	Congenital	1–9 years
Final acuity	20/20–1/60	Severe loss	10/200	20/100 to severe	Severe loss	20/60 to 10/200
Nystagmus	No	No	No	Yes	Yes	Possible
Fundus picture	Temporal optic atrophy	Total optic atrophy	Optic disc edema followed by optic atrophy	Total optic atrophy	Total optic atrophy	Temporal optic atrophy
Visual fields	Relative centrocecal scotoma, inversion of peripheral color field	N/A	Central scotoma, normal peripheral fields	Constricted peripheral, possible scotoma	Constricted peripheral, possible scotoma	Central scotoma, normal peripheral fields
Color vision	Blue–yellow defect	N/A	Red–green defect	Red–green defect	Red–green defect	Red–green defect
Associated systemic signs and symptoms	N/A	Diabetes? Auditory problems?	Headaches, vertigo, nervousness	N/A	N/A	Increased deep tendon reflex, positive Romberg sign, ataxia, muscle rigidity, mental debilitation
Clinical course	Usually stabilizes but may present a slow progression	N/A	Acute loss that may regress or after years of delay may progress	May have slow progression	May have slow progression	Neurologic signs and symptoms evolve years after, then stabilize, optic atrophy stabilizes

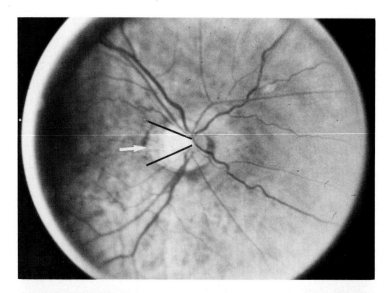

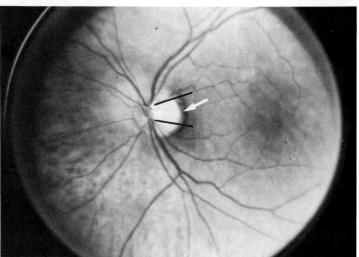

Figure 1–63. Top and Bottom. Classic presentation of autosomal dominant juvenile optic atrophy. There is a triangular sector of temporal optic atrophy in both eyes.

> **AUTOSOMAL DOMINANT JUVENILE OPTIC ATROPHY—PEARLS**
>
> - Variable optic nerve pallor often temporal in presentation
> - Insidious loss of vision ages 6 to 12 years, with variable final acuity and fields that usually stabilize with age
> - Usually associated with a blue–yellow defect
> - Management includes
>   - Rule out any neurologic cause
>   - Patient education
>   - Provision of best possible prescription
>   - Routine yearly examinations

Autosomal Recessive Congenital Optic Atrophy

Autosomal recessive congenital optic atrophy is very rare and is characterized by poor vision and nystagmus at birth. The inheritance pattern implicates consanguinity of parents.

Leber's Hereditary Optic Atrophy

Appearance, Signs, and Symptoms. Leber's hereditary optic atrophy is a bilateral disease of unknown etiology other than the proposed inherited inability to detoxify cyanide. It usually occurs as an acute to subacute disease in males between ages 10 and 40 years. Inheritance is a factor, but the precise pedigree fits no established pattern. Pedigree analysis is nonetheless important. At the onset of the acute attack, optic disc edema often is accompanied by circumpapillary telangiectactic microangiopathy that does not leak on fluorescein angiography. Visual acuity quickly reduces to the 20/200 level. Both eyes usually are affected simultaneously, but this is not an absolute rule.

In some patients, there is a dropout of retinal nerve fibers, an alteration of the Farnsworth-Munsell 100-hue test and altered visually evoked potential before the acute attack. During the active phase, there may be associated headaches, vertigo, and general nervousness.

As the condition progresses, the nerve heads become atrophic, resulting in central scotomas, color vision loss, and stabilization of vision in the 20/200 range.

Prognosis and Management. The prognosis for Leber's hereditary optic atrophy is grim. There are reports of spontaneous recovery of vision as well as spontaneous further reduction in vision.

Early recognition and establishment of pedigree are important in the management of Leber's hereditary optic atrophy. Genetic counseling is important, keeping in mind the following characteristics of the disease:

1. Men are affected (6.7/1) more often than women
2. The age of onset in men is 18 to 30 years, and it is 10 to 40 years in women
3. Affected males cannot transmit the disease
4. The sister of an affected male is a carrier
5. Affected females have nonaffected fathers
6. A heterozygous female can transmit the trait to a son and the carrier state to a daughter

There are some advocates of medical intervention in this disease based on the hypothesis that the cause is a defect in cyanide metabolism. It has been suggested that vitamin B_{12A} and vitamin B_{12} given 1 mg parenterally daily for 7 days may be effective in treatment of the acute phase. There is no proof as to its efficacy. Vitamin therapy is used in the treatment of Leber's hereditary optic atrophy because it cannot create a problem and it may be beneficial.

The end result of Leber's atrophy becomes a problem best solved with an optimal prescription often accompanied by low vision rehabilitation.

LEBER'S HEREDITARY OPTIC ATROPHY—PEARLS

- Usually acute presentation at ages 10 to 40 years affecting primarily males
- Optic disc edema accompanied by circumpapillary telangiectatic microvasculopathy followed by optic atrophy and severe loss of vision
- May be associated systemic signs of headaches, vertigo, and nervousness
- Management includes
  - Genetic counseling
  - Consultation with neuro-ophthalmology for possible medical intervention if in the acute stages
  - Provision of best possible refraction and low vision rehabilitation

---

ACQUIRED OPTIC NERVE DISEASE

Acquired optic nerve disease can be the result of numerous afflictions. Such terms as "optic neuritis" and "papilledema" have been applied erroneously in past discussions of optic neuropathy. This discussion considers all acquired diseases of the optic nerve under the terminology of optic neuropathy. Terminology is applied that specifically defines the pathologic process. The suffix *itis* refers only to proven inflammatory processes, and the term "optic disc edema" refers to any swelling of the nerve fibers of the optic nerve. **Table 1–8 summarizes the general categories of etiology of optic neuropathy and Table 1–9 summarizes many of the causes of optic disc edema. Table 1–10 is a simplified summary of typical causes of optic neuropathy by age.**

Inflammatory Optic Neuropathy

Appearance and Layers Involved. In the case of inflammatory optic neuropathy, there is initially optic disc edema, with the possibility of accompanying hemorrhage, vascular changes, vitritis, and circumpapillary choroiditis. The affliction is an inflammatory reaction to an infection. The appearance of optic atrophy depends on the interval between genesis and therapeutic intervention. This condition usually occurs in younger patients (under 20 years) and often is referred to as "papillitis" (Fig. 1–64).

Papillitis is the most common form of optic neuropathy in children. **Table 1–11 summarizes the common etiologic factors associated with optic neuropathy secondary to inflammatory processes.** The vision loss in papillitis is similar to other forms of optic neuropathy in that there is a rapid decrease in acuity over the first 2 to 3 days, followed by stabilization over 7 to 10 days, ultimately resulting in a slight improvement. Optic atrophy occurs 4 to 8 weeks after the inflammation.

Two distinctive types of papillitis may occur. The papillitis associated with viral infections in children exhibits dirty-yellow globular exudates

---

TABLE 1–8. ETIOLOGY OF OPTIC NEUROPATHY

Hereditary or familial optic neuropathy
Inflammatory optic neuropathy
Demyelinizing optic neuropathy
Toxic optic neuropathy
Ischemic optic neuropathy
Compressive optic neuropathy

TABLE 1–9. SOME OF THE MORE COMMON CAUSES OF OPTIC DISC EDEMA

Anterior ischemic optic neuropathy
Carotid cavernous fistula
Cavernous sinus thrombosis
Central retinal vein occlusion
Demyelinizing optic neuropathy
Diabetic papillopathy
Drusen of the nerve head
Foster-Kennedy syndrome
Hemicentral retinal vein occlusion
Leukemic infiltrates of the optic nerve

Orbital cellulitis
Papilledema secondary to intracranial mass or hemorrhage
Papilledema secondary to benign intracranial hypertension
Papillitis (inflammatory optic neuropathy)
Papillophlebitis
Primary optic nerve tumors
Primary orbital tumors
Thyroid eye disease

scattered throughout the papillomacular bundle. These exudates may coalesce to form a macular star or wing. Retinal edema accompanies the process. This variety of papillitis may resolve spontaneously without treatment.

The other variety of papillitis (neuroretinitis) is characterized by a yellow, swollen disc obscuring vessels and spreading far into the retina. Linear hemorrhages may appear adjacent to the disc. This form usually results in poor vision, gliosis, perivascular sheathing, and optic atrophy.

Signs and Symptoms. Inflammatory optic neuropathy occurs as a unilateral mild to severe loss of vision and visual field. Field defects vary depending on the location and severity of the inflammation. There is usually an associated Marcus-Gunn pupillary defect as well as other signs of optic nerve conduction compromise, including a red desaturation defect. There may be ocular pain or tenderness as well as some pain on motion of the globe. **See color plate 11.**

Prognosis and Management. Prognosis for inflammatory optic neuropathy varies considerably. Reduction of the inflammation by ACTH or corticosteroid usage has proponents and opponents. Diagnosis of the underlying causative agent or condition is crucial to specify the proper therapeutic

TABLE 1–10. TYPICAL CAUSES OF OPTIC NEUROPATHY CLASSIFIED BY AGE OF ONSET

Age (years)	Typical Cause
1–10	Inflammatory disease
11–20	Postinfectious disease
21–40	Demyelinizing disease
50–70	Atherosclerotic anterior ischemic optic neuropathy or toxic optic neuropathy
60–80	Temporal arteritic optic neuropathy

Modified from Alexander LJ: Diseases of the optic nerve. In Bartlett JD, Jaanus SD (eds): *Clinical Ocular Pharmacology.* Boston, Butterworth, 1989.

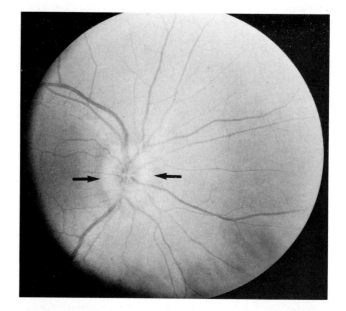

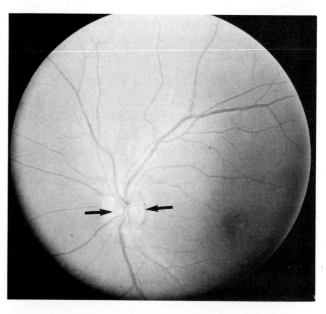

Figure 1–64. Top and Bottom. Unilateral optic disc edema with reduced vision in a young person. This is referred to as inflammatory optic neuropathy, or papillitis.

TABLE 1–11. SOME OF THE COMMON ETIOLOGIC FACTORS ASSOCIATED WITH INFLAMMATORY OPTIC NEUROPATHY		
Toxoplasmosis	Presumed ocular histoplasmosis	Crohn's disease
Toxocariasis	Chickenpox	Ulcerative colitis
Meningitis	Herpes zoster	Poliomyelitis
Measles	Cat scratch fever	Mononucleosis
Mumps	Behcet's disease	Reiter's disease
Syphilis	Postvaccination reaction	Bacterial infections
Tuberculosis	Pharmacologic idiosyncrasies	Fungal infections
Collagen vascular disease		

Modified from Alexander LJ: Diseases of the optic nerve. In Bartlett JD, Jaanus SD (eds): *Clinical Ocular Pharmacology.* Boston, Butterworth, 1989.

intervention. The sooner the resolution, the better the prognosis for return of vision function.

The most important aspect of management of inflammatory optic neuropathy is rapid diagnosis, with emphasis placed on attempting to ascertain the etiology. Basic adjunct diagnostic tests should be run on patients and should be supplemented by others when a specific etiologic agent is suspected. Basic tests should include erythrocyte sedimentation rate (to rule out temporal arteritis), complete blood count (CBC), fluorescent treponemal antibody absorption test (FTA-ABS) (to rule out syphilis), collagen vascular screen, computed axial tomography (CT), or magnetic resonance imaging (MRI). Supplementary tests may include specific antibody titer tests (such as toxoplasmosis titer) for infection.

Therapeutic intervention must be applied as soon as the etiologic factor has been determined. The therapy may be insufficient in reducing the inflammation, necessitating incorporation of corticosteroids into the treatment regimen. All arguments that support initiation of corticosteroid or ACTH therapy must be tempered by the associated inherent risk factors.

INFLAMMATORY OPTIC NEUROPATHY—PEARLS

- Optic disc edema, hemorrhage, vitritis, and peripapillary choroiditis usually in younger patients
- Rapid decrease in vision over 2 to 3 days, followed by stabilization over 7 to 10 days. Optic atrophy occurs in 4 to 8 weeks
- May be accompanying pain and tenderness of globe
- Often a central scotoma
- Associated optic nerve conduction defects
- Associated with a wide variety of inflammatory processes
- Management includes
  - Ascertain etiology
  - Immediate consultation with neuro-ophthalmology

Demyelinizing Optic Neuropathy

Appearance and Layers Involved. Demyelinizing optic neuropathy (Fig. 1–65) is best known as "retrobulbar neuritis" and is classically described as "the patient sees nothing and the doctor sees nothing." The patient presents with a sudden unilateral loss of vision. The patient with demyelinizing optic neuropathy is usually 20 to 40 years of age.

Very often there are no appreciable ophthalmoscopic nerve head changes, but optic disc edema secondary to axoplasmic stasis may occur. After the acute process runs it course, optic atrophy may appear.

The process is thought to be secondary to a reaction of the nerve fibers to a demyelinizing process. The fibers lose function because the nerve-conducting sheath is compromised.

Signs and Symptoms. The patient with demyelinizing optic neuropathy presents with an impairment of visual acuity or visual field that progresses to a maximum loss at the end of about 1 week. Other signs and symptoms that may be associated with vision loss are pain or tenderness of the globe near the insertion of the superior rectus, pain on gross excursions of the eye, a Marcus-Gunn pupil, color desaturation, light comparison variation, Pulfrich's stereo phenomenon, Uhthoff's and L'Hermitte's symptoms, and an altered visually evoked potential. Systemic manifestations include Romberg's sign as well as other indications of poor balance (cerebellar dysfunction). The patient may complain of mobility problems associated with the onset of the optic neuropathy.

Visual field defects associated with demyelinizing optic neuropathy vary considerably. The highest percentage of defects is central, but peripheral defects as well as generalized depressions can occur. It should be noted that these fields can fluctuate depending on the activity of the disease process. **See color plate 12.**

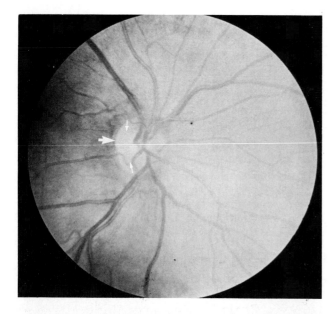

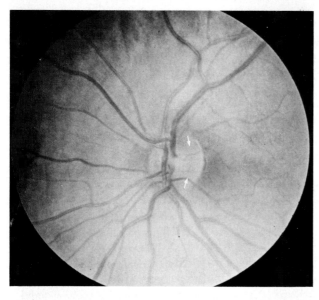

Figure 1–65. Top. The large arrow points to a zone of optic atrophy secondary to demyelinizing optic neuropathy. The zone of atrophic neuroretinal retinal rim is difficult to discern unless one makes a simultaneous comparison to the fellow eye **(bottom).** The small arrows demarcate the zone for comparison.

TABLE 1–12. DIAGNOSTIC CLASSIFICATION CRITERIAE FOR MULTIPLE SCLEROSIS

Classification	Criteria
Proven	Pathologic proof
Clinically definite	Some physical disability, remissions and relapses greater than two episodes
Early or probable	Signs of lesions at two or more sites, age of onset 10–50 years, no better explanation, lesions predominantly in white matter, remissions and relapses, early single episode suggesting MS with signs of multiple lesions, slight or no disability

Modified from Alexander LJ: Diseases of the optic nerve. In Bartlett JD, Jaanus SD (eds): *Clinical Ocular Pharmacology.* Boston, Butterworth, 1989.

Of acute importance is the differential diagnosis of cause. Although most optic neuropathy in the 20 to 40 year age category can be attributed to a demyelinizing disease, it is important that the clinician rule out other potential causes, such as Guillain-Barré syndrome, carbon monoxide poisoning, and metabolic factors.

Multiple sclerosis does not always occur systemically after demyelinizing optic neuropathy. Reports in the literature vary from zero percent to 85 percent of cases of multiple sclerosis developing after a case of retrobulbar neuritis. Some of the discrepancy probably revolves around an inappropriate diagnosis of either demyelinizing optic atrophy or multiple sclerosis (MS).

The criteria for the diagnosis of MS are very controversial. The Medical Research Council Committee developed a set of criteria for classification of MS that are shown in Table 1–12.

A CT scan may be of some assistance in discovering a cortical plaque, but MRI has been proven to be more effective. The myelin basic protein test may be run on cerebrospinal fluid to evaluate the possibility of MS. Regardless of the controversy about diagnosis, any patient suspected of having demyelinizing optic neuropathy should have a neurological consultation.

Treatment of the optic neuropathy is also very controversial. Corticosteroid therapy has been demonstrated to reduce optic disc edema associated with demyelinizing optic neuropathy. This reduction in edema is thought to minimize scarring and destruction of the nerve fibers. There are as many opponents as proponents of therapeutic intervention by corticosteroids. Therapy may be provided via a parenteral route with ACTH. This modality does not have the negative side effect of suppression of adrenal function but does require hospitalization.

Oral corticosteroid therapy in the form of high doses of prednisone tapered over time may be

Prognosis and Management. Prognosis for return of at least some vision function is good. Visual acuity or fields usually begin to improve within 2 to 3 weeks of the attack and stabilize in 4 to 5 weeks. Some patients improve rapidly to a moderate acuity level, stabilize, then return to better vision over a more prolonged period of time. Recurrences can occur and usually cause a further reduction in acuity or an enlargement of the visual field defects. Each attack has the potential to produce irreversible optic atrophy.

TABLE 1–13. ACTH PARENTERAL REGIMEN

ACTH 20 units/ml to 80 units IV q6–8h in 500 ml of 5% dextrose in water for 3 days. Then ACTH gel (40 units/ml) IM 40 units q12h for 7 days. Then the dose is reduced by 10 units every 3 days as follows:

35 units bid × 3 days
30 units bid × 3 days
50 units qid × 3 days
40 units qid × 3 days
30 units qid × 3 days
20 units qid × 3 days
10 units qid × 3 days

TABLE 1–15. SUBTENON INJECTION OF CORTICOSTEROID REGIMEN

A sterile, disposable 1 ml tuberculin syringe with a 27-gauge, ½-inch needle is used. One ml of Kenalog is loaded into the syringe. The lower lid is gently wiped with an alcohol sponge, the patient is instructed to look up and to the opposite side, and the injection is given through the lower lid at the junction of the outer and middle third in the same direction as for a routine retrobulbar anesthetic. The needle is pushed snugly to its base, and the medication is injected moderately slowly. Covering the eye for about 30 minutes until the bolus of the drug is absorbed is helpful in avoiding transient diplopia. A semipressure eye patch can be applied for 1 to 2 hours if desired. The effect of the injection usually lasts for 1 to 2 weeks.

used. If therapy is instituted it needs to be done early in the disease process. Tables 1–13 to 1–15 summarize treatment modalities. Good conservative advice about demyelinizing optic neuropathy is to secure a neuro-ophthalmological consultation as soon as possible.

DEMYELINIZING OPTIC NEUROPATHY—PEARLS

• Sudden unilateral loss of vision or visual field in 20 to 40-year-old patients; loss progresses to maximum in about one week
• Associated optic nerve conduction defects
• May have associated optic disc edema but often no ophthalmoscopic signs
• Visual acuity or fields start to improve in 2 to 3 weeks and stabilize in 4 to 5 weeks, often accompanied by some optic atrophy
• Usually have associated cerebellar (balance) signs
• Management includes
  • Ascertain cause
  • Consult with neuro-ophthalmology for institution of therapy
  • Provision of best refraction
  • Regular eye examinations

■ Clinical Note: Neuromyelitis Optica

Neuromyelitis optica (Devic's disease) is a demyelinizing disease occurring in children and young adults.

TABLE 1–14. ORAL PREDNISONE THERAPY REGIMEN

100 mg day 1
80 mg day 2
60 mg days 3–5
30 mg days 6–7

Assess benefit at end of day 7; if positive, taper slowly

This disease is characterized by a rapid-onset bilateral loss of vision with a poor prognosis for recovery.

Ischemic Optic Neuropathy

Ischemic optic neuropathy (ION) (Figs. 1–66 and 1–67) is a disease of sudden onset with variable vision and visual field loss. There is usually an absence of identifiable inflammatory cause, an absence of demyelinization, and an absence of an identifiable cranio-orbital mass. Many classifications have been assigned to ischemic optic neuropathy, but this discussion categorizes the affliction into (1) arteriosclerotic–hypertensive ION, (2) temporal arteritic ION, and (3) diabetic ION. With the exception of diabetic ION, most ION occurs in patients over 50 years of age, although there are isolated reports of its occurrence in younger patients.

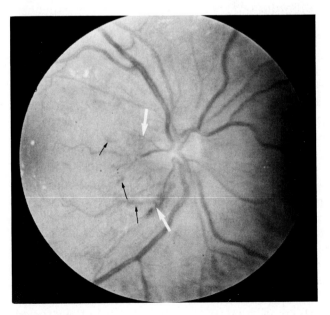

Figure 1–66. The white arrows demarcate the edematous zone of ischemic optic neuropathy. The black arrows point to flame-shaped hemorrhages.

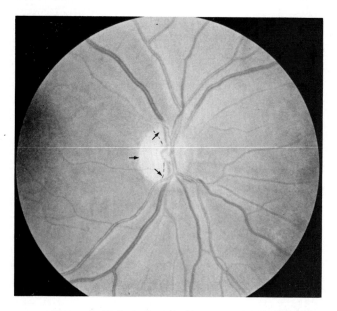 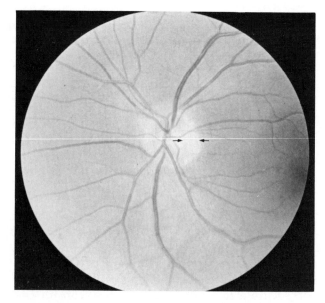

Figure 1–67. Left. The small arrows point to the extent of the zone of atrophy in ischemic optic neuropathy. **Right.** The fellow eye also has a smaller zone of atrophy of the neuroretinal rim.

Arteriosclerotic–Hypertensive ION

Appearance and Layers Involved. Arteriosclerotic–hypertensive ION (AHION) (also known as anterior ischemic optic neuropathy) is a small vessel disease of the optic nerve head creating an imbalance in the pressure/perfusion ratio. Sudden systemic hypotension and high incidences of systemic hypertension are associated with AHION and lend credence to the hypothesis that there is an acute alteration of the pressure/perfusion ratio within the nerve head. The alteration of pressure/perfusion also occurs in glaucoma (both chronic and low tension) only over a prolonged period of time. It should be noted that a patient with a chronically lowered pressure/perfusion ratio, as in glaucoma, has a greater chance of developing AHION. Fluorescein angiography confirms the presence of an occlusive disorder of the short posterior ciliary arteries. There is delayed to absent filling associated with this affliction; however, it is known that the vessels need not be totally occluded to produce the effect. The occlusion usually affects only isolated sections of the nerve.

AHION usually occurs in patients over 50 years of age, with equal sex distribution. It may become bilateral after a time delay. Reports vary from 14 percent to 73 percent regarding bilaterality in AHION.

The optic disc changes can be variable, from isolated sectoral optic disc edema to full-blown areas of optic atrophy. Small, linear, flame-shaped hemorrhages may occur on the disc margin. These hemorrhages disappear in 3 to 5 weeks. Eventually, activity subsides, and optic atrophy appears in about 3 months.

Signs and Symptoms. Prodromal signs and symptoms can occur with AHION (25 percent of patients). Prodromata consist of transient blurring of vision and sectors of visual field loss. In addition, blurring, flashing, and flickering of vision may occur.

With the onset of the attack, vision is decreased, and visual field loss may occur over 24 hours to 4 weeks without remission. A Marcus-Gunn pupil can occur as well as other optic nerve conduction defects. The classic visual field defect is a variety of an altitudinal loss, usually inferior, but any defect is possible.

There often is a family history of hypertension or diabetes in the patient with AHION, but usually there is no strong history of transient ischemic attacks, cerebral infarction, or cardiac disease. Table 1–16 illustrates the differential diagnosis between ION and Foster Kennedy syndrome. **See color plates 13 through 16.**

Prognosis. Visual acuity usually stabilizes at 20/60 or better in 45 to 50 percent of cases of AHION and is worse than 20/200 in about 40 percent. The incidence of development in the fellow eye averages about 25 percent. There is some concern about the possibility of secondary central and branch retinal artery occlusion, but this is not well documented. Cupping of the disc, that is erosion of disc tissue, may occur secondary to the AHION.

TABLE 1–16. DIFFERENTIAL DIAGNOSIS BETWEEN FOSTER KENNEDY SYNDROME AND ISCHEMIC OPTIC NEUROPATHY

Characteristic	Ischemic Optic Neuropathy	Foster Kennedy Syndrome
Onset	Sudden vision loss or field defect in one eye, followed by stabilization	Insidious progression of reduced vision with papilledema in fellow eye
Fields	Altitudinal hemianopsia, arcuate scotoma, central scotoma	Central scotoma in atrophic eye and enlarged blind spot in fellow eye
Fundus picture	Sector optic disc edema followed by sector atrophy	Uniform optic atrophy with optic disc edema in fellow eye
Associated systemic signs and symptoms	May be a family or personal history of hypertension, diabetes, or stroke	Hemiplegia, loss of smell, personality change

Modified from Alexander LJ: Diseases of the optic nerve. In Bartlett JD, Jaanus SD (eds): *Clinical Ocular Pharmacology.* Boston, Butterworth, 1989.

In some instances, patches of chorioretinal degeneration may occur in the periphery after an incident of AHION. This chorioretinal breakdown may be physical evidence of further choroidal vascular compromise.

Management. Recognition and management of any underlying systemic condition is imperative. Table 1–17 lists some of the systemic diseases of concern.

When considering therapeutic intervention of AHION, two schools of thought exist, the treaters and the nontreaters. If treatment is employed, it is in the form of corticosteroids or intraocular pressure-lowering drugs. There are reports of improvement in 75 percent of patients treated compared to 17 percent of patients not treated.

The successful treatment of AHION by corticosteroids depends on rapid diagnosis and immediate institution of therapy. It is proposed that the corticosteroid reduces capillary permeability in the optic nerve, reducing swelling and improving circulation. This process, coupled with a reduction of intraocular pressure, improves the pressure-perfusion ratio to minimize atrophy. The recognized treatment is 60 to 80 mg of oral prednisolone for 10 to 14 days tapered over a 2-month period until edema subsides. There are some reports that advocate initiation of anticoagulant or antiplatelet therapy as well, but there are no controlled studies to validate this proposed modality.

ARTERIOSCLEROTIC–HYPERTENSIVE ISCHEMIC OPTIC NEUROPATHY—PEARLS

- Small vessel disease of the optic nerve vascular supply
- Usually occurs in patients over 50 years with some chance of bilaterality
- Optic disc edema accompanied by hemorrhage in active phase, which eventually subsides with ensuing optic atrophy
- Optic nerve conduction defects, visual field compromise (altitudinal), and possible vision reduction
- Management includes
  - Attempt to ascertain underlying systemic disease
  - If resolved, educate patient and use home monitoring reevaluating yearly
  - If active, consult with neuro-ophthalmology for possible initiation of therapy *(Controversial)*

TABLE 1–17. SYSTEMIC DISEASES ASSOCIATED WITH ARTERIOSCLEROTIC–HYPERTENSIVE ISCHEMIC OPTIC NEUROPATHY

Generalized atherosclerosis and arteriosclerosis	Polyarteritis nodosa
Carotid artery disease	Systemic lupus erythematosus
Systemic hypertension	Blood loss
Systemic hypotension	Vasomotor problems (migraine)
Myocardial infarction	Syphilis
Cardiac emboli	Allergic disorders
Mitral valve prolapse	Hematologic disorders (polycythemia, sickle cell)
Diabetes	Glaucoma

Temporal Arteritic ION

Appearance and Layers Involved. Temporal arteritic ischemic optic neuropathy (TAION) is a blood vessel disease of the optic nerve head creating an imbalance in the pressure/perfusion ratio in a fashion similar to AHION. The primary differences are the degree of involvement and prognosis. The cause is unknown; the disease appears as inflammation of arteries (Fig. 1–68). Any large or medium-sized artery may be involved. TAION is an

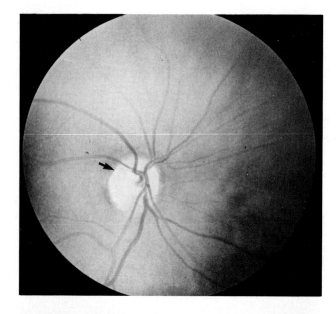

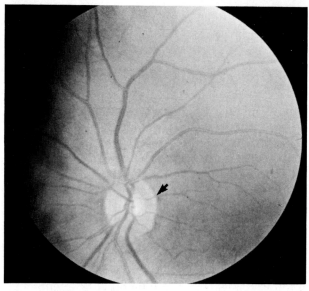

Figure 1–68. Example of total atrophy of the optic nerve head **(top)** compared to **(bottom)** in a case of temporal arteritic ischemic optic neuropathy.

ocular emergency necessitating immediate therapeutic intervention to prevent contralateral involvement.

TAION usually occurs in patients over 65 years of age (75 ± 9 years) and affects females more than males. The condition can be bilateral (25 to 33 percent), with variable intervals of onset in the second eye. It has been reported that if the second eye is not involved within 6 to 8 weeks, the prognosis is good for that eye.

The ophthalmoscopic picture at onset varies between two common presentations. In 50 percent of patients, the discs appear chalky white, with an apparent white mass lying deep in the disc with a circumpapillary white zone. Hemorrhages usually are absent in this variety. In 50 percent, the disc is edematous and pale pink. Edema spreads to the circumpapillary area, with superficial flame-shaped hemorrhages. When viewed with a fundus lens, a layer of pallor exists in the prelaminar region. Optic atrophy eventually occurs secondary to the infarct.

Signs and Symptoms. Prodromal symptoms occur in approximately 75 percent of patients with TAION about 1 to 2 weeks before the acute attack. These symptoms include trouble in focusing, loss of vision with return to normal, flashing or flickering, color disturbances, headaches (50 percent), weight loss, suboccipital neck pain, scalp tenderness on the affected side, and jaw aches associated with mastication (50 percent).

The attack of TAION is heralded by an acute vision loss of 20/60 to no light perception (NLP), with poor vision being the rule. All nerve conduction defects are present. As stated previously, TAION can affect the fellow eye (25 to 33 percent) at variable intervals. I have seen onset occur within 2 days in the second eye in spite of massive doses of corticosteroids.

Leukocytosis, elevated erythrocyte sedimentation rate (ESR usually above 50 mm), and a hard, nonpulsating temporal artery also occur. The symptom complex of polymyalgia rheumatica may occur, consisting of pain and stiffness in the shoulders and neck and in the hips and thighs, marked morning stiffness, and pain increasing with motion (joint pain). **See color plate 17.**

Prognosis. Visual acuity rarely improves with TAION. In spite of long-term corticosteroid therapy, loss can occur in the fellow eye. From a management standpoint, it should be assumed that the fellow eye will become involved. Even if both eyes are involved to the point of loss of vision, discontinuing corticosteroid therapy can allow for further compromise of visual field. Mortality rates associated with giant cell arteritis average about 20 percent. Death is associated with cerebrovascular disease. Optic disc cupping occurs over a time in temporal arteritic ischemic optic neuropathy.

Management. In any elderly patient suspected of having ischemic optic neuropathy, an immediate ESR determination should be made. Although reports vary concerning normal ranges for ESRs in elderly patients, it can be said that any patient suspected of having ischemic optic neuropathy with an ESR above 40 mm in the first hour Westergren test should be considered as having temporal arteritis until proven otherwise. An emergency neuro-ophthalmology consultation is then necessary.

Temporal artery biopsy is the definitive diagnostic test for TAION. Therapy should not, however, be withheld while awaiting the results of the biopsy. Systemic corticosteroids should be given immediately on suspicion of TAION to prevent involvement in the contralateral eye. The corticosteroids act as anti-inflammatory agents to decrease arterial inflammation. The initial dosages of oral prednisolone are high (80 to 120 mg/day). The dosage is adjusted downward according to signs, symptoms, and reduction of the ESR. Therapy is often continued at 5 to 10 mg/day for several years while the patient's ESR is monitored.

The use of anticoagulants and vasodilators may be indicated if hematologic disorders accompany the giant cell arteritis. Inherent risks in this therapy necessitate constant monitoring by a hematologist.

TEMPORAL ARTERITIC ISCHEMIC OPTIC NEUROPATHY—PEARLS

- Small vessel disease of the optic nerve vascular supply
- Occurs in patients over 65, with strong possibility of bilaterality
- Prodromal symptoms include
  - Transient monocular blindness, trouble focusing
  - Flashing or flickering, color vision disturbances
  - Headaches, weight loss, neck pain
  - Scalp tenderness and jaw aches
- Attack is a sudden loss of vision
- Management includes
  - ESR immediately in all suspected cases
  - Emergency neuro-ophthalmology referral for immediate institution of corticosteroid therapy
  - Temporal artery biopsy
  - Monitoring of corticosteroid therapy with ESR

Diabetic ION

Appearance and Layers Involved. Ischemic optic neuropathy can occur in any patient with diabetes, since diabetes is a small vessel disease. Diabetic ION or diabetic papillopathy, however, refers to optic neuropathy in a young Type 1 patient with diabetes, whereas the classic ION secondary to small vessel disease occurs in older patients. Diabetic ION can be characterized as neither AHION nor papilledema because it lacks some characteris-

tics of both processes. Diabetic ION is considered to be the result of diffuse microangiopathy.

The clinical appearance of diabetic ION is optic disc edema that may be sectoral or total (Fig. 1–69). There may be associated circumpapillary superficial hemorrhages. There usually is associated background diabetic retinopathy, although disc neovascularization has been reported along with diabetic ION. **See color plate 18.**

Signs and Symptoms. There are often no reported signs or symptoms associated with diabetic ION. Visual field loss varies from enlarged blind spots to isolated scotomas. Vision loss may occur but is typically mild to moderate.

Prognosis and Management. Vision loss or visual field compromise usually resolves over a few months without therapeutic intervention. If the condition is extensive, residual optic atrophy may occur.

Proper diagnosis is crucial. The clinician must rule out optic disc edema secondary to a space-occupying lesion as well as ruling out neovascularization of the disc. This usually necessitates a consultation with neuro-ophthalmology. Fluorescein angiography will demonstrate leakage with both diabetic ION and neovascularization of the disc. Certainly, one must investigate the current status of control of the diabetes as well as the possibility of other types of hematologic or blood vessel disease.

In general, corticosteroid therapy should be avoided in diabetic patients because of the potentiation of diabetes by these therapeutic agents.

DIABETIC ISCHEMIC OPTIC NEUROPATHY—PEARLS

- Small vessel disease of the optic nerve head
- Occurs in young Type 1 patients with diabetes
- Optic disc edema that may be accompanied by hemorrhages
- Vision loss is typically minimal, but visual field loss may be variable
- Usually resolves without damage
- Management includes
  - Rule out other causes of optic disc edema; a neuro-ophthalmology consultation
  - Evaluate control of diabetes
  - Standard eye examination follow-up

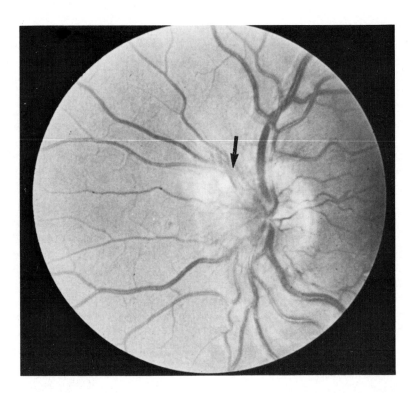

Figure 1–69. The arrow points to a nasal zone of disc edema in a case of diabetic ischemic optic-neuropathy.

Papillophlebitis

Appearance and Layers Involved. Papillophlebitis (Figs. 1–70 and 1–71) is a relatively minor affliction of the optic nerve occurring in otherwise healthy young adults 20 to 40 years of age. Males and females are affected equally.

The condition appears as optic disc edema supposedly secondary to inflammatory occlusion of the central retinal vein. There are two distinctive ophthalmoscopic presentations: (1) gross unilateral optic disc edema with no retinal vascular changes and (2) unilateral optic disc edema with hemorrhages on and surrounding the disc, accompanied by grossly dilated and tortuous retinal veins.

Signs and Symptoms. A patient with papillophlebitis usually has visual acuity reduced to the 20/30 level. This complaint is, however, often vague. There may be enlarged blind spots and variable central scotomas.

Prognosis. Papillophlebitis is considered self-limiting, with none of the sequelae commonly identified with central retinal vein occlusion, papilledema, inflammatory optic neuropathy, or ischemic optic neuropathy. The condition is a hybrid, resolving untreated over a 6 to 18 month period. Mild vision reduction may occur associated with macular pigmentary changes. Perivenous sheathing of large veins may occur, as may persistent dilated venules in and around the disc. An optociliary shunt may form to drain the vascular congestion of the nerve head.

Management. As with all other optic nerve diseases, management is controversial in papillophlebitis. Intervention with corticosteroid therapy is advocated by some who point to the inflammatory nature of the disease. Opponents of therapy note the fact that the disease is basically benign and self-limited and institution of therapy may mask the true underlying cause. Of primary concern in this disease is the ruling out of other causes of optic disc edema. To rule out other causes of optic disc edema, the clinician may order skull films and CT scans, chest x-rays, blood work including complete blood count, Lupus erythematosus (LE) preparation, antinuclear antibody (ANA), ESR, Fluorescent Treponemal Antibody Absorption (FTA-ABS), and possibly a lumbar puncture. Always remember, however, that in most cases of papillophlebitis these tests are nonproductive.

The neuro-ophthalmology consultation can best rule out the cause of unilateral optic disc edema. In the case of suspected papillophlebitis, the consultation is not an emergency as it is in TAION.

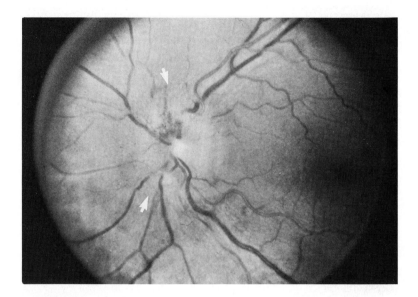

Figure 1–70. Optic disc edema, hemorrhage, and venous tortuosity in a case of papillophlebitis.

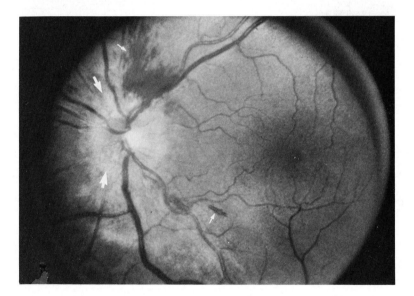

Figure 1–71. Variant of papillophlebitis characterized by scattered hemorrhaging.

PAPILLOPHLEBITIS—PEARLS

- Optic disc edema secondary to affectation of the disc veins
- May be accompanied by hemorrhages and dilated tortuous veins
- Usually in otherwise healthy young adults (20 to 40 years of age) with slight reduction in vision
- Resolves untreated in 6 to 18 months
- Usually no strong relationship to systemic disease
- Management includes
  - Rule out other causes of optic disc edema
  - Rule out possible systemic disease
  - Corticosteroid therapy is controversial, but a neuro-ophthalmology consultation is prudent

Toxic Optic Neuropathy

Appearance and Layers Involved. Toxic optic neuropathy (Fig. 1–72) can occur as a result of nerve fiber reaction to toxins or deficiencies of nutrition. The atrophy occurs secondary to exogenous metabolic stimuli. The affectation of the nerve fibers appears to be the result of alteration in adenosine triphosphate (ATP) formation. This alteration seems to cause a stasis of axoplasmic flow, with secondary optic disc edema and eventual axonal atrophy. **See color plate 19.**

Initially there is optic disc edema with the possibility of splinter hemorrhages. As the condition progresses unchecked, optic atrophy occurs.

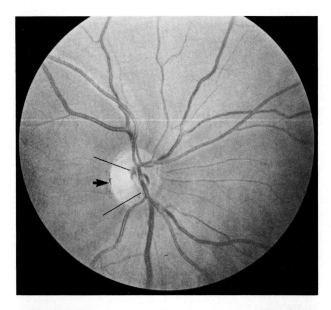

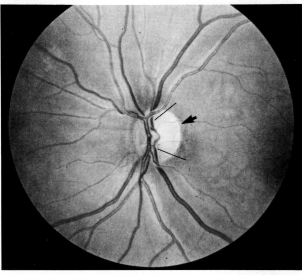

Figure 1–72. In both the right eye **(top)** and the left eye **(bottom),** there is a zone of optic atrophy secondary to alcohol toxicity.

Signs and Symptoms.

With toxic optic neuropathy, there is a gradual bilateral loss of visual acuity. Centrocecal scotomas are the classic presentation, but there is some variability. Concentric contraction of the visual fields occurs with tryparsamide poisoning. The field changes are progressive but may be reversed with therapeutic intervention. There is color vision loss, as well. The condition is insidious in its onset and progression.

Prognosis and Management.

Toxic optic neuropathy progresses to permanent irreversible vision loss if intervention does not occur. Even with intervention, permanent loss of vision or visual field may occur.

Toxic optic neuropathy is reversible if the toxic agent or nutritional problem is discovered and elim-

TABLE 1–18. SUBSTANCES RESPONSIBLE FOR TOXIC OPTIC NEUROPATHY

Alcohol	Hydroxychloroquine
Antabuse	Iodide
Barbiturates	compounds
Carbon monoxide	Iodochlorhydroxyquin
Chloramphenicol	Isoniazid
Chloroquine	Lead
Corticosteroids	Placidyl
Cyanide	Phenothiazines
Digitalis	Streptomycin
Diiodohydroxyquin	Tobacco
Ethambutol over	Tryparsamide
15 mg/kg	Vitamin D
Heavy metals	Disulfiram
Hexamethonium	Ethchlorvynol

Modified from Alexander LJ: Diseases of the optic nerve. In Bartlett JD, Jaanus SD (eds): *Clinical Ocular Pharmacology*. Boston, Butterworth, 1989.

inated. Table 1–18 lists some of the substances responsible for the genesis of toxic optic neuropathy.

Certain drugs will alter zinc serum levels and precipitate optic atrophy. These include ethambutol, diiodohydroxyquin, and iodochlorhydroxyquin. Serum zinc levels should be evaluated in these patients, with 100 to 250 mg of zinc sulfate (three times a day) given if the initial signs of neuropathy develop. The dosage of oral zinc sulfate depends on the individual's ability to absorb the drug as well as the appearance of side effects, such as nausea, vomiting, diarrhea, and gastric bleeding. Zinc sulfate therapy is currently under investigation by the Food and Drug Administration.

Should isoniazid be implicated in toxic optic neuropathy, pyridoxine (vitamin B_6) may be used, with 25 to 100 mg/day as the standard dosage. This therapy has been recommended prophylactically in all patients placed on isoniazid therapy.

Toxic neuropathy secondary to tobacco or alcohol use usually is associated with vitamin B_{12} deficiencies. Treatment for this condition involves removal of the violating dietary agent and adjunctive vitamin therapy. Because often there is poor intestinal absorption of vitamin B_{12} in these conditions, the therapy must be given intramuscularly. The standard dosage is 1000 μg of intramuscular hydroxocobalamin each week for 3 weeks, often supplemented by 300 mg of oral thiamine each week. It should be noted that vitamin B_{12} deficiency also can cause megaloblastic anemia, which would appear as hemorrhages and cotton wool spots in the posterior pole. A complete blood count will confirm the diagnosis of associated anemia. Serum folate levels may need to be checked as well as serum vitamin B_{12} levels.

In the management of toxic optic neuropathy, prevention is the most effective tool. Although prevention is not always possible because of the nature of the disease, prevention can be a part of the plan when known violating drugs are used in patients for therapeutic purposes. With the initiation of any drug therapy known to cause optic neuropathy, it is important to use routine eye examination as well as some form of patient home monitoring. The sooner the optic neuropathy is discovered, the better the potential for reversal.

TOXIC OPTIC NEUROPATHY—PEARLS

- Optic disc edema followed by optic atrophy as the result of toxins or nutritional deficiencies
- Gradual bilateral loss of vision with classic presentation of central scotomas
- If diagnosed early enough, possible to reverse the process by elimination of the toxic agent or nutritional supplementation
- Patients taking known toxic substances should have routine eye examinations and should employ home monitoring to prevent irreversible changes

---

Papilledema

Appearance and Layers Involved. Papilledema (Figs. 1–73 to 1–76) is best defined as optic disc edema secondary to increased intracranial pressure. The primary cause of disc swelling is the blockage of axoplasmic transport in the prelaminar portion of the ganglion cell axons. The blockage occurs at the lamina cribrosa, with accumulation of mitochondria and other axoplasmic particles in the nerve head. The nerve head swells forward into the vitreous as well as laterally, causing the retina to buckle inward. This buckling is known as Paton's folds and affects the function of the circumpapillary photoreceptors, creating the enlarged blind spot. The patient may notice metamorphopsia in the area of the blind spot as well. Figure 1–77 outlines the proposed etiopathogenesis of papilledema.

Optic disc edema is considered the first observable clinical sign of papilledema. The disc edema can occur 1 to 7 days after an increased intracranial pressure but even sooner (2 to 48 hours)

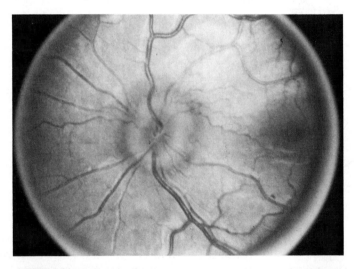

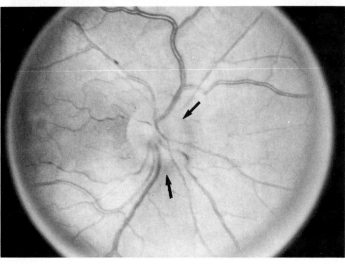

Figure 1–73. Top. Considerable disc swelling is the characteristic in this left optic nerve head. This compensated papilledema was secondary to benign intracranial hypertension. **Bottom.** The fellow eye, with moderate swelling confined to the areas of the disc indicated by the arrows.

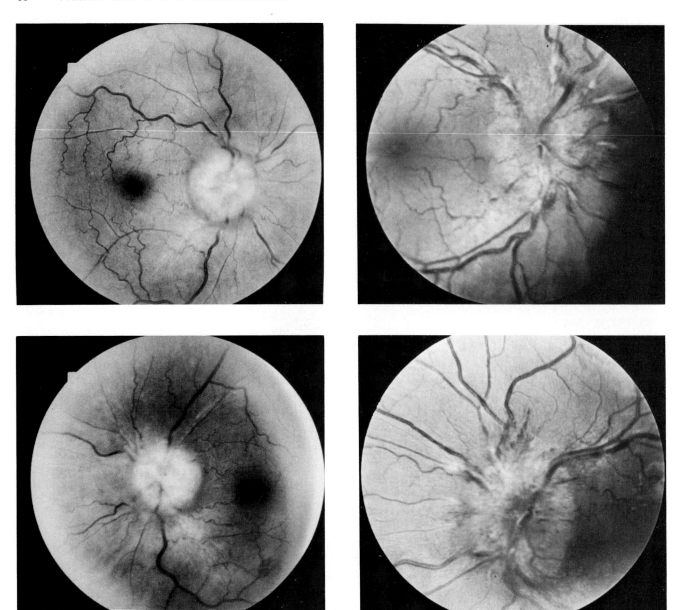

Figure 1–74. Top and Bottom. Bilateral compensated papilledema. Note the severe disc swelling and venous tortuosity but absence of hemorrhage and cotton wool spots.

Figure 1–75. Top and Bottom. Bilateral noncompensated papilledema characterized by significant disc edema, venous tortuosity, flame-shaped hemorrhages, and cotton wool spots.

as the consequence of abrupt intracranial hemorrhage. The swelling of the nerve fibers and subsequent debris accumulation occur initially in the inferior aspect of the disc, followed by the superior, nasal, and temporal aspects. The swelling spreads into the surrounding retina. Disc vessel involvement then occurs. The condition is usually bilateral but may be asymmetrical. **See color plates 20 and 21.**

Clinically, one may consider two distinct varieties of papilledema, compensated and noncompensated. Acute noncompensated papilledema is representative of a rapid rise in intracranial pres-

sure that does not allow for compensatory measures by the disc vasculature. This results in grossly swollen discs with flame-shaped hemorrhages and cotton wool spots. Initially, vision is intact but blind spots are enlarged. Chronic compensated papilledema is characterized by gross disc-into-retina swelling with minimal vascular changes because the disc vessels have had time to compensate for the rise in pressure.

Absence of venous pulsation is of questionable value in differentiating papilledema from pseudopapilledema. The often reported sign of reddish

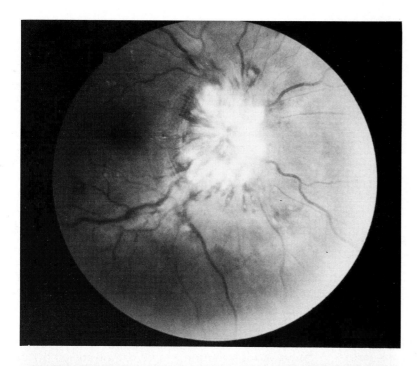

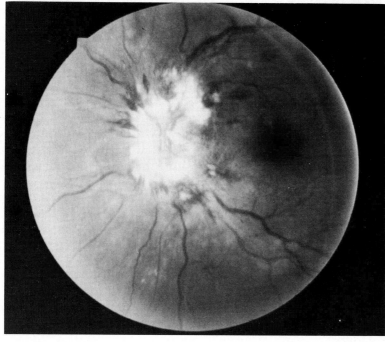

Figure 1–76. Top and Bottom. Bilateral noncompensated papilledema with a predominance of cotton wool spots overlying severely swollen nerve heads.

disc coloration may be due solely to a smaller than average scleral canal. A hyperemic disc does not equate to acquired papilledema.

Signs and Symptoms. Transient obscurations or 5 to 30 second blurring or loss of vision associated with postural changes may occur as prodromal symptoms of papilledema. Visual symptoms are rare in the early phases of papilledema because axoplasmic stasis will not alter the transmission of the nerve impulse along the outer membrane of the

nerve fibers. Reduction in vision does occur with ischemia secondary to compression of optic nerve vasculature.

Visual field defects appear as an enlarged blind spot. The blind spot may then spread out to involve the macular area. As nerve destruction continues, variable field defects occur.

Focal neurological signs associated with increased intracranial pressure may occur associated with papilledema. In addition, benign intracranial hypertension (pseudotumor cerebri) is another im-

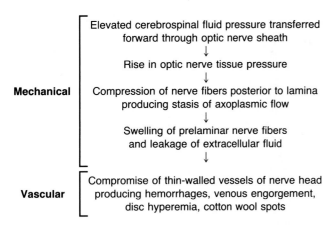

Figure 1–77. The mechanical theory of etiopathogenesis of papilledema.

portant cause of papilledema. Benign intracranial hypertension is characterized by bilateral papilledema associated with headache, altered blind spot, sudden increased obesity, occasional sixth nerve palsy with the absence of frank neurological signs, and depressed plasma corticosteroid levels. Benign intracranial hypertension occurs most frequently in females age 10 to 50 years. Benign intracranial hypertension is not life-threatening, but optic atrophy can occur secondary to the longstanding disc edema. Benign intracranial hypertension may be secondary to otitis media, minor head injury, or such toxic conditions as hypervitaminosis A (especially in children), tetracycline, or nalidixic acid toxicity. In over 50 percent of the patients, the etiology of benign intracranial hypertension is unknown.

Should vitamin A intoxication be suspected as the cause of papilledema, other signs may appear. Vitamin A intoxication is characterized by dry rough skin, fissuring of the angles at the mouth, loss of hair, migratory bone pain, headache, blurred vision or diplopia, and nausea with vertigo.

Complications of papilledema that may lead to reduction of visual acuity include choroidal neovascularization, preretinal macular hemorrhage, choroidal folds, and macular star formation. Another sign of long-standing papilledema is an optociliary shunt vessel on the nerve head occurring secondary to optic nerve compression. These shunt vessels often are associated with sphenoid ridge meningiomas.

Prognosis. When considering papilledema, the clinician must realize that untreated papilledema can result in optic atrophy, but the underlying condition may cause death. It is imperative that the cause of increased intracranial pressure be determined and eliminated or controlled.

Management. After differentiating papilledema from pseudopapilledema, it is important to determine the cause of increased intracranial pressure (Table 1–19).

If the underlying cause cannot be determined readily, medical or surgical intervention must be undertaken to prevent continuing compromise resulting in optic atrophy.

Medical treatment must be initiated only after ruling out space-occupying lesions because papilledema may resolve but the causative agent may remain. Medical therapy is instituted to control or eliminate cerebral edema. Medical control can be achieved by using 2 to 4 g of acetazolamide plus 40 to 100 mg of oral prednisolone per day. Should this not achieve control, surgical intervention by lumbar puncture, neurosurgical shunting procedures, or optic nerve decompression must be employed. Surgical intervention can be compromised by infection and must be undertaken with great care.

Treatment of benign intracranial hypertension is determined by cause. Since benign intracranial hypertension is considered a self-limiting process, intervention is necessary only in cases of severe headaches or papilledema threatening to progress. There are advocates of the standard prednisolone–acetazolamide therapy and advocates of dehydration therapy. In any case, if increased intracranial pressure threatens vision, intervention must occur even to the point of neurosurgical shunting or optic nerve decompression.

Should a patient have suspect papilledema, take care to make a careful differential diagnosis from other causes of optic disc edema. Immediate consultation with neurology, neuro-ophthalmology, or neurosurgery is indicated to discern the cause of the papilledema and initiate therapy or surgical intervention as soon as possible.

Table 1–20 provides a summary of the characteristics of optic neuropathy.

TABLE 1–19. POSSIBLE CAUSES OF INCREASED INTRACRANIAL PRESSURE

Space-occupying lesion
Aqueductal stenosis
Obstruction of cerebrospinal fluid resorption
Intracerebral hemorrhage
Subarachnoid hemorrhage
Tumors of the spinal cord
Inflammatory polyneuritis
Infectious disease
Toxic metabolic diseases
Trauma
Lithium carbonate at therapeutic doses

TABLE 1-20. CHARACTERISTICS OF OPTIC NEUROPATHY

Characteristic	Inflammatory Optic Neuropathy	Demyelinizing Optic Neuropathy	Arteriosclerotic–Hypertensive Ischemic Optic Neuropathy	Temporal Arteritic Ischemic Optic Neuropathy	Diabetic Ischemic Optic Neuropathy	Papilledema
Age	Usually under age 20	20–40 years	50–70 years	60–80 years	Young diabetics	No specific age
Laterality	Usually unilateral in adults, may be bilateral in children	Unilateral initially	Unilateral but may become bilateral	Starts unilateral	Variable	Typically bilateral but asymmetrical
Vision loss	Moderate to severe	Variable but worsens with repeated attacks	Minimal to severe	Usually severe	None to minimal	Usually none
Visual field	Usually central scotoma	Variable but often central scotoma	Altitudinal, arcuate, central scotoma or generalized field constriction	Altitudinal, arcuate, central scotoma or field constriction	Enlarged blind spot	Enlarged blind spot
Pupillary findings	Positive Gunn sign	Positive Gunn sign	Positive Gunn sign	Positive Gunn sign	Usually normal	Normal
Other signs	Pain on ocular movement in addition to a tender globe, plus orbit or brow ache	Pain on gross excursions, cerebellar signs, remissions, and exacerbations	Elevated blood pressure possible, diabetes possible, prominent temporal migraine possible, occlusive artery disease possible	Fever, weakness, muscle pain, head pain, jaw pain, weight loss, artery nonpulsatile and tender to palpation, transient blackouts	Type 1 diabetes	Headache, nausea, vomiting, transient obscurations
Fundus	Often exudates near disc; disc swelling and flame hemorrhages; optic atrophy occurs	Usually retrobulbar and nothing is seen; may have optic disc edema; optic atrophy is the result	Segmental or diffuse disc swelling, splinter hemorrhages; optic atrophy segmental	Disc swelling and chalky appearance to disc; ultimately optic atrophy	Disc edema plus other signs of diabetes possible	Variable disc edema with flame hemorrhages and cotton wool spots
Treatment	Controversy, but possible corticosteroid therapy; discern cause	Controversial, but possible corticosteroid therapy	No specific treatment but monitor vascular status; corticosteroid use often attempted	Aggressive corticosteroid therapy	None, but assess systemic health and assure that there is no neurologic cause	Referral to neuroophthalmologist or neurosurgeon for further testing to uncover underlying etiology
Visual prognosis	Poor prognosis unless therapy instituted to prevent optic atrophy	Unpredictable and highly variable, with exacerbations	Poor prognosis for recovery	Poor prognosis with chance of fellow eye involvement	Usually returns to normal or near normal	Good vision if pressure is relieved

OPTIC NERVE HEAD TUMORS

Both primary and secondary tumors may occur within the confines of the optic nerve. Primary tumors of the optic nerve head include vascular tumors, astrocytic hamartomas, melanocytomas, and medulloepitheliomas. Secondary tumors, such as retinoblastoma, uveal melanoma, metastatic carcinoma, and meningiomas, may extend into the optic nerve head. **Differential diagnosis and clinical pearls are listed in Table 1–21.**

Vascular tumors are discussed in the section on retinal vascular disease.

Melanocytoma

A melanocytoma of the optic nerve head is a primary tumor that occurs as an elevated black (may be gray to dark black) lesion on the nerve head that can involve the nerve fiber layer and present flayed edges (Fig. 1–78). It actually can appear as the photographic negative of myelinated nerve fibers. Usually 50 percent or less of the disc is covered, but in approximately 10 percent of cases, most of the disc is covered. The melanocytoma may grow beyond the borders of the disc. Growth can occur over 5 to 20 years, and there may be potential for malignant transformation. Optic disc edema, sheathing of retinal vessels, and subretinal edema may occur associated with the tumor.

Vision may become reduced with melanocytoma, but over 75 percent of eyes maintain an acuity of 20/15 to 20/30. Field defects and pupillary defects may occur. Melanocytomas occur in blacks as well as whites, but uveal melanomas are very rare in blacks.

The melanocytoma is composed of pigmented polyhedral cells that readily block fluorescence throughout a fluorescein angiogram.

Management of melanocytoma of the optic disc consists of proper diagnosis and follow-up to ensure that there is no progression to malignancy.

Astrocytic Hamartoma

Astrocytic hamartomas are considered to be congenital and have variable presentation. The lesions may appear anywhere in the retina but tend to occur on or near the optic nerve head. These lesions have an association with tuberous sclerosis and, less commonly, neurofibromatosis. In fact, over 50 percent of patients with tuberous sclerosis have astrocytic hamartomas of the retina or optic nerve. Tuberous sclerosis presents other signs and symptoms to assist in the differential diagnosis, including adenoma sebaceum (butterfly shape on nose and cheeks), seizures, cutaneous patches, mental retardation, and intracranial calcifications.

The tumor may appear as a dirty white lesion that is oval with a relatively smooth surface. It also may appear as a whitish yellow multilobulated mulberry lesion. It has been suggested that the multilobulated lesion may be an aged version of the smooth variety. The lesions may autofluoresce.

Vision may be decreased, and visual fields may be affected. The lesion is very slow growing or may remain stable. An astrocytic hamartoma is highly vascularized and hyperfluoresces in all stages of fluorescein angiography.

The astrocytic hamartoma is composed of benign astrocytes, calcium, and collections of other materials. Management of an astrocytic hamartoma consists of ruling out systemic disease associated with the lesion as well as patient education about the condition. **See color plate 22.**

Retinoblastoma. Retinoblastoma is a malignant tumor that may extend from the retina to occupy the optic nerve head. Retinoblastoma is a tumor of the young in that almost all cases are diagnosed before 4 years of age. The mean age of diagnosis is 18 months.

Some families with the inherited form (autosomal dominant with variable penetrance) of retinoblastoma do not show high penetrance and demonstrate retinal lesions, called retinomas, that do not show progression. Retinomas are characterized by a translucent grayish mass protruding into the vitreous that may have cottage cheese calcifications or retinal pigment epithelium migration and proliferation. Virtually all bilateral cases of retinoblastoma are hereditary, whereas 10 to 15 percent of unilateral cases are hereditary.

The retinoblastoma of the optic nerve head is an elevated, dull, chalky lesion that usually is present also in the adjacent retina. The tumor has a

TABLE 1-21. OPTIC NERVE HEAD TUMORS—PEARLS

Tumor	Age of Onset	Laterality	Progression	Ophthalmoscopic Picture	Associated Systemic Conditions	Prognosis and Management
Angiomatosis retinae (autosomal dominant)	15–40 years	Bilateral in 50%	Yes	Reddish orange elevated, well circumscribed	25% with CNS hemangioblastomas; some have pheochromocytoma	Loss of vision, tough to photocoagulate, genetic counseling, neurology consult
Cavernous hemangioma (possible autosomal dominance)	First to second decade	Unilateral	Rare	Grape clusters of aneurysmal dilations with preretinal membrane	Neurocutaneous or oculocutaneous lesions	Education, rare progression, genetic counseling
Melanocytoma	Variable	Unilateral	Common but rare loss of vision	Elevated gray to black lesion eccentric on the nerve head, flayed edges	None	May grow over the years to two disc diameters; Monitor for conversion to malignancy
Astrocytic hamartoma	Congenital	Unilateral	Possible	Dirty white oval, smooth lesion; multilobullated mulberry yellowish lesion	Tuberous sclerosis, neurofibromatosis	Rule out systemic disease, patient education, possible field loss or reduced vision
Retinoblastoma (autosomal dominant)	0–4 years	Either	Yes	Retinomas (nonmalignant), elevated dull chalky lesion with evidence of calcium	Only subsequent possibility of metastasis to intracranial, bone, and liver.	Deadly without intervention; 90% survival with intervention
Spread of diffuse choroidal melanoma	Variable	N/A	Yes	Subretinal yellowish brown area with optic nerve swelling and variable pigmentation	Metastasis to other organs	Five-year mortality rate of 75%; no effective intervention
Metastatic carcinoma	Variable	Bilateral in 20%	Yes	Swollen nerve head associated with yellowish structure; often choroidal metastases as well	Metastasis from breast, lung, stomach, sarcoma	Mean survival time 10 months; symptomatic treatment with radiation and chemotherapy
Leukemic nerve head infiltration	Variable most often in acute cases	Variable	Yes, several	Optic disc edema, hemorrhage, surround of subretinal fluid	Leukemia	Survival rate usually less than 12 months; irradiation may delay vision loss

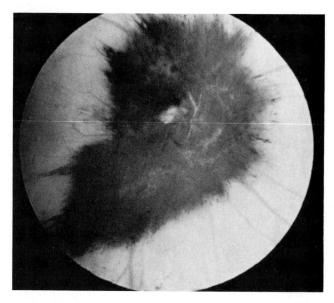

Figure 1–78. Melanocytoma of the optic nerve head spreading to involve the surrounding retina.

high calcium content and is, therefore, very reflective on ultrasonography. Calcium deposits may be visible within the tumor. Fluorescein angiography shows hyperfluorescence throughout, indicating that the tumor is vascularized. Leukokoria, strabismus, and iris neovascularization also are common.

Early identification is crucial, since retinoblastoma can metastasize to the brain, bones, and liver. Enucleation is indicated when the lesion is unilateral and acuity is severly impaired. When bilateral, the lesions may be treated by irradiation, photocoagulation, or cryotherapy. Survival rates for patients with retinoblastoma are above 90 percent when the lesions are treated.

Pedigree analysis and genetic counseling are crucial in cases of retinoblastoma.

Choroidal Melanoma

Choridal melanomas of the optic nerve head result from intrusion from the choroid. The diffuse variety of choroidal melanoma may actively infiltrate the optic nerve area and is highly malignant. The 5-year mortality rate associated with this tumor approaches 75 percent.

The diffuse choroidal melanoma of the optic nerve head is a subretinal yellowish brown area with variable surface pigmentation. As the tumor invades, the optic nerve head swells. Fluorescence with fluorescein angiography is variable depending on the degree of pigmentation.

Management of diffuse choroidal melanoma of the optic nerve head is somewhat controversial, but enucleation usually is performed because of the strong association with metastasis.

Metastatic Carcinoma

Carcinomas usually metastasize to the choroid, but occasionally the optic nerve head may be involved. When a carcinoma metastasizes to the optic nerve head, it occurs bilaterally in almost 20 percent of patients. Often, there will be coincident choroidal metastasis, which appears as a placoid yellow subretinal lesion with overlying sensory retinal primary detachment. The primary lesion often occurs in the breast, lung, or stomach or occurs as a sarcoma.

Carcinomas of the optic nerve head usually cause loss of vision, a swollen nerve head, and a yellowish structure above normal anatomic structures. Venous tortuosity or central retinal vein occlusion often are present.

The mean survival time after the metastasis to the nerve head is under 10 months. Radiation and chemotherapy may be of symptomatic benefit.

Leukemic Nerve Head Infiltration

There is a high rate of ocular involvement in patients who die of leukemia. Acute forms usually create more ocular involvement than do chronic forms. The choroid is the site of greatest involvement, and the optic nerve head is affected at about the same rate as it is with metastatic carcinoma. Optic nerve head involvement usually occurs only in acute cases.

Leukemic infiltration of the nerve head occurs as optic disc edema and may have associated hemorrhaging. Subretinal fluid may surround the infiltrated area. As the leukemic cells replace normal nerve tissue, vision drops significantly to a point where it is not amenable to therapy. Survival rates after nerve head infiltration usually are less than 12 months, but irradiation may delay or abort nerve head destruction and vision loss.

REFERENCES

Alexander LJ: Diseases of the optic nerve, in Bartlett JD, Jaanus SD (eds): *Clinical Ocular Pharmacology*, Boston, Butterworths, 1984, chap 25.

Alexander LJ: The tilted disc syndrome. *J Am Optom Assoc* 1978;49:1060–1062.

Alexander LJ, Jackson JE: Congenital optic nerve hypoplasia. The importance of differential diagnosis. *SJO* 1983;1:16–20.

Alexander LJ, Jones WL, Potter J: *Retina, Retina, Retina. Primary Eye Care*. Philadelphia, 1985.

Alexander LJ, Wilson SM: The macular photostress test. *SJO* 1983;9:5–10.

Anderson DR, Davis EB: Retina and optic nerve after posterior ciliary artery occlusion. *Arch Ophthalmol* 1974;92:422–426.

Appen RE, Chandra SR, Klein R, Meyers FL: Diabetic papillopathy. *AM J Ophthalmol* 1980;90:203–209.

Bird AC, Sanders MO: Choroidal folds in association with papilledema. *Br J Ophthalmol* 1973;57:89–97.

Boddie HG, Banna M, Bradley WG: "Benign" intracranial hypertension: A survey of the clinical and radiological features, and long-term prognosis. *Brain* 1974;97:313–326.

Boghen DR, Glaser JS: Ischemic optic neuropathy. *Brain* 1975;98:689–708.

Boke W, Voigt CJ: Circulatory disturbances of the optic nerve. *Ophthalmologia* 1980;180:88–100.

Brown GC, Augsburger JS: Congenital pits of the optic nerve head and retinochoroidal colobomas. *Can J Ophthalmol* 1980;15:144–146.

Brown GC, Shields J: Tumors of the optic nerve head. *Surv Ophthalmol* 1985;4:239–262.

Brown GC, Shields JA, Goldberg RE: Congenital pits of the optic nerve head. II. Clinical studies in humans. *Ophthalmology* 1980;87:51–65.

Brown GC, Tasman W: *Congenital Anomalies of the Optic Disc.* New York, Grune & Stratton, 1983.

Cogan DG: Coloboma of optic nerve with overlay of peripapillary retina. *Br j Ophthalmol* 1978;62:347–350.

Corbett JJ, Savino PJ, Schatz NJ, Orr LS: Cavitary developmental defects of the optic disc. *Arch Neurol* 1980;37:210–213.

Dorrell D. The tilted disc. *Br J Ophthalmol* 1978;62:16–20.

Eggers HM, Sanders MD: Acquired optociliary shunts vessels in papilloedema. *Br J Ophthalmol* 1980;64:267–271.

Ellenberger C, Messner KH: Papillophlebitis: Benign retinopathy resembling papilledema or papillitis. *Anns Neurol* 1978;3:438–440.

Francois J. Hereditary optic atrophy. *Int Ophthalmol Clin* 1968;8:1016–1054.

Fraunfelder FT, Roy FH: *Current Ocular Therapy.* Philadelphia, Saunders, 1980.

Galbraith JFK, Sullivan JH: Decompression of the perioptic meninges for relief of papilledema. *Am J Ophthalmol* 1973;76:687–692.

Galvin R, Sanders MD: Peripheral retinal hemorrhages with papilloedema. *Br J Ophthalmol* 1980;64:262–266.

Glaser JS: Neuro-ophthalmic examination: General considerations and special techniques, in Duane TD (ed): *Clinical Ophthalmology.* Philadelphia, Harper and Row, 1981, chap 2.

Goldstein JE, Cogan DG: Exercise and the optic neuropathy of multiple sclerosis. *Arch Ophthalmol* 1964;72:168–170.

Griffin JF, Wray SH: Acquired color vision defects in retrobulbar neuritis. *Am J Ophthalmol* 1978;86:193–201.

Gupta DR, Strobas RJ: Bilateral papillitis associated with Cafergot therapy. *Neurology* 1972;22:793–797.

Hayreh MS, Hayreh SS, Baumbach GL, et al: Methyl alcohol poisoning. III. Ocular toxicity. *Arch Ophthalmol* 1977;95:1851–1858.

Hayreh SS: *Anterior Ischemic Optic Neuropathy.* New York, Springer-Verlag, 1975.

Hayreh SS: Anterior ischemic optic neuropathy. III. Treatment, prophylaxis, and differential diagnosis. *Br J Ophthalmol* 1974;58:981–989.

Hayreh SS: Optic disc edema in raised intracranial pressure. *Arch Ophthalmol* 1977;95:1553–1565.

Hayreh SS: *Anterior Ischemic Optic Neuropathy.* New York, Springer-Verlag, 1975.

Hayreh SS: Optic disc vasculitis. *Br J Ophthalmol* 1972;56:652–670.

Herring R: How to perform and interpret the Amsler grid. *SJO* 1983;1:8–17.

Hotchkiss ML, Green WR: Optic nerve aplasia and hypoplasia. *J Pediatr Ophthalmol Strabismus* 1979;16:225–240.

Hoyt CS: Autosomal dominant optic atrophy. *Ophthalmology* 1980;87:245–250.

Jamison RR: Subretinal neovascularization and papilledema associated with pseudotumor cerebri. *Am J Ophthalmol* 1978;85:78–81.

Jefferson A, Clark J: Treatment of benign intracranial hypertension by dehydrating agents with particular reference to the measurement of the blind spot area as a means of recording improvement. *J Neurosurg Psychiatry* 1976;39:627–639.

Johnson I, Paterson A: Benign intracranial hypertension. I. Diagnosis and prognosis. *Brain* 1974;97:289–300.

Johnson I, Paterson A: Benign intracranial hypertension. II. CSF pressure and circulation. *Brain* 1974;97:301–312.

Kline LB, Glaser JS: Dominant optic atrophy. *Arch Ophthalmol* 1979;97:1680–1686.

Krill AE: *Hereditary Retinal and Choroidal Diseases. Clinical Characteristics.* Hagerstown, Harper and Row, 1977, vol. 2.

Laibovitz RA: Presumed phlebitis of the optic disc. *Ophthalmology* 1979;86:313–319.

Leopold IH: Zinc deficiency and visual impairment? (Editorial), *AM J Ophthalmol* 1978;85:871–878.

Lobo A, Pilek E, Stokes PE: Papilledema following therapeutic dosages of lithium carbonate. *J Nerv Ment Dis* 1978;166:526–529.

Martin-Amat G, Tephly TR, McMartin KE, et al: Methyl alcohol poisoning. II. Development of a model for ocular toxicity in methyl alcohol poison using the rhesus monkey. *Arch Ophthalmol* 1977;95:1847–1850.

Miller NR: Anterior ischemic optic neuropathy: Diagnosis and management. *Bull NY Acad Med* 1980;56:643–654.

Mosher HA: The prognosis in temporal arteritis. *Arch Ophthalmol* 1959;62:641–644.

Nikoskelainen E: Symptoms, signs and early course of optic neuritis. *Acta Ophthalmol* 1975;53:254–271.

Perkin GD, Rose FC: *Optic Neuritis and Its Differential Diagnosis.* New York, Oxford University Press, 1979.

Perkin GD, Rose FC: Uhthoff's syndrome. *Br J Ophthalmol* 1976;60:60–63.

Perrine JM: Drusen of the optic nerve head. *SJO* 1983;1:17–21.

Quigley H, Anderson DR: Cupping of the optic disc in ischemic optic neuropathy. *Trans Am Acad Ophthalmol Otolaryngol* 1977;83:755–762.

Rosenberg MA, Savino PJ, Glaser JS: A clinical analysis of pseudopapilledema. I. Population, laterality, acuity, refractive error, ophthalmoscopic characteristics, and coincident disease. *Arch Ophthalmol* 1979;97:65–70.

Savino PJ, Glaser JS: Pseudopapilledema versus papilledema. *Int Ophthalmol Clin* 1977;17:115–137.

Savino PJ, Glaser JS, Rosenberg MA: A clinical analysis of pseudopapilledema. II. Visual field defects. *Arch Ophthalmol* 1979;97:71–75.

Seedorff T: Leber's disease. V. *Acta Ophthalmol* 1970;48:186–213.

Seedorff T: Leber's disease. IV. *Acta Ophthalmol* 1969;47:813–821.

Smith JL: *The Optic Nerve.* Miami, Neuro-Ophthalmology Tapes, 1977.

Smith JL, Hoyt WF, Susac JO: Ocular fundus in acute Leber optic neuropathy. *Arch Ophthalmol* 1973;90:349–354.

Sokol S: The Pulfrich stereo-illusion as an index of optic nerve dysfunction. *Surv Ophthalmol* 1976;20:432–434.

Spalton DJ, Hitchings RA, Hunter PA: *Atlas of Clinical Ophthalmology.* London, Gower, 1984.

Spencer WH: *Ophthalmic Pathology. An Atlas and Textbook.* Philadelphia, Saunders, 1986.

Spoor TC: *Modern Management of Ocular Diseases.* Thorofare, NJ, Charles Slack, 1985.

Steahly LP: A colobomatous optic disc anomaly and associated retinal detachment. *J Pediatr Ophthalmol Strabismus* 1977;14:103–105.

Steinkuller PG: The morning glory disc anomaly: Case report and literature review. *J Pediatr Ophthalmol Strabismus* 1980;17:81–87.

Theodossiadis G: Evolution of congenital pit of the optic disc with macular detachment in photocoagulated and nonphotocoagulated eyes. *Am J Ophthalmol* 1977;84:620–631.

Walsh FB, Hoyt WF: *Clinical Neuro-ophthalmology,* 3rd ed. Baltimore, Williams & Wilkins, 1969.

Wirtschafter JD, Rizzo FJ, Smiley BC: Optic nerve axoplasm and papilledema. *Surv Ophthalmol* 1975;20:157–189.

Yanoff M, Fine BS: *Ocular Pathology. A Text and Atlas.* Hagerstown, MD, Harper and Row, 1975.

2

Retinal Vascular Disorders

RETINAL VASCULAR ANATOMY AND PHYSIOLOGY

The retinal tissue has the highest consumption of oxygen by weight of any tissue in the human body. The outer third of the retina is supplied by the choroidal–choriocapillaris system, and the inner two thirds of the retina is supplied by branches of the central retinal artery system. The choroidal system is characterized by fenestrated vessels that allow for a free exchange of fluids, creating a spongelike tissue layer. This system is nutritive but also serves as a cooling system for the retina. The retinal circulation is characterized by vessels that do not leak readily except in diseased conditions.

Basic Embryologic Development
The hyaloid vascular system supplies the eye structures until the fourth month. At that stage, spindle (mesenchymal) cells of Bergmeister's papilla form vascular channels that grow into the nerve fiber layer. This cellular proliferation continues toward

69

the ora serrata in the form of endothelial cords. Clefts then develop in these cords by endothelial cell proliferation. These clefts expand into a profusion of very small vascular channels that spread throughout the retina. The channelization reaches the nasal ora at about the same time as it reaches the temporal equator.

As development continues, larger caliber vessels are created by redirection of blood flow combined with selective atrophy of a large number of endothelial cords. There remains a vascular-free zone around the larger vessels in adulthood, wider around arteries than around veins. The retinal vasculature is the last of retinal structures to develop and does not stop until about 3 months after full gestation. Retinal capillaries do not attain maturity for several years, as evidenced by the fact that intramural pericytes only begin to appear at birth.

The Arteries

The central retinal artery along with a cilioretinal artery (25 percent of the population) serves as the blood supply to the inner retina. The central retinal artery is a branch of the ophthalmic artery derived from the internal carotid system. The central retinal artery has a smooth muscle layer as it passes through the optic nerve and can be affected by diseases of other muscular arteries, such as cranial arteritis. The central retinal artery loses the internal elastic lamina as it passes into the retina. Arteriosclerosis that involves intimal and endothelial hyperplasia may occur within the optic nerve and retinal portion of the arteries. As the artery passes through the lamina cribrosa, there is a focal constriction that can serve as a site for embolic occlusion.

As mentioned previously, the arteries within the retina are devoid of elastic lamina but have well-developed smooth muscle. The vessels diminish in caliber toward the retinal periphery to come within about 1.5 mm of the ora. Throughout the retinal tissue, the arteries maintain a strong barrier to perfusion of blood components. Diseased vascular states alter this tight-walled construction, allowing for leakage and intraretinal edema. Intraretinal arteries are not affected by either sympathetic or parasympathetic innervation.

Arteries lie in the nerve fiber or ganglion cell layer, with strong connections to the internal limiting membrane. This strong adhesion may become an important factor in the genesis of retinal hemorrhage. The arteries are insulated from retinal tissue by the glial perivascular limiting membrane of Kruckmann.

Grossly, the arteries appear less tortuous and of a smaller diameter than the veins. The blood column is a brighter red because of the oxygenation of the blood. The central retinal artery typically enters nasally to the central retinal vein and bifurcates above the nerve head. Arteries typically cross over veins and find their deepest penetration into retinal tissue at this point. There are supposedly no arteriovenous shunts in the retina, and, with the exception of the congenital macrovessel, the arteries and veins usually do not cross the horizontal raphé.

The Veins

The veins are all thin walled with abundant elastic tissue and are very subject to compression. Near the nerve head, the vein walls contain muscle cells that disappear toward the periphery, being replaced by pericytes. The lack of definitive wall structure allows for the variable appearance (sausaging and distention) in diseased conditions. The veins have isolated attachments to retinal structure, contributing to the serpentine appearance in vaso-occlusion. The same glial insulating structure exists with veins as with arteries. An anatomic variation may occur in which the central retinal vein bifurcates retrolaminarly and enters the intraocular region as two separate vessels. This anatomic variation is thought to be one explanation for hemi-central retinal vein occlusions.

The central retinal vein represents the drain for the retinal vascular watershed. When this drain is closed at the lamina or retrolaminarly, a shunt may develop between the central retinal vein and the choroidal system, which is known as an optociliary shunt. At the lamina, as with the central retinal artery, there is compression of the vein or a stricture during passage. This compression is an area for potential turbulence and thrombus deposition.

At artery–vein crossings, there is a merging of arterial adventitia and venous glial coverings. This sharing of tissue results in compression of the vein wall when the arterial wall develops atherosclerotic changes. The compression is variously interpreted as artery–vein crossing changes, with the ultimate example being branch retinal vein occlusion. The venous system extends to within about 1.5 mm of the ora serrata.

The Capillaries

The capillaries spread throughout the retina in two networks. The superficial network runs in the superficial nerve fiber layer and the ganglion cell layer. The superficial network is of a loose arrangement and is considered the postarteriolar network. It most often is affected in arterial-based diseases. The deep network runs primarily in the inner nuclear layer, is tightly packed, and is considered

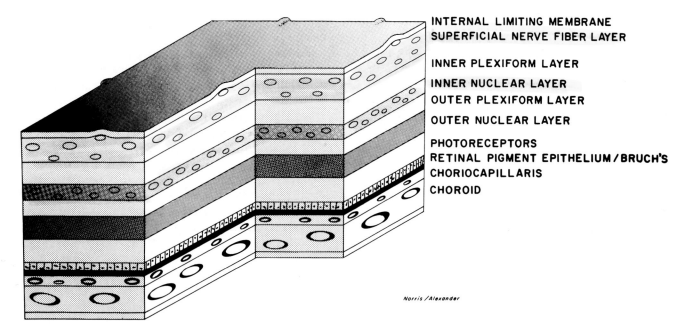

INTERNAL LIMITING MEMBRANE
SUPERFICIAL NERVE FIBER LAYER

INNER PLEXIFORM LAYER
INNER NUCLEAR LAYER
OUTER PLEXIFORM LAYER
OUTER NUCLEAR LAYER

PHOTORECEPTORS
RETINAL PIGMENT EPITHELIUM / BRUCH'S
CHORIOCAPILLARIS
CHOROID

Norris / Alexander

Figure 2–1. A schematic cross-section of the normal retina with representation of vascular locations.

prevenular. The deep capillary layer most often is affected in congestive venous-based diseases (Fig. 2–1). Three zones of the retina are known to vary from this basic scheme. In the circumpapillary zone, there may be four capillary layers, the most superficial of which is the radial peripapillary capillaries, which originate from precapillary retinal arterioles and drain into intraretinal venules on the nerve head. These capillaries are long and pursue a straight path along the superior and inferior temporal arcades out 2 disc diameters but not involving the macula. Figure 2–2 demonstrates the distribution pattern of the radial peripapillary arteries. There is no anastamosis of the radial peripapillary bed with other capillary beds, implying that infarction in this area could create a scotoma. The radial peripapillaries have been implicated in the genesis of glaucomatous field defects, flame-shaped hemorrhages, and cotton wool spots. In the zone near the ora and in the perifoveal region, the capillary net thins to one layer.

Three areas of the retina are devoid of capillaries. Near the ora serrata, there are no capillaries. There is a capillary-free zone 0.5 mm wide centered at the fovea. There is also a capillary-free perivascular zone throughout the retina that is larger around the arteries.

The basic capillary structure is that of endothelial cells, intramural pericytes, and basement membrane. Even with a simplistic structure, the walls form a tight barrier to passage of fluids (blood–retinal barrier) such that metabolic transfer is achieved through pinocytotic vesicle transfer. The pericytes display necrosis in some ischemic vascular disorders, such as diabetes. This loss of pericytes may be the initiating step in microaneurysm formation and possibly shunt formation.

With age, peripheral vessels lose endothelial cells and pericytes. When both are compromised, the capillary shuts down. Dilatation of adjacent capillaries, shunts, and microaneurysms forms as a

RADIAL PERIPAPILLARY DISTRIBUTION

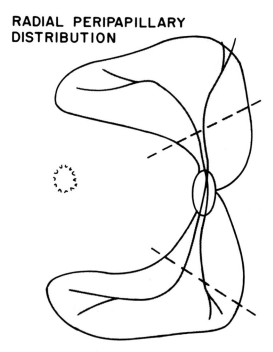

Figure 2–2. A schematic representing the proposed distribution pattern of the superficial radial peripapillary arteries.

normal aging process in the peripheral retina secondary to capillary death. Often this will appear as isolated hemorrhaging in the aged peripheral retina.

The Choroid and Choriocapillaris

Any discussion of the choroid–choriocapillaris complex must include the retinal pigment epithelium and Bruch's membrane.

Retinal Pigment Epithelium. The retinal pigment epithelium (RPE) is a single layer of heavily pigmented cuboidal cells extending from the optic nerve head to the ora serrata. Anterior to the ora, the layer continues but becomes the pigmented epithelium of the ciliary body. The density of the intracellular melanin determines the relative degree of pigmentation. There is a space between the RPE and the photoreceptors filled with mucopolysaccharide glue that can be altered by liquefied vitreous. The RPE is loosely adherent to the overlying sensory retina. The pigment cells are tightly adherent to one another in an area known as the zonula occludens. The basement membrane of the RPE and the fibers of the inner collagenous zone of Bruch's membrane form a very strong bond.

The RPE serves as a barrier between the sensory retina and the choroid. It processes metabolites for the retina and absorbs light. A break in the RPE can cause sensory retinal detachments.

Bruch's Membrane. Bruch's membrane extends from the optic nerve head to the ora serrata as a multilayered structure. It continues beyond the ora with modification characterized by absence of the elastic layer. The innermost layer is the basement membrane of the RPE. The inner collagenous zone is the thickest layer covered by the elastic layer. The outer collagenous zone becomes continuous with the choroidal zone to become a structural framework for the choriocapillaris. The basement membrane of the choriocapillaris envelops the structure. With age, Bruch's membrane develops vesicles, holes, and calcific foci that may evolve into senile maculopathy.

Choriocapillaris. The choriocapillaris is the capillary bed of the choroidal system. The vessels are of larger caliber than retinal capillaries and are fenestrated, which creates a wet sponge effect under Bruch's membrane. The short posterior ciliary arteries, the recurrent branches of the long posterior ciliary arteries, and branches of the anterior ciliary arteries feed this system. Drainage of the system is

provided by venules that eventually drain into the vortex vein ampulla scattered about the equator.

The greatest hemodynamic activity in the retina occurs at the foveal area. As a result, the choriocapillaris is densest in this area. It is important to realize that the choriocapillaris blood supply in this area is compartmentalized as it is in the periphery. A feeder vessel supplies a particular zone, and there is limited anastomosis. An infarct of this vessel creates a window defect and loss of photoreceptor function. This is known as Elschnig spots (Fig. 2–3). The histopathologic equivalent in the peripheral retina is chorioretinal atrophy, or pavingstone degeneration.

Choroid. The choroid proper is composed of larger blood vessels, nerves, melanocytes, immune system cells, and extensions of the collagenous supporting tissue of Bruch's membrane. The larger blood vessels are branches of feeder arteries and drainage veins that support the choriocapillaris. Again, as with the choriocapillaris, there is limited anastomosis of vessels. There is a nervous supply to this vascular system that has been identified as sympathetic-like cells. The immunologic cells represent a source for the genesis of inflammatory retinal disease, such as presumed ocular histoplasmosis.

The choroid supplies nutrition to the RPE and outer third of the retina and serves as a method of dispersion of heat generated by light absorption of the RPE and metabolic activity of the retina.

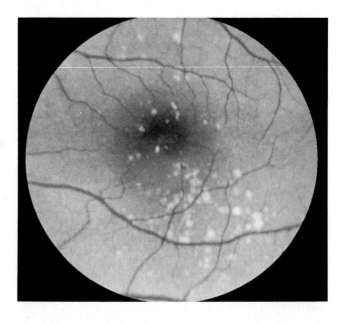

Figure 2–3. Photograph of focal infarcts of the choriocapillaris (Elschnig spots).

Basic Physiology of Retinal Vessels

The ophthalmic artery has sympathetic innervation up to the eye, but there is no sympathetic retinal vessel control within the eye. Retinal vascular changes occur secondary to local metabolic regulation. Adult retinal vessels are narrowed when exposed to excessive oxygen, whereas vasodilatation and hemorrhaging occur at low oxygen concentrations.

The flow of blood within the vessels is faster at the center of the vessels than at the walls. In veins, the blood returning from the periphery flows along the walls, whereas blood from the posterior pole flows through the center of the vein. This gives rise to the laminar flow apparent in fluorescein angiography.

Venous pulsation is present in most adult eyes, and its incidence increases with age because of increased intraocular pressure as well as increased systemic blood pressure. Venous pulsation is determined by the ventricular rate and can, therefore, show alterations during cardiac arrythmia. Venous pulsation may be diminished or absent with (1) decreased intraocular pressure, (2) central retinal vein occlusion, (3) mechanical elevation of venous pressure, and (4) increased intracranial pressure.

Arterial pulsation is an unusual finding in the adult eye. For arterial pulsation to occur, intraocular pressure must be raised above ophthalmic artery pressure (glaucoma) or ophthalmic artery pressure must be lowered below intraocular pressure (internal carotid stenosis). In any case, arterial pulsation at the nerve head often is indicative of an underlying disease condition. A serpentine pulsation—rhythmic lateral arterial movements—may be seen in retinal vessels and is not necessarily indicative of vascular disease.

THE BASICS OF PHOTOCOAGULATION

Laser (light amplification by stimulated emission of radiation) photocoagulation is used to treat retinal vascular disease by its effect on the alteration of ocular tissue. The tissue is altered by varying wavelength and intensity of radiation and is dependent on the absorption characteristics of the retinal tissue and the scatter of that light by the ocular media.

High-energy (short wavelength) photons in the laser dissociate or ionize, disrupting DNA and RNA, which leads to cell death. Photons in the longer wavelengths (low energy) cause vibration and bending of molecules and thermal changes, resulting in cell death. Visible wavelength photons cause thermal damage to the incident cell, resulting in vaporization of intracellular and extracellular fluid and cell death. In all wavelengths, the surrounding tissue is spared as the thermal change is localized, and heat dissipates rapidly when proper burns have been applied.

Pulsed laser energy also is effective in altering structure because a dramatic increase in tissue temperature occurs over a short time frame. The target tissue is treated without altering the surrounding structures. Optical breakdown is the microexplosion that results from pulsed photocoagulation. This can create tissue destruction without thermal change and protein destruction.

Proper photocoagulation depends on effective transmission through the ocular media. It is well known that in the aging eye transmission in all wavelengths is severely depressed. This reduction in transmission is especially apparent in the shorter wavelengths. To offset the scattering and achieve therapeutic effect at the retinal site, the laser intensity and spot size must be increased. Any time a spot size is increased, however, there is the chance of damaging surrounding retinal tissue. This is of special importance near the fovea, since the presence of the yellowish xanthophyll pigment naturally attracts blue wavelengths, enhancing the chances of photochemical and thermal damage to the photoreceptors.

Absorption of the laser wavelengths assists in the therapeutic effect. Most absorption occurs within the melanin-containing retinal structures and blood vessels containing hemoglobins. Figure 2–4 summarizes absorption characteristics of different lasers within the retina. **Table 2–1 summarizes the characteristics of the lasers used in retinal work.** Figures 2–5 through 2–7 illustrate the characteristics of the tissues affected by the application of laser to the retina. New work in dye lasers offers the possibility of improved success rates in laser treatment.

THE BASICS OF FLUORESCEIN STUDIES

Fluorescein angiography and oral fluorography are gaining importance as diagnostic tools now that new developments are being made in laser treatment of retinal vascular disease. Laser modifications and a better understanding of ocular vasculopathy are allowing for earlier therapeutic intervention, treatment closer to the macula (foveal

TISSUE PENETRATION BY LASER LIGHT OF VARIOUS WAVELENGTHS (SHADING INDICATES SITE OF BURN)

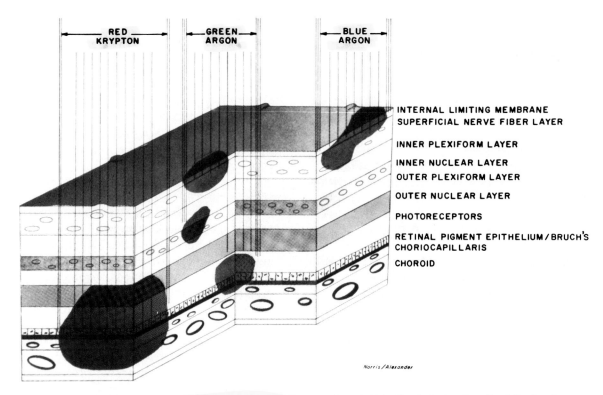

Figure 2–4. Tissue penetration by laser light of various wavelengths (shading indicates the site of the burn).

avascular zone, FAZ), and better visual results. All recent studies point to the importance of early diagnosis of retinal and choroidal vascular disease. In general, the earlier a disease process is discovered and treated, the better the clinical results.

Fluorescein has been used in vision care for over 100 years. The use of fluorescein by the oral route of administration to study the retinal vasculature was attempted in 1910. The first use of intravenous fluorescein was reported in 1930, and sev-

TABLE 2–1. CHARACTERISTICS OF LASERS USED IN OPHTHALMIC DISEASES

Commonly Used Lasers in Retinal Vascular Disease	Wavelength	Molecule and Tissue Absorption Characteristics	Clinical Use
Green argon	514.5 nm	Hemoglobin Oxyhemoglobin Melanin Pigment epithelium	Penetration of media and retina without thermal damage Minimal xanthophyll absorption Problem with blood vessel absorption Used in hemorrhagic retinal disease Retinal tears and holes Retinoschisis
Blue argon	488 nm	Vitreous Crystalline lens Hemoglobin Oxyhemoglobin Melanin Pigment epithelium Xanthophyll pigment	Used to treat retinal hemorrhagic disease Retinoschisis Retinal tears or holes
Red krypton	647. 1 nm	85% choroid 15% retinal pigment epithelium	Penetrates cataracts and cloudy media Passes through hemorrhage and retinal vessels Passes through xanthophyll Treatment of choroidal neovascularization Treatment of retinal tears

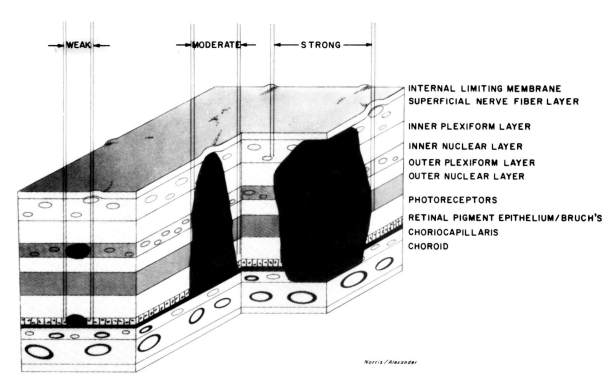

Figure 2–5. Retinal tissue effects of varying intensities of blue—green argon laser burns.

RETINAL TISSUE EFFECTS OF VARYING INTENSITIES OF GREEN ARGON LASER BURNS

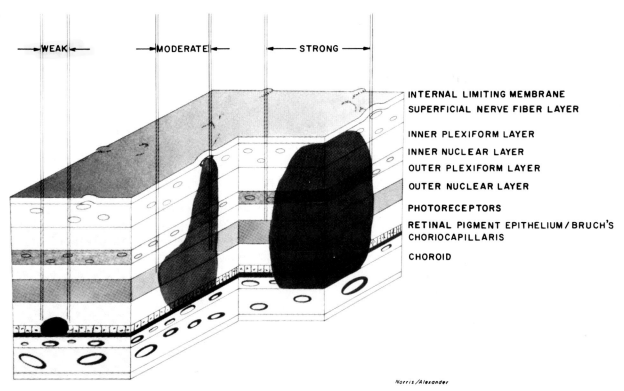

Figure 2–6. Retinal tissue effects of varying intensities of green argon laser burns.

RETINAL TISSUE EFFECTS OF VARYING INTENSITIES OF KRYPTON LASER BURNS

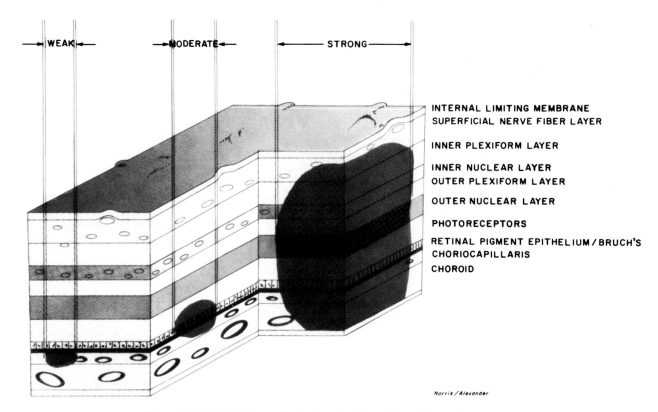

Figure 2–7. Retinal tissue effects of varying intensities of krypton laser burns.

eral other reports followed over the next 30 years. The most significant work, however, came in 1961, with photodocumentation of fluorescein studies. The photographs allowed a more detailed logical approach to understanding fluorescein angiography. The first comprehensive text on fluorescein studies was published in 1977 and was soon followed by other works.

The concept of oral fluorography was resurrected in 1979 to conduct fluorescein studies without the potential systemic side effects. Further studies in oral fluorography established the technique as a viable alternative in diagnosis of retinal vascular diseases. The Oral Fluorescein Study Group was formed in 1984 to further evaluate the orally administered fluorescein technique. The report in 1985 concluded that oral fluorography was not a substitute for the diagnostic capabilities of intravenous fluorescein angiography but was a significant diagnostic tool, especially for fundus disorders that demonstrated fluorescein leakage. It was concluded that minimal side effects occurred with oral administration, whereas it is known that intravenous fluorescein administration carries risks.

Why Perform Fluorescein Angiography?

There must be justification for any diagnostic procedure that has an inherent risk to the patient. Is it safe to assume that a careful dilated fundus examination with state of the art instrumentation is sufficient for maximal patient care? Unfortunately, this assumption is not always valid. It is reasonable to assume that the more diagnostic input that is available, the more efficient and effective is patient management.

Fluorescein angiography is especially useful in detection of subclinical retinal changes in diabetic patients. One study reported that of 272 eyes of 166 patients with no ophthalmoscopically visible vascular changes, fluorescein angiography demonstrated diabetic vascular changes in 66.5 percent. Others report angiographic changes in diabetic children that were not observed by ophthalmoscopy alone. Fluorescein studies have demonstrated significant vascular changes in the midperiphery that were overlooked previously. Prudent clinical judgment would dictate that fluorescein studies should be performed in diabetic patients with any unexplained reduction in macular function, with encroachment of diabetic retinopathy into the macular area, with any sign of proliferative retinopathy, with the appearance of intraretinal microvascular abnormalities (IRMA), and with the appearance of three or more signs of preproliferative diabetic retinopathy. Table 2–2 outlines some ocular disease processes that indicate the need for fluorescein angiography to assist in the differential diagnosis.

The one fact that the clinician must always remember is that a very high percentage of vision-threatening ocular disease has associated leaking retinal or choroidal vessels. Leaking retinal and choroidal vessels are best seen with fluorescein angiography. Edema is most difficult to see with ophthalmoscopy alone.

Technique of Intravenous Fluorescein Angiography

Fluorescein studies may be performed with or without an appropriate fundus camera. If performed with a binocular indirect ophthalmoscopy, the technique is known as fluorescein angioscopy. To successfully perform fluorescein angioscopy, the binocular indirect must be equipped with a high-intensity light source and appropriate filters.

If fluorescein photographic studies are desired, it is necessary to use an appropriately equipped fundus camera. This camera must have a high-intensity flash system with a rapid recycle time as well as appropriate blue excitation and yellow–green barrier filters. The excitation filter should be either the Baird Atomic B4 470 or Kodak Wratten 47 to create a light to stimulate fluorescence. The standard cobalt blue filter is ineffectual. The barrier filter should be either an Ilford 109 Delta Chromatic 3 or Kodak Wratten G15 to block the exciting light from the film plane, allowing only visualization of the fluorescing blood. It should be noted that both barrier and excitation filters lose specificity (fade) with age and should be replaced according to manufacturer's guidelines. It is advisable to fit the camera back with a power winder, since the early phases of fluorescein studies necessitate rapid-fire photography.

Several films and developing processes are available to enhance the results of the studies. Although it is easy to advise the use of any high-speed 200-400 ASA black and white film, it is difficult to advise on processing. It is probably best to contact a local film-processing laboratory or someone else in the community who routinely performs fluorescein studies regarding the optimal processing and film usage. There are some studies that advocate color film because of the ability of the stud-

TABLE 2–2. THE MORE COMMON OCULAR DISEASE CONDITIONS INDICATING THE NEED FOR FLUORESCEIN ANGIOGRAPHY TO ASSIST IN DIFFERENTIAL DIAGNOSIS AND MANAGEMENT

Acute posterior multifocal placoid pigment epitheliopathy (APMPPE)

Angiomatosis retinae

Anterior ischemic optic neuropathy

Bechet's disease

Branch retinal vein occlusion

Cavernous hemangioma of the retina

Choroidal rupture (when developing choroidal neovascularization)

Coat's disease (retinal telangiectasia)

Cystoid maculopathy (Irvine–Gass)

Diabetic retinopathy: If near macula, if proliferative, if intraretinal microvascular abnormalities

Eales' disease

Fuch's spot (degenerative myopia)

Hemicentral retinal vein occlusion

Idiopathic central serous choroidopathy

Iris neovascularization

Maculopathy of angioid streaks

Malignant choroidal melanoma

Preretinal macular fibrosis

Presumed ocular histoplasmosis (macular changes)

Proliferative peripheral retinal disease

Retinal capillary hemangioma

Retinal macroaneurysm

Retinal pigment epithelial dystrophies (central)

Retinal pigment epithelial detachment

Retinal tumors

Sensory retinal detachments

Tumors of iris and ciliary body

ies to eliminate autofluorescence, but adoption of this technique has met with resistance.

Although other dyes have been tried, sodium fluorescein is still the accepted standard. Sodium fluorescein for intravenous injection is available in 5 percent, 10 percent, and 25 percent concentrations. Generic brands are available at considerably reduced prices and may be used without fear. One study, however, reports the presence of a toxic substance, dimethyl formamide, an industrial solvent, in commercially prepared sodium fluorescein for injection. Outdated fluorescein carries the potential for side effects, such as an increase in the incidence of nausea.

Sodium fluorescein is considered pharmacologically inert and fluoresces when stimulated by an excited light source. Fluorescein is injected into a suitable vein in the antecubital space or on the hand. It reaches ocular circulation bound to serum albumin and in a free unbound state. This then fluoresces, allowing for easy visualization of vascular alterations and leakage out of altered vasculature. Factors affecting the quality of the results include clarity of the media, maximal dilation of the patient, and most of all the concentration of sodium fluorescein reaching the retinal–choroidal vascular system. Improper injection is the most significant factor contributing to decreased retinal–choroidal concentration. The injection must be into the vein and performed in a 10 to 15 second time frame.

A crash cart (cardiopulmonary resuscitation unit) must be available on site to handle any potential side effects. Before the procedure, the clinician must ensure that (1) a release form has been read and signed, (2) the patient is aware of what is about to transpire, (3) the patient is maximally dilated, (4) color photographs of the fundus have been taken, (5) red-free photographs of the fundus have been taken on the black and white angiographic film, (6) the fundus camera and patient are adjusted to appropriate comfortable height, (7) the filters are placed in the camera, (8) the proper flash settings are made, and (9) an appropriate intravenous line has been established and maintained with heparinized saline. Then, with 5 ml of 10 percent sodium fluorescein ready in a syringe to replace the heparinized saline, situate the patient in front of the camera and have an assistant attach the syringe of fluorescein. When behind the camera with the appropriate area of the patient's fundus in focus and the filters in place, have the assistant rapidly (over 10 to 15 seconds) inject the bolus of fluorescein. The photography usually begins within about 15 seconds, which is the choroidal flush phase, before which, nothing can be seen in the fundus. Rapid sequence photographs are taken within the first few minutes, then intermittently for the next 10 to 20 minutes. Late-phase photographs will pick up leakage problems, such as sensory retinal detachments associated with choroidal neovascular nets. Specific timing sequences depend on the suspected disease being investigated.

Complications Associated with Intravenous Fluorescein Angiography

Complications are inherent in any procedure, such as fluorescein angiography. Fortunately, the more common complications can be managed easily without aborting the diagnostic procedure. One study reported adverse reactions in 4.82 percent of 5000 procedures. Of these, nausea was most frequent (2.24 percent), followed by vomiting (1.78

percent) and urticaria or pruritus (0.34 percent). It was also found that there was no higher rate of side effects when 25 percent sodium fluorescein was used than when 10 percent sodium fluorescein was used. The itching and hives are thought to be associated with a change in the plasma complement level associated with a rise in the histamine level. In another study of 2631 procedures, it was found that males and young patients experienced side effects at a higher rate. In this study, 1 life-threatening situation, acute pulmonary edema, was reported. Attempts have been made to provide prophylaxis against the histaminic side effects of fluorescein angiography, but statistically significant positive results were not achieved. The author has found that the primary side effect of nausea or warm flush occurs within the first 30 seconds after injection and is very transient in nature. Advising the patient of this potential side effect and assuring the patient that it is very quick to leave has allowed me to take the patient through the problem without aborting the procedure. It is wise to advise patients that their skin and urine will be discolored for a few days after the procedure.

Technique of Oral Fluorography

Oral fluorography can give results similar to those obtained with intravenous fluorescein angiography without the potential side effects. Oral fluorography is especially useful in cases where late dye leakage is expected. It can be performed using either USP Bulk & Powder Sodium Fluorescein or commercially available 5 ml vials of 10 percent injectable sodium fluorescein. The powdered form is difficult to obtain, but using two to three 5 ml vials of 10 percent fluorescein usually is sufficient to obtain good results. The fluorescein is mixed with a powdered flavored citrus drink and allowed to cool in crushed ice. The patient fasts about 8 hours before the test. The patient then is asked to remove any dentures, since the solution will discolor these devices. Before the procedure it must be ensured that (1) a release form has been read and signed, (2) the patient is aware of what is about to transpire, (3) the patient is maximally dilated, (4) color photographs of the fundus have been taken, (5) red-free photographs have been taken, (6) the fundus camera has been adjusted, and (7) the proper film has been loaded, filters put in place, and flash settings set. The patient is then asked to drink the solution rapidly through a straw to prevent staining of the lips.

Photography begins at the first sign of retinal circulation (15 to 30 minutes), with the late phase showing in about 1 hour. As with intravenous studies, the skin and urine will be slightly discolored for a few days.

Reported complications of oral fluorography are few and minor. It has been suggested that it would take ingestion of 90 g of fluorescein by a 100-pound person to produce a toxic effect.

The technique has been reported useful in children and certainly has potential in patients with cardiovascular compromise who may be at risk for an intravenous procedure.

Interpretation of Fluorescein Angiography

A good basic understanding of retinal–choroidal anatomy and vasculature is crucial for interpretation of fluorescein angiography. Some basic features of the retinal and choroidal system create the diagnostic capabilities of fluorescein angiography. These features are (1) healthy retinal vessels do not leak fluorescein because the vessel walls are not fenestrated, (2) healthy choriocapillaris vessels are fenestrated and freely leak, creating a spongelike tissue, (3) in a healthy retina, the fluid in the choriocapillaris is kept away from the sensory retina by an intact RPE–Bruch's membrane barrier. The RPE also serves as a filter to allow only part of the choroidal glow to show through. If the RPE is absent, more glow (hyperfluorescence) will be visible, and if there is an excess of RPE, less glow (hypofluorescence) will be visible. Dense RPE and xanthophyl mask the choroidal flush in a healthy macula.

In addition to the basic anatomic characteristics, there is the consideration of the time-related stages of the angiogram. The stages are classically described as the choroidal flush (prearterial phase), the arterial–venous phase, and the late phase. The choroidal flush occurs within seconds postinjection. The posterior ciliary arteries supply the choroidal system in a patchy pattern that is quickly masked by the fluorescein leaking into the choroidal swamp through fenestrated vasculature. This fluorescein will stay within the swamp if the RPE–Bruch's membrane barrier is healthy. Observation of the choroidal flush stage is especially useful in the determination of diseases of the choroidal vasculature or the RPE–Bruch's membrane barrier, such as the choroidal neovascularization in age-related maculopathy.

Within a few more seconds, the retinal arteries start to fill in a laminar flow pattern. The central core of the artery glows first, followed by filling to the limits of the walls. The capillaries then fill, followed by the laminar filling of the veins. With the veins, the area of the blood column near the walls glows first, followed by filling to the center. The walls of the arteries, capillaries, and veins in the healthy retina are not fenestrated and, as such, should demonstrate no leakage. Any disease condition that creates breakdown of vessel walls with subsequent leakage or neovascularization would be most apparent in this stage. An example is leaking microaneurysms in diabetic retinopathy.

The late stages of fluorescein angiography usually occur about 10 minutes postinjection. During this stage, the arteries and veins have almost emptied of fluorescein, and the underlying choroidal flush is minimized. The optic nerve remains hyperfluorescent as the dye adheres to the nerve tissue. During this stage, leakage of choroidal and retinal vessels becomes more apparent by the diffusely spreading staining pattern overlying the vascular lesion. Late staining also occurs in sensory retinal detachments and RPE detachments because of leakage through Bruch's membrane from underlying choroidal structures.

Application of the time stages of fluorescein angiography and the basic retinal–choroidal anatomy allow for effective fluorescein angiogram interpretation. Two basic situations occur in diseased conditions: (1) hypofluorescence or a blockage of the glow where you would normally expect it and (2) hyperfluorescence or an excessive glow where you would not normally expect it.

Disease Conditions That Create Hypofluorescence or Hyperfluorescence

Fluorescein angiography is an invaluable tool for the differential diagnosis of retinal vascular disease. Table 2–3 outlines conditions that create hypofluorescence or hyperfluorescence.

Example 1. Preretinal hemorrhages lie on top of the retina, blocking the view of both the choroid and retinal structure. A scotoma is created in this area. Figure 2–8 is a clinicopathologic cross section of the retina with a preretinal hemorrhage. The dark arrows represent the fluorescein pattern of the choroidal flush coming toward the observer, and the open arrows represent the choroidal flush that is actually seen. The preretinal hemorrhage blocks the choroidal flush. Figure 2–9 is an arteriovenous stage fluorescein angiogram demonstrating a hemorrhage around the disc that blocks choroidal fluorescence but does not block retinal vessel fluorescence. This means that the hemorrhage is between the retinal vessels and the choriocapillaris, or subretinal. Figure 2–10 is an arteriovenous stage fluorescein angiogram demonstrating a hemorrhage

TABLE 2–3. COMMON OCULAR CONDITIONS CREATING HYPOFLUORESCENCE OR HYPERFLUORESCENCE

Site	Hypofluorescence	Site	Hyperfluorescence
Retinal pigment epithelium (RPE)–Bruch's membrane	APMPPE,[a] Early Congenital hypertrophy of RPE RPE hyperplasia	RPE–Bruch's membrane	Age-related maculopathy, dry Angioid streaks APMPPE, late Choroidal folds Chorioretinal scars Drusen ICSC (cystoid maculopathy) Retinal hole RPE detachment RPE window defects Serous sensory RD
Choroid	Benign choroidal melanoma with no overlying serous detachment	Choroid	Choroidal neovascularization Malignant choroidal melanoma
Retina	Branch retinal artery occlusion Central retinal artery occlusion Cotton wool spots Preretinal hemorrhages Retinal exudates Subretinal hemorrhages	Retina	Angiomatosis retinae Capillary hemangioma Cavernous hemangioma, stasis Leaking compromised veins Macroaneurysms Microaneurysms Neovascularization, retina Periphlebitis Telangiectasia
		Optic nerve	Anterior–ischemic optic neuropathy Neovascularization, disc Papilledema

[a]APMPPE, Acute posterior multifocal placoid pigment epitheliopathy; ICSC, idiopathic central serous choroidopathy; RD, Retinal detachment.

PRE-RETINAL HEMORRHAGE

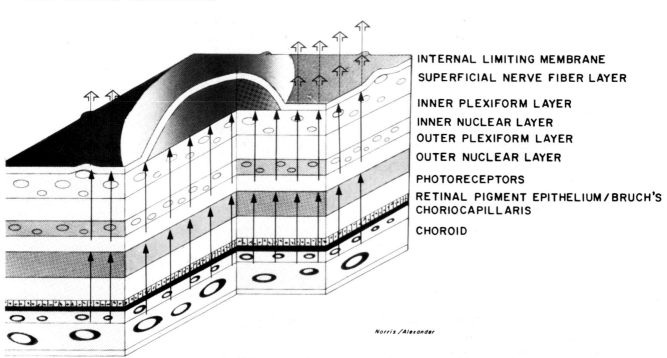

Figure 2–8. A clinicopathologic cross-section of the retina with a preretinal hemorrhage. (*See* text Example 1.) *(Reprinted with permission from Alexander LJ: How to perform and interpret fluorescein angiography. Rev Optom, 1988; 125:72–82.)*

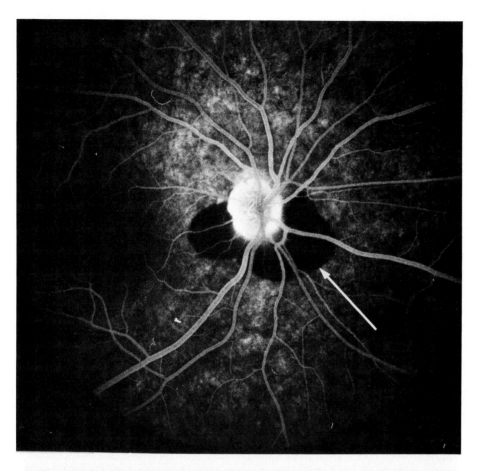

Figure 2–9. An arteriovenous stage fluorescein angiogram of a subretinal hemorrhage. (*See* text Example 1.)

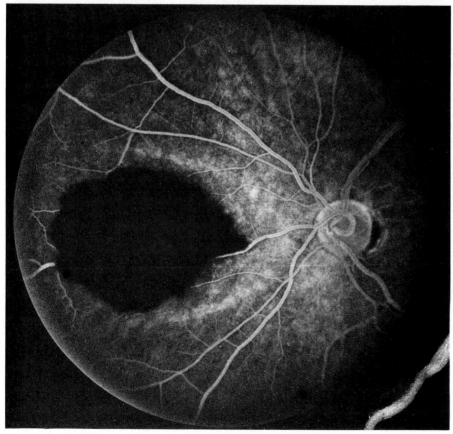

Figure 2–10. An arteriovenous stage fluorescein angiogram of a preretinal hemorrhage. (*See* text Example 1.)

DOT/BLOT HEMORRHAGES

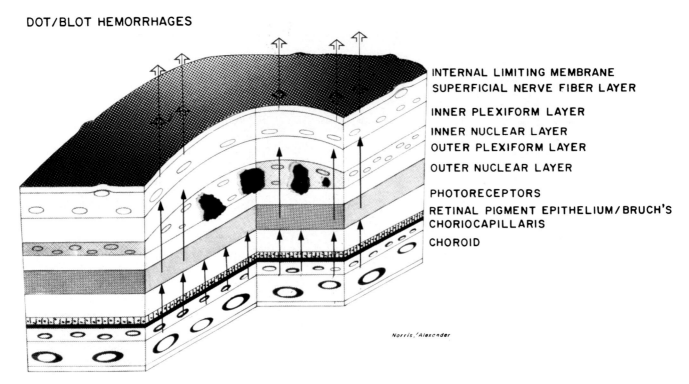

INTERNAL LIMITING MEMBRANE
SUPERFICIAL NERVE FIBER LAYER

INNER PLEXIFORM LAYER
INNER NUCLEAR LAYER
OUTER PLEXIFORM LAYER
OUTER NUCLEAR LAYER

PHOTORECEPTORS
RETINAL PIGMENT EPITHELIUM/BRUCH'S
CHORIOCAPILLARIS
CHOROID

Norris/Alexander

Figure 2–11. A clinicopathologic cross section of the retina with a dot hemorrhage. (*See* text Example 2.) *(Reprinted with permission from Alexander LJ. How to perform and interpret fluorescein angiography. Rev Optom, 1988; 125: 72–82.)*

that blocks both choroidal and retinal vessel fluorescence. This is interpreted as the hemorrhage being above the choroid and the retinal vessels, or a preretinal hemorrhage.

Example 2. Dot–blot hemorrhages lie within the retina near the inner nuclear layer blocking the photoreceptors and the underlying choroid but not the retinal vessels. Figure 2–11 illustrates dot–blot hemorrhages in a clinicopathologic cross section. The dark arrows represent the fluorescein pattern of the underlying choroidal flush coming toward the observer, and the open arrows represent the choroidal flush that is actually seen. The dot–blot hemorrhage blocks the choroidal flush. Figure 2–12 is an arteriovenous phase angiogram demonstrating an isolated area of blockage of the choroidal flush secondary to a dot–blot hemorrhage.

Example 3. Cotton wool spots represent areas of ischemia in the superficial nerve fiber layer. As such they lie above retinal and choroidal structures. Figure 2–13 is a clinicopathologic cross section of a cotton wool spot. The dark arrows represent the fluorescein pattern of the underlying choroidal flush, and the open arrows represent the choroidal flush that actually is seen. The cotton wool spot blocks the choroidal flush and retinal vessel glow. Figure 2–14 is a photograph of cotton wool spots (small arrows) and disc neovasculariza-

tion (large arrows). Figure 2–15 is the venous phase, with the large arrows pointing to the enlarging disc neovascularization and the small arrows pointing to the area of blockage of background choroidal fluorescence secondary to a cotton wool spot. It should be noted that the vessels surrounding the cotton wool spot are compromised and leaking.

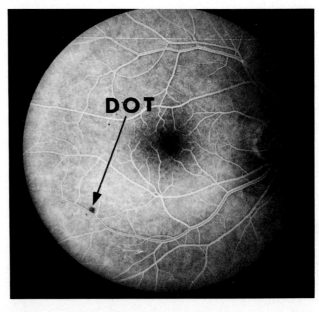

Figure 2–12. An arteriovenous stage fluorescein angiogram of a dot hemorrhage. (*See* text Example 2.)

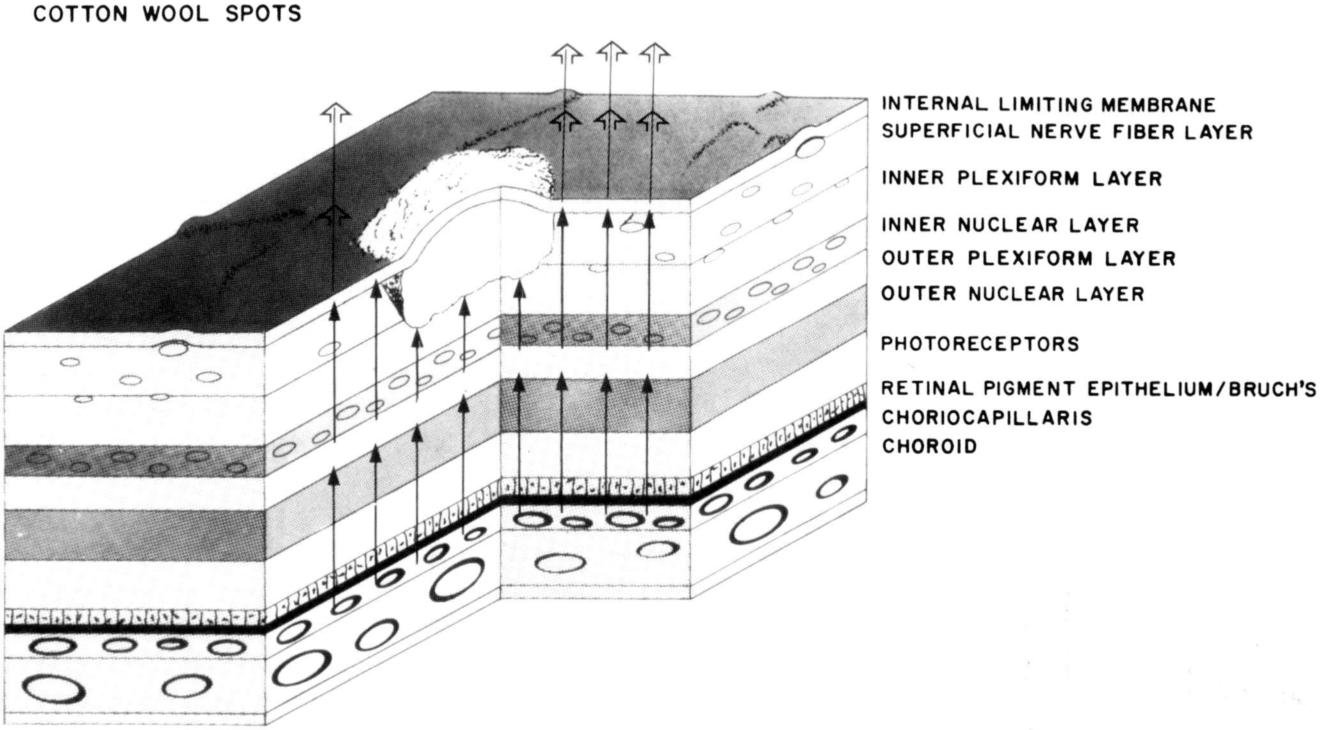

COTTON WOOL SPOTS

INTERNAL LIMITING MEMBRANE
SUPERFICIAL NERVE FIBER LAYER

INNER PLEXIFORM LAYER

INNER NUCLEAR LAYER
OUTER PLEXIFORM LAYER
OUTER NUCLEAR LAYER

PHOTORECEPTORS

RETINAL PIGMENT EPITHELIUM/BRUCH'S
CHORIOCAPILLARIS
CHOROID

Norris / Alexander

Figure 2–13. A clinicopathologic cross section of the retina with a cotton wool spot. (*See* text Example 3.) *(Reprinted with permission from Alexander LJ: How to perform and interpret fluorescein angiography. Rev Optom, 1988; 125: 72–82.)*

Example 4. Hard exudate formation occurs secondary to a breakdown in retinal tissue and blood vessels. This breakdown occurs when microaneurysms leak, creating intraretinal edema in which a lipid soup is cooked. Figure 2–16 illustrates a clinicopathologic cross section of the retina in which microaneurysms are leaking. The dark arrows represent the fluorescein pattern of the underlying choroidal flush, and the open arrows represent the flush that actually is seen. Hard exudates lie deep

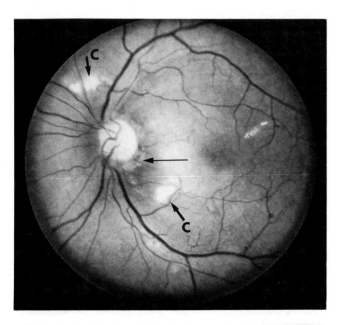

Figure 2–14. Photograph demonstrating areas of cotton wool spots and disc neovascularization. (*See* text Example 3.)

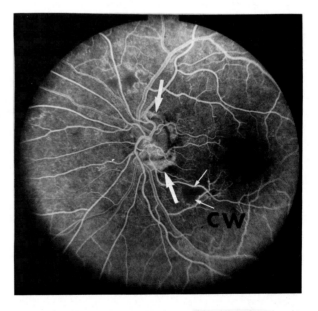

Figure 2–15. Fluorescein angiogram of cotton wool spots and disc neovascularization shown in Figure 2–14. Large arrows point to leaking disc neovascularization and the small arrows to the hypofluorescence created by the cotton wool spots. (*See* text Example 3.)

HARD EXUDATE FORMATION

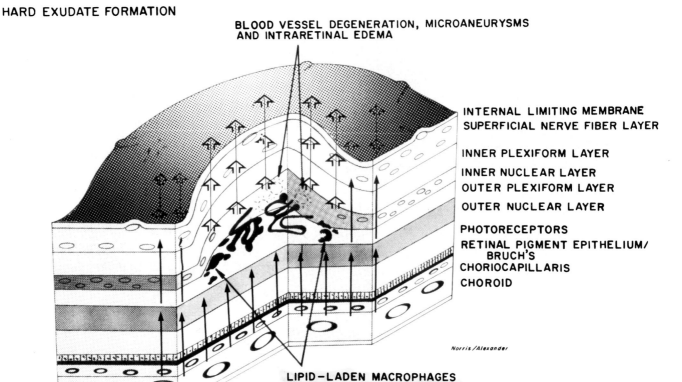

Figure 2–16. A clinicopathologic cross section of the retina with leaking microaneurysms. (*See* text Example 4.) *(Reprinted with permission from Alexander LJ: How to perform and interpret fluorescein angiography. Rev. Optom, 1988; 125: 72–82.)*

within the retina blocking underlying choroidal fluorescence. The leaking microaneurysms that contribute to the problem will hyperfluoresce. Figures 2–17 and 2–18 show a patient with hard exudates in the macula secondary to leaking microaneurysms. The ensuing edema compromises the retina, creating reduced visual acuity.

With this basic description of the clinicopathologic process, further case presentations will enhance the understanding of fluorescein angiogram interpretation.

Example 5. Figures 2–19 to 2–22 illustrate the differentiation of benign drusen and/or RPE window defects from microaneurysms. Figures 2–19 and 2–20 are of the same patient, Figure 2–19 being an early phase (note that the vein is just starting laminar filling) and Figure 2–20 being a later phase. In both instances, the macular area pigment blocks background choroidal fluorescence, but isolated areas of glow occur within the hypofluorescence (black arrows). These isolated areas of glow do not spread with time, implying no leakage. When there

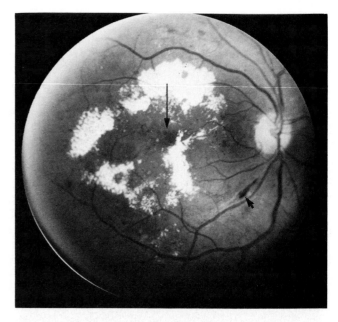

Figure 2–17. Photograph of hard exudates surrounding the macula **(long arrow).** The short arrow points to a flame-shaped hemorrhage. (*See* text Example 4.)

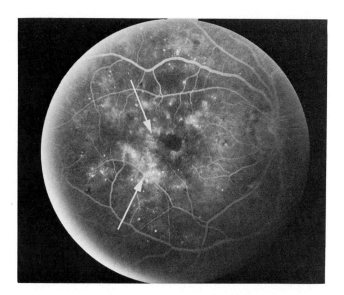

Figure 2–18. Fluorescein angiogram of patient in Figure 2–17 demonstrating areas of significant edema **(arrows)** secondary to leaking microaneurysms. (*See* text Example 4.)

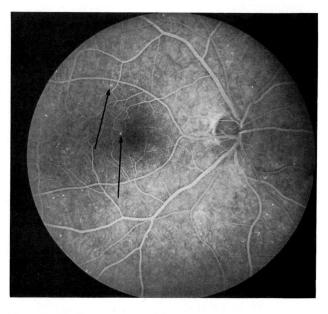

Figure 2–20. The late stage of the patient shown in Figure 2–19, showing no spread of hyperfluorescence. This is indicative of a benign defect in the retinal pigment epithelium. (*See* text Example 5.)

is hyperfluorescence that does not enlarge over time, it is safe to assume that there is a benign defect in the RPE, such as a drusen or an RPE window defect. Figure 2–21 demonstrates hyperfluorescence at the early stages of the angiogram, with an enlargement of the area of hyperfluorescence over time (Fig. 2–22). When this occurs, there is spread of edema, with a resultant direct threat to vision.

Example 6. Another situation that can create edema with a threat to vision is idiopathic central serous choroidopathy (ICSC). ICSC results from a break in the RPE–Bruch's barrier, allowing for seepage of the choriocapillaris fluid into the retina. Figure 2–23 illustrates an area of hyperfluorescence in the normally dark macular area that enlarges slightly and becomes more diffuse in the later stages (Fig. 2–24). This is a case of ICSC in a 45-

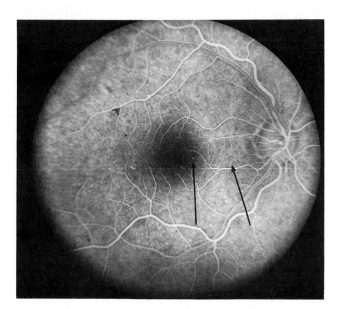

Figure 2–19. An early-stage fluorescein angiogram with arrows pointing to hyperfluorescence. (*See* text Example 5.)

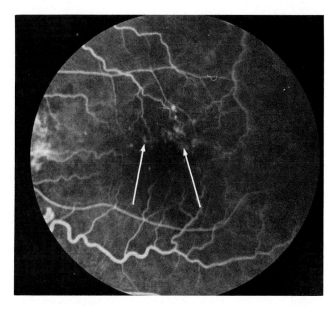

Figure 2–21. An early-stage angiogram demonstrating areas of focal hyperfluorescence (arrows). (*See* text Example 5.)

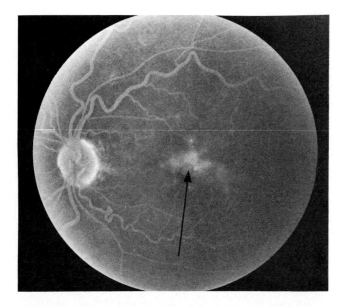

Figure 2–22. The late stage of Figure 2–21, showing a spread of hyperfluorescence. In this case, it is indicative of leaking microaneurysms. (*See* text Example 5.)

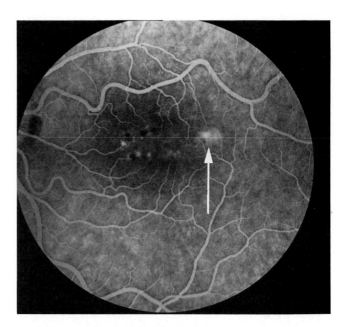

Figure 2–24. The late-stage angiogram of the patient in Figure 2–23 demonstrating the actively leaking zone **(long arrow)** characterized by a spread of hyperfluorescence. (*See* text Example 6.)

year-old man. Figures 2–25 and 2–26 demonstrate the progression of this case over a 5-year period. Metamorphopsia had increased significantly over the years.

Example 7. One of the most dangerous ocular conditions that can develop is a choroidal neovascular net in the macular area. It can be devastating

to vision because of the possibility of hemorrhage and/or scar formation. The neovascularization develops because of a combination of a break in the RPE–Bruch's barrier and the presence of oxygen starvation (hypoxia). This condition can occur in age-related maculopathy, angioid streaks, degenerative myopia, and presumed ocular histoplasmosis, among other conditions. The factor that makes

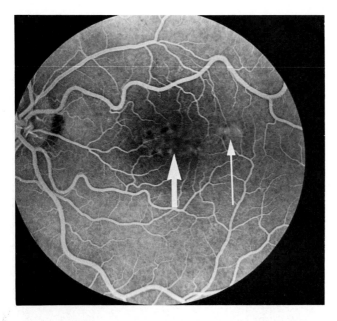

Figure 2–23. Areas of hyperfluorescence and hypofluorescence in the macular area characteristic of idiopathic central serous choroidopathy. (*See* text Example 6.)

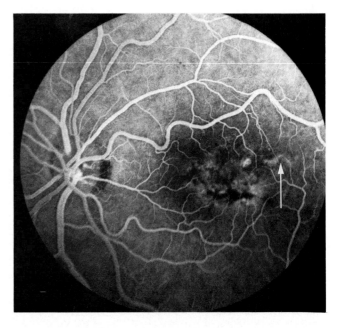

Figure 2–25. An early-stage angiogram of the patient shown in Figure 2–23 only 5 years later. (*See* text Example 6.)

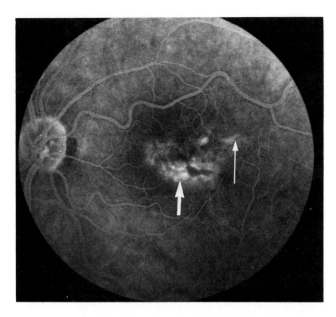

Figure 2–26. A late-stage angiogram of the patient shown in Figure 2–25 demonstrating the degree of destruction that can occur over time in idiopathic central serous choroidopathy. (*See* text Example 6.)

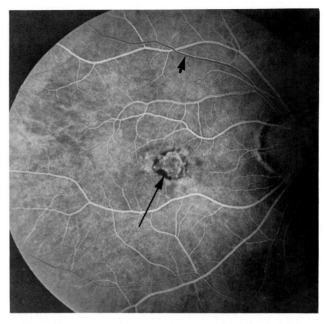

Figure 2–28. An area of hyperfluorescence in a normally dark macular area in an early-stage angiogram. The small arrow points to laminar flow in the vein. (*See* text Example 7.)

this condition so dangerous is that these developing nets are extremely difficult to see ophthalmoscopically in the early stages of development. If patients are elderly, or if they have other conditions lending to the development of choroidal neovascular nets and they report with reduced vision or metamorphopsia, it is prudent to assume the presence of a neovascular net until proven otherwise. *Order fluorescein angiography!*

Figure 2–27 illustrates a healthy eye, with the arrow pointing to the normally dark macular area in a fluorescein study. Figures 2–28 and 2–29 represent early and later fluorescein studies, respectively, with hyperfluorescence in the normally dark macular area. Figure 2–28 is the early venous phase (small arrow pointing to laminar venous flow), with the large arrow pointing to a choroidal neovascular net. All neovascularization leaks, as is

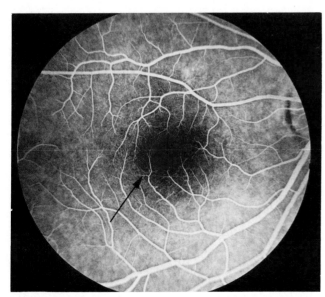

Figure 2–27. A normal eye with a dark macular area **(arrow)** in a fluorescein study.

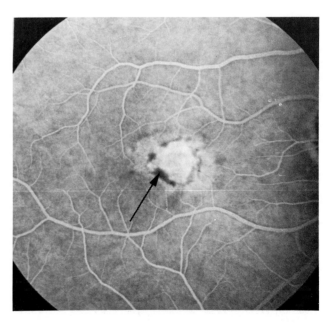

Figure 2–29. The late-stage angiogram of the eye in Figure 2–28 showing a spread of hyperfluorescence secondary to a neovascular net. (*See* text Example 7.)

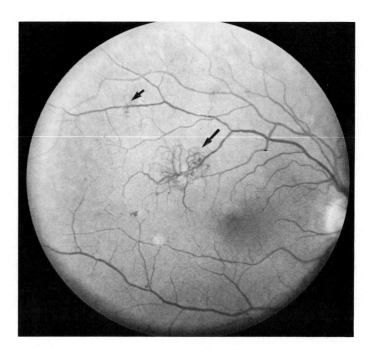

Figure 2–30. A photograph of two patches of neovascularization elsewhere in the retina **(arrows).** (*See* text Example 8.)

demonstrated by the expanding area of edema in the late stage of Figure 2–29 (large arrow). This patient had presumed ocular histoplasmosis (20/200).

It is extremely important to diagnose choroidal neovascular nets as soon as possible, since laser photocoagulation may be able to seal the nets and abort progressive vision loss.

Example 8. Retinal and disc neovascularization also can be diagnosed earlier by fluorescein angiography than by ophthalmoscopic observation. Disc

and retinal neovascularization is very fine and may be difficult to observe with ophthalmoscopy. The staining pattern with fluorescein angiography is, however, classic.

Figure 2–30 is a black and white photograph of neovascularization of the retina (arrows). The large net is easily observable, but the small net offers a challenge. Figure 2–31 is an early-phase angiogram of this area, demonstrating the characteristic leakage from the nets (arrows). Figure 2–32 illustrates the late-stage staining pattern (arrows).

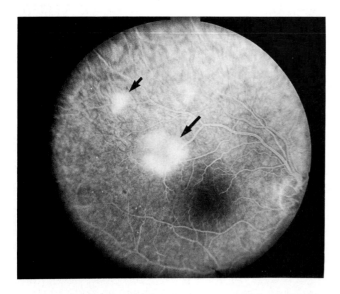

Figure 2–31. Early-phase angiogram of the neovascularization shown in Figure 2–30. (*See* text Example 8.)

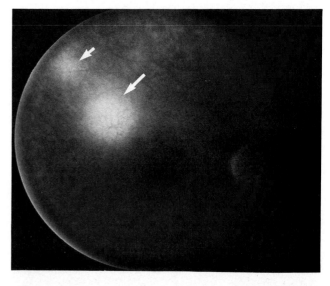

Figure 2–32. Late-phase angiogram of the neovascularization shown in Figure 2–30. (*See* text Example 8.)

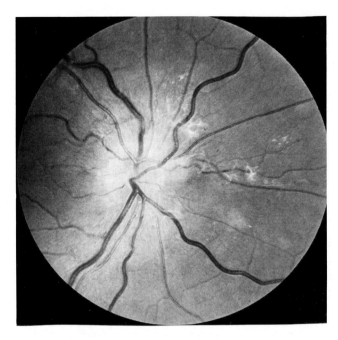

Figure 2–33. Black and white photograph of a right optic disc with subtle disc neovascularization. (*See* text Example 8.)

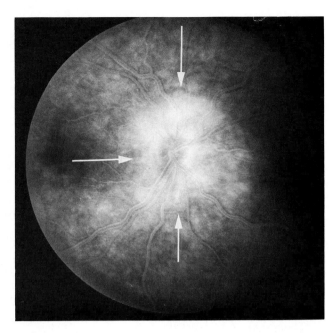

Figure 2–35. Late-phase angiogram of the eye in Figure 2–34 showing considerable new leakage. (*See* text Example 8.)

Figures 2–33 to 2–38 illustrate the right and left eyes of a person with diabetes who had no observable diabetic retinopathy by ophthalmoscopy. Black and white photographs of both optic nerves show areas of suspicion (white arrows) that are confirmed as neovascularization of the disc by fluorescein angiography. The time-sequenced angiogram of the right eye demonstrates a spreading of the staining pattern characteristic of neovascularization of the disc (white arrows). The left eye angiograms demonstrated a similar pattern.

Figures 2–39 and 2–40 give another example of hyperfluorescence of the disc (arrow), but in this case the condition was anterior ischemic optic neuropathy (AION) in an insulin-dependent diabetic patient.

Early diagnosis of neovascularization is extremely important because of the imminent threat to vision. The earlier the diagnosis, the better the cure rate.

Example 9. Disc neovascularization can occur in other conditions that create a hypoxic stimulus in the retina. Figure 2–41 is a photograph of a hemicentral retinal vein occlusion (hemi-CRVO). This is characterized by retinal vascular changes in either the superior or inferior portion of the retina. Figures 2–42 and 2–43 are of another patient, illustrating the potential sequela to a hemi-CRVO, disc neovascularization. Figure 2–42 is the early stage, illustrating the frilly net on the nerve head, and Figure 2–43 illustrate the late-stage leaking of that neovascularization. This is of particular significance because of the likelihood of vitreous hemorrhage.

Example 10. Branch retinal artery occlusion (BRAO) and branch retinal vein occlusion (BRVO) also create classic fluorescein angiography patterns. Figures 2–44 and 2–45 illustrate a combined BRAO

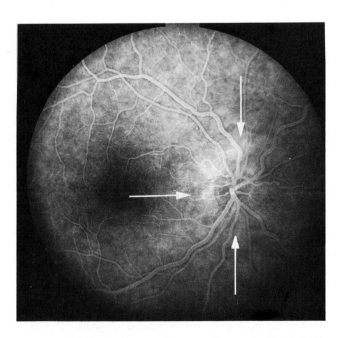

Figure 2–34. Early-phase angiogram of the eye in Figure 2–33 showing leakage (**arrows**) from the disc neovascularization. (*See* text Example 8.)

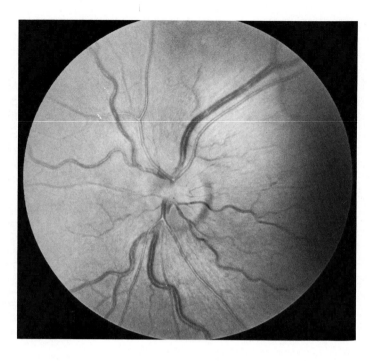

Figure 2–36. Black and white photograph of very subtle disc neovascularization in the fellow left eye to that in Figure 2–33. (*See* text Example 8.)

and BRVO. Figure 2–44 is a photograph of the combination, with white arrows pointing to the area of BRVO and black arrows outlining the retinal infarct of the BRAO. Large intraretinal hemorrhages appear superiorly as black spots, and a long white arrow pinpoints the site of the vein occlusion. The long white arrow in Figure 2–45 points to the hypofluorescent area created by the BRAO. The site of the BRAO is pinpointed in Figure 2–45 by the black arrow. In most cases of BRVO, the

area of stasis is characterized by leaking microaneurysms and intraretinal edema.

Example 11. RPE–Bruch's membrane barrier changes also can influence the angiogram pattern. Figures 2–46 to 2–49 are examples of these alterations. Figures 2–46 and 2–47 illustrate dominant drusen and the effect on the macular area. Hyperfluorescence is the characteristic feature. Figure 2–

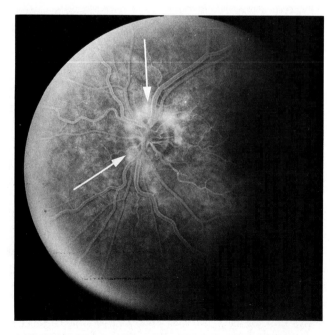

Figure 2–37. Early-phase angiogram of the eye in Figure 2–36 showing leakage **(arrows).** (*See* text Example 8.)

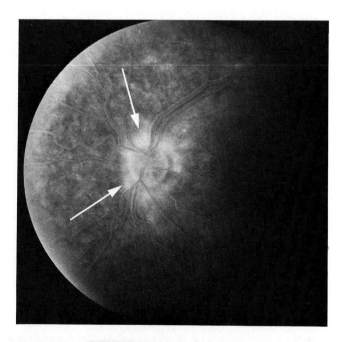

Figure 2–38. Late-stage staining of the eye in Figure 2–36. (*See* text Example 8.)

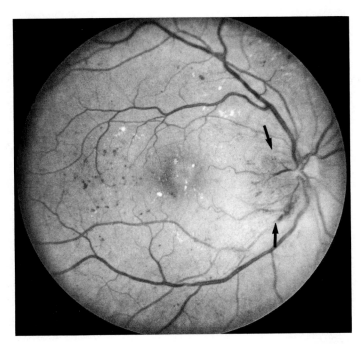

Figure 2–39. Black and white photograph of a patient with background diabetic retinopathy and active anterior ischemic optic neuropathy (**arrows**). The affected disc area is elevated. (*See* text Example 8.)

48 shows angioid streaks in the right eye (arrows). Figure 2–49 is a fluorescein angiogram of the left eye of the same patient, with an exudative macular scar secondary to trauma. Fluorescein angiography is invaluable in diagnosing RPE–Bruch's membrane disorders.

Illustrations and examples of the benefits of fluorescein angiography are endless. The technique of fluorescein angiography gives an added dimension to differential diagnosis. Often, fluorescein an-giography is the only diagnostic technique that will reveal an underlying smoldering disease process. The technique is easy to understand if the doctor visualizes the clinicopathologic process as disease that is nothing more than an alteration of retinal structure at specific layers. Fluorescein angiography enhances and often pinpoints the specific clinicopathologic alteration. The more tools, the better the understanding; the better the understanding, the better the patient management.

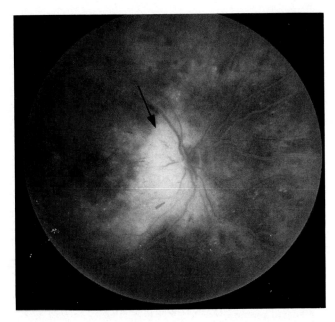

Figure 2–40. The late stage angiogram of the disc area in Figure 2–39 demonstrating leakage associated with active anterior ischemic optic neuropathy. (*See* text Example 8.)

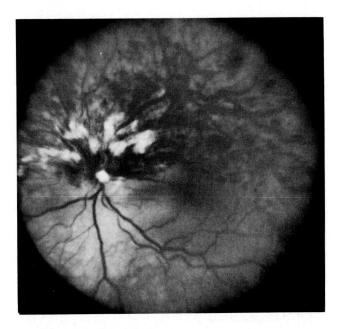

Figure 2–41. Black and white photograph of an ischemic hemicentral retinal vein occlusion. The cotton wool spots indicate severe hypoxia. (*See* text Example 9.)

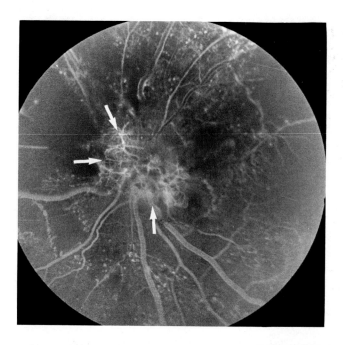

Figure 2–42. Early-stage angiogram of disc neovascularization **(arrows)** secondary to the hypoxia of hemicentral retinal vein occlusion. (*See* text Example 9.)

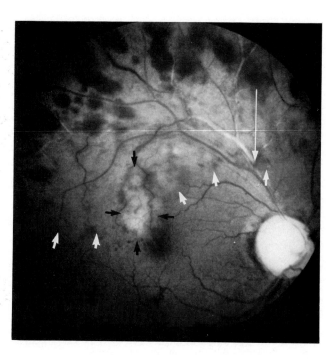

Figure 2–44. Black and white photograph of a combined branch retinal artery occlusion (BRAO) and branch retinal vein occlusion (BRVO). The white arrows point to the effects of the BRVO, the long white arrow points to the site of the occlusion, and the black arrows outline the zone of arterial infarct. (*See* text Example 10.)

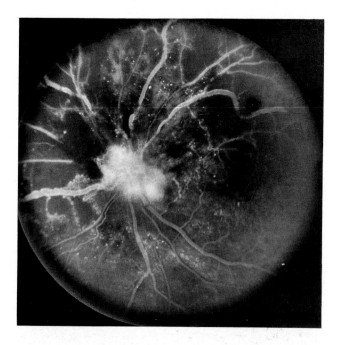

Figure 2–43. Late-stage angiogram of the disc in Figure 2–42 demonstrating significant spread of hyperfluorescence from the disc neovascularization. (*See* text Example 9.)

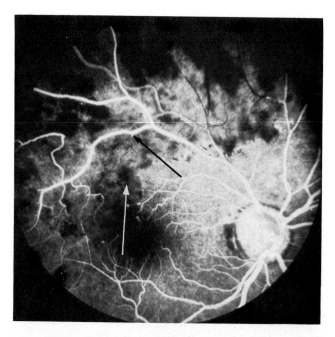

Figure 2–45. Fluorescein angiogram of the eye shown in Figure 2–44. The black arrow points to the site of the arterial occlusion, and the white arrow points to the zone of infarct. The zone of the branch retinal vein occlusion dims the background choroidal fluorescence. (*See* text Example 10.)

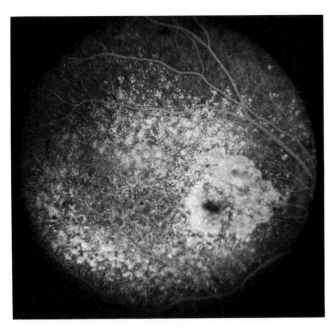

Figure 2–46. Fluorescein angiogram of right eye of approximately 30-year-old patient with dominant drusen. (*See* text Example 11.)

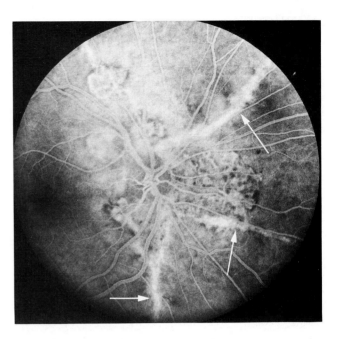

Figure 2–48. Fluorescein angiogram of angioid streaks indicating severe retinal pigment epithelium dropout in the circumpapillary region, with spokes (**arrows**) radiating outward. (*See* text Example 11.)

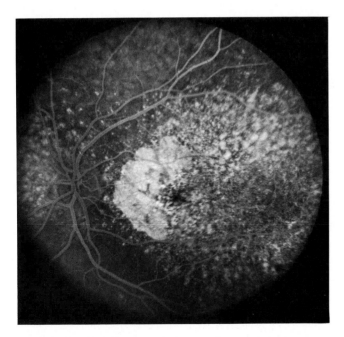

Figure 2–47. Fluorescein angiogram of same patient as in Figure 2–46. The characteristic feature is widespread hyperfluorescence. (*See* text Example 11.)

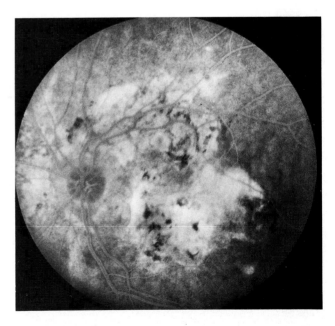

Figure 2–49. Fluorescein angiogram of the left eye of patient in Figure 2–48. The angioid streaks in this eye allowed for choroidal neovascularization, with the development of the massive disciform scar. (*See* text Example 11.)

CLINICOPATHOLOGICAL BASIS OF RETINAL VASCULOPATHY

Retinal Hemorrhages

Retinal hemorrhages are not an ocular disease process but rather an ocular manifestation of underlying vascular or blood disease. Hemorrhages are a sign to the clinician that an evaluation of the systemic health of the patient is indicated.

Retinal hemorrhages are discussed here with specific emphasis on cause and management. It is useful to remember that the superficial capillary layer in the retina is considered to be postarteriolar and, as such, is most often affected by artery-based diseases. Superficial hemorrhages, such as flame-shaped and preretinal hemorrhages, may then be considered as artery-based hemorrhages. The deeper capillary bed is considered prevenular and is affected most often by vein-based or congestive diseases. Dot–blot hemorrhages are deep in the retina and are considered to be related to congestive retinal diseases, such as central retinal vein occlusion.

Preretinal Hemorrhages. Preretinal hemorrhages (Figs. 2–50 to 2–53) lie just under the internal limiting membrane and in front of the nerve fiber layer. **See color plate 23.** The hemorrhages arise from the superficial capillary system or the radial peripapillary system. Preretinal hemorrhages typically occur in the posterior pole and create a positive scotoma. Vision may be severely reduced if preretinal hemorrhages occur in front of the macula. The typical preretinal hemorrhage is about 1 to 2 disc diameters in size, with gravity affecting the appearance. Gravity causes the blood to settle, resulting in darker blood at the bottom of the D-shape or keel-shape and a horizontal clear line demarcating the top of the hemorrhage. With resolution, the thinner layer at the top clears first. Resolution demonstrates a very specific color change, going from red to yellow to white and often leaving no trace of the hemorrhage and no compromise of retinal function. The rapidity of resolution depends on the amount of blood within the pocket. The hemorrhage will appear black with fluorescein angiography.

A variation of preretinal hemorrhages occurs in what has been called a "thumbprint" pattern. These thumbprint hemorrhages occur in the posterior pole and are about 1 disc diameter in size. They are darkest centrally, with flayed edges and a small central reflex that moves with the viewing angle. Although not specific to any disease, the thumbprint hemorrhage often is associated with pernicious anemia.

PRE-RETINAL HEMORRHAGE

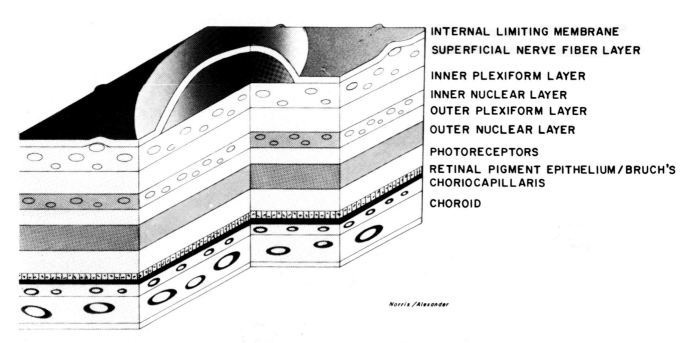

INTERNAL LIMITING MEMBRANE
SUPERFICIAL NERVE FIBER LAYER

INNER PLEXIFORM LAYER
INNER NUCLEAR LAYER
OUTER PLEXIFORM LAYER
OUTER NUCLEAR LAYER

PHOTORECEPTORS
RETINAL PIGMENT EPITHELIUM/BRUCH'S
CHORIOCAPILLARIS

CHOROID

Norris/Alexander

Figure 2–50. Schematic cross section of the retina demonstrating the clinicopathology of preretinal hemorrhages.

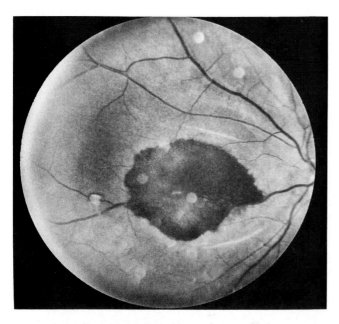

Figure 2–51. Black and white photograph of a large preretinal hemorrhage nasal to the optic nerve head.

Preretinal hemorrhages may be caused by many factors, and it is important to determine the precipitating factor because of systemic disease associations. Table 2–4 shows common causes of preretinal hemorrhages. Determination of the cause is the primary treatment for the preretinal hemorrhage.

PRERETINAL HEMORRHAGES—PEARLS

- Occur between internal limiting membrane and nerve fiber layer
- Create a positive scotoma
- Gravity creates D-shape
- Changes red to yellow to white on resorption
- Usually related to artery-based diseases
- May occur associated with a posterior vitreous detachment
- Do not leak
- Management includes ascertaining the underlying cause and allowing time for resorption

Superficial Flame-Shaped Hemorrhages. Superficial flame-shaped hemorrhages (Figs. 2–54 and 2–55) originate from the postarteriolar superficial capillary bed or the radial peripapillary capillary system. The flayed or flame-shaped edges result from the blood seeking lines of least resistance in the contour of the nerve fiber layer. These hemorrhages vary in size, configuration, and color. Often they have a white center and are called Roth's spots. Superficial flame-shaped hemorrhages are short-lived, lasting but a few weeks, and have no particular effect on vision. During resorption, there is a color change to dull red, with fragmentation and disappearance. A scotoma will occur at threshold levels if carefully investigated. The hemorrhage appears black on fluorescein angiography.

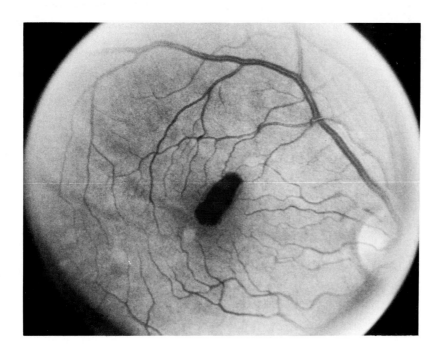

Figure 2–52. Black and white photograph of a small preretinal hemorrhage over the macula creating 20/200 vision. The hemorrhage cleared, with resultant 20/20 visual acuity.

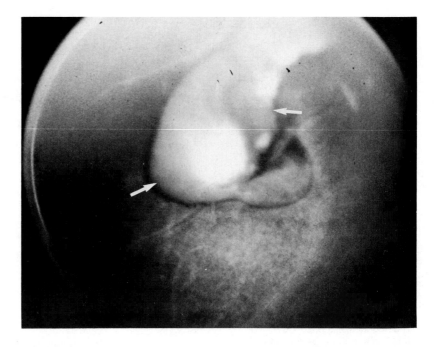

Figure 2–53. A large preretinal hemorrhage in the stage of color change.

Superficial flame-shaped hemorrhages usually are confined to the posterior pole, most commonly occurring in the radial peripapillary distribution area. These hemorrhages represent an area of localized retinal hypoxia as the oxygenated arterial supply is compromised. As such, the hemorrhage may be a sign that neovascularization is a potential problem.

Roth's spots represent hemorrhage surrounding a white center. This white center may represent any of the following: (1) focal accumulations of white blood cells in inflammatory vascular disease, (2) cotton wool spots surrounded by hemorrhage, (3) leukemic cell foci surrounded by hemorrhage, or (4) fibrin surrounded by hemorrhage. As with

superficial hemorrhages, the clinician must attempt to ascertain the cause of the arterial capillary compromise. Table 2–5 lists the common causes of superficial flame-shaped hemorrhages, and Table 2–6 outlines the diseases associated with white-centered flame-shaped hemorrhages. **See color plate 24.**

SUPERFICIAL FLAME-SHAPED HEMORRHAGES—PEARLS

- From the postarteriolar superficial capillary bed
- Possible radial peripapillary capillary bed
- Occur in nerve fiber layer in posterior pole
- Usually related to arterial-based diseases—hypoxia
- Do not leak
- Management includes ascertaining the underlying cause, allowing time for resorption, and watching for other signs of hypoxia

---

TABLE 2–4. TYPICAL CAUSES OF PRERETINAL HEMORRHAGES

Posterior vitreous detachment, near optic nerve head
Subdural hemorrhage in children
Subarachnoid hemorrhage in adults and children
Pernicious anemia, thumbprint
Hypertension
Diabetes
Emboli
Blood dyscrasias
Anemias
Leukemias
Bacterial endocarditis
Trauma
Idiopathic

TABLE 2–5. CONDITIONS COMMONLY ASSOCIATED WITH SUPERFICIAL FLAME-SHAPED HEMORRHAGES

Ocular	Systemic
Papilledema	Hypertension
Papillitis	Diabetes
Ischemic optic neuropathy	Blood dyscrasias
Papillophlebitis	Anemias
Low-tension glaucoma	Leukemias, large fan-shaped
Glaucoma	Oral contraceptives
Branch retinal vein occlusion	Idiopathic
Central retinal vein occlusion	

SUPERFICIAL FLAME-SHAPED HEMORRHAGE

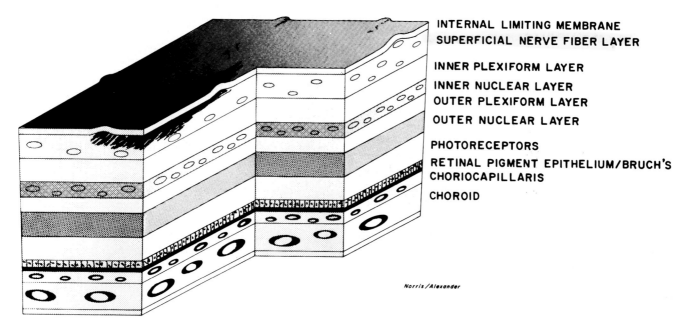

INTERNAL LIMITING MEMBRANE
SUPERFICIAL NERVE FIBER LAYER

INNER PLEXIFORM LAYER

INNER NUCLEAR LAYER
OUTER PLEXIFORM LAYER

OUTER NUCLEAR LAYER

PHOTORECEPTORS
RETINAL PIGMENT EPITHELIUM/BRUCH'S
CHORIOCAPILLARIS

CHOROID

Norris/Alexander

Figure 2–54. Schematic cross section of the retina, demonstrating the clinicopathology of superficial flame-shaped hemorrhages.

Dot–Blot Hemorrhages.
Dot–blot hemorrhages (Figs. 2–56 and 2–57) also are known as deep retinal hemorrhages. Dot–blot hemorrhages occur in the inner nuclear layer, outer plexiform layer, and

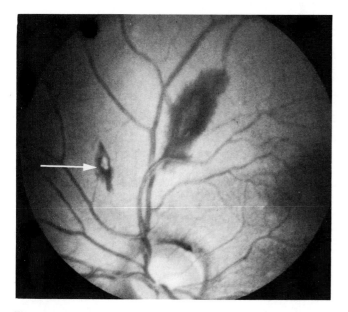

Figure 2–55. Black and white photograph of a flame-shaped hemorrhage and a white-centered flame-shaped hemorrhage **(arrow)**. These hemorrhages were secondary to bacterial endocarditis.

at times outer nuclear layer. They originate from the prevenular deep capillary bed and, as such, are most often associated with venous-based congestive disease. Their configuration results from the compression deep in the retina, confining the hemorrhages to specific localities. Dot–blot hemorrhages typically follow vertical lines of cleavage within the retina. Retinal structure is displaced in the area of the hemorrhage, but there is no necrosis of tissue. A dot–blot hemorrhage usually is indicative of deep retinal edema, although this is difficult to appreciate clinically. The deep retinal edema is a by-product of the stasis.

Dot–blot hemorrhages may persist longer than a superficial flame-shaped hemorrhage but eventually disappear, leaving no evidence of their existence. A visual compromise in the form of thresh-

TABLE 2–6. SYSTEMIC DISEASES ASSOCIATED WITH ROTH'S SPOTS

Diabetes

Leukemias

Bacterial endocarditis

Disseminated lupus erythematosus

Dysproteinemia

Aplastic anemia

old field defects may occur in areas with dot–blot hemorrhages, or vision reduction can occur if the hemorrhages occur in the macula. The vision compromise is, however, a manifestation of the stasis in the involved retina rather than directly related to the hemorrhage. The hemorrhage is an indicator of intraretinal compromise. Dot–blot hemorrhages do not leak into the retina. **See color plate 25.**

Dot–blot hemorrhages may be isolated in such conditions as localized diabetic retinopathy. They may, however, involve a total sector of the retina, as in BRVO, or the entire retina out to the periphery, as in CRVO. They are easy to distinguish from microaneurysms, since microaneurysms are smaller than the resolution power of the direct ophthalmoscope. The differential from macroaneurysms is more difficult, and the clinician may have to rely on observation or fluorescein angiography for differential diagnosis. On fluorescein angiography, dot–blot hemorrhages block background choroidal fluorescence, whereas microaneurysms and macroaneurysms typically leak. Microaneurysms are almost always present when there are dot–blot hemorrhages.

Management of dot–blot hemorrhages can become a complicated matter. It is important to ascertain the underlying cause (Table 2–7). The clinician must remember that the dot hemorrhage is a sign of venous stasis and retinal edema. Should this

TABLE 2–7. CONDITIONS ASSOCIATED WITH DOT–BLOT HEMORRHAGES

Diabetes
Blood dyscrasias
Venous occlusive disease
Hypertension
Estrogen-based pharmaceutical agents
Ipsilateral internal carotid stenosis in periphery

edema and hemorrhage appear in the macular area or encroach on the macular area, fluorescein angiography is indicated to determine if photocoagulation can be applied to assist in regression of the edema.

DOT–BLOT HEMORRHAGES—PEARLS

- Occur in inner nuclear to outer nuclear layer
- Originate from prevenular deep capillary bed
- Associated with deep retinal edema but do not leak
- Most often a sign of venous stasis retinopathy
- Management
  - Ascertain cause
  - Fluorescein angiography if encroaching on or within the macula

---

DOT/BLOT HEMORRHAGES

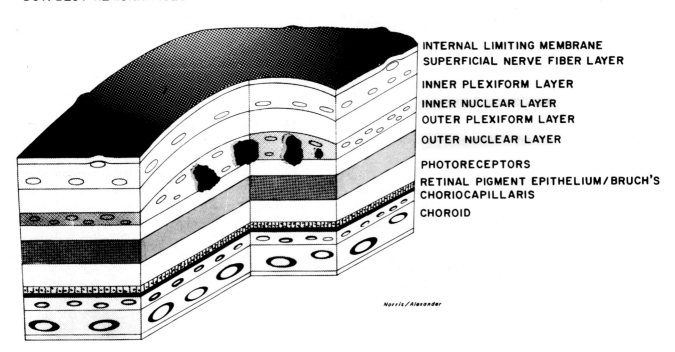

INTERNAL LIMITING MEMBRANE
SUPERFICIAL NERVE FIBER LAYER

INNER PLEXIFORM LAYER
INNER NUCLEAR LAYER
OUTER PLEXIFORM LAYER
OUTER NUCLEAR LAYER

PHOTORECEPTORS
RETINAL PIGMENT EPITHELIUM/BRUCH'S
CHORIOCAPILLARIS
CHOROID

Norris/Alexander

Figure 2–56. Schematic cross section of the retina demonstrating the clinicopathology of dot–blot hemorrhages.

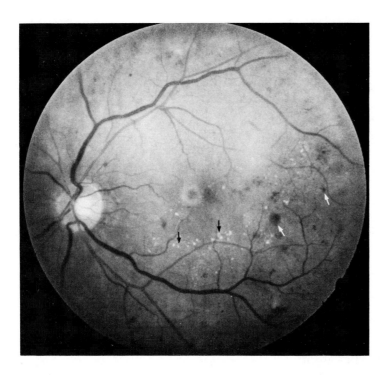

Figure 2–57. Black and white photograph of background diabetic retinopathy, with white arrows pointing to dot–blot hemorrhages and black arrows pointing to hard exudates.

Subretinal Hemorrhages. Most subretinal hemorrhages in the clinical population are secondary to choroidal neovascular membranes (Figs. 2–58 and 2–59). Subretinal hemorrhages can, however, occur as an extension of deep retinal hemorrhages breaking through to lie underneath the retina. This can occur in conditions such as Coat's disease, sickle cell disease, leukemia, retinopathy of prematurity, angiomatosis retina, and severe diabetic retinopathy.

Subretinal hemorrhages secondary to retinal vascular disease appear between the retinal pigment epithelium and sensory retina. They usually occur in the posterior pole, are large, and have lobulated borders. When they are fresh, they are usually dark red, often darker at the bottom. With age, subretinal hemorrhages show yellowish exudative accumulations eventually being replaced by scar tissue and pigment mottling. They resorb from the area of thinnest hemorrhage, which is often superior. Subretinal hemorrhages are very destructive, resulting in permanent scotomas with vision loss. Sub-RPE hemorrhages are gray-green in color, with the same devastating effects.

Should a subretinal hemorrhage occur, the clinician must ascertain the cause. If the cause is choroidal neovascularization, laser photocoagulation may be beneficial. Control of the systemic condition may prevent involvement of the fellow eye. Photocoagulative intervention may be beneficial if the macula is not involved. If the macula is involved, little can be done to reverse the process and restore vision. **See color plates 45 and 46.**

SUBRETINAL HEMORRHAGES—PEARLS

- Usually secondary to choroidal neovascular network
- Large with lobullated borders
- If subretinal, they are red
- If sub-RPE, they are gray-green
- Visually devastating
- Management
  - Fluorescein angiography to ascertain cause
  - Retinology consultation

Vitreous Hemorrhage. Vitreous hemorrhage (Figs. 2–60 and 2–61) can occur either out into the vitreous body or between the detached vitreous face and the internal limiting membrane (retrovitreous). The blood in the vitreous is the result of a break in the internal limiting membrane, allowing for retinal bleeding to flow forward. This process occurs in diseases with associated periphlebitis, allowing for inflammatory breakdown of the overlying internal limiting membrane. This bleeding can occur also from a fragile neovascular network emanating from the optic nerve head where there is no true internal limiting membrane or from preretinal neovascularization.

The appearance of a vitreous hemorrhage depends on extent and elapsed time since the event. In the early phase of a hemorrhage out into the vitreous body, the retina may not be visible. The red blood cells may persist for a few weeks if the hemorrhage is small or may remain for years.

THE POSSIBLE CONSEQUENCES OF CHOROIDAL NEOVASCULARIZATION

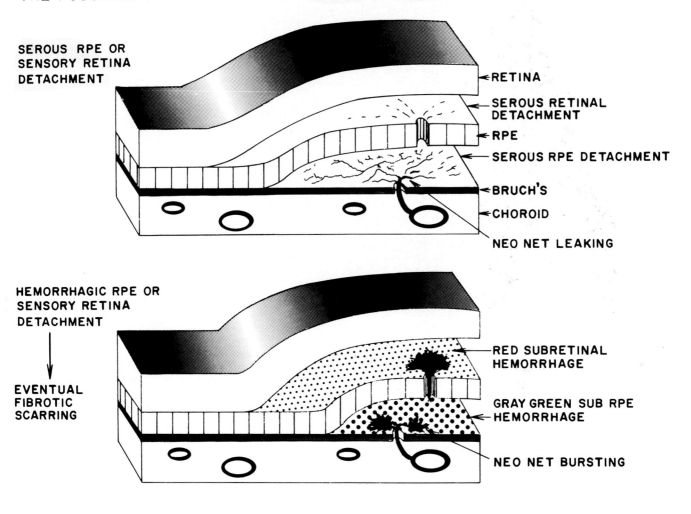

SEROUS RPE OR SENSORY RETINA DETACHMENT

- RETINA
- SEROUS RETINAL DETACHMENT
- RPE
- SEROUS RPE DETACHMENT
- BRUCH'S
- CHOROID
- NEO NET LEAKING

HEMORRHAGIC RPE OR SENSORY RETINA DETACHMENT

↓

EVENTUAL FIBROTIC SCARRING

- RED SUBRETINAL HEMORRHAGE
- GRAY GREEN SUB RPE HEMORRHAGE
- NEO NET BURSTING

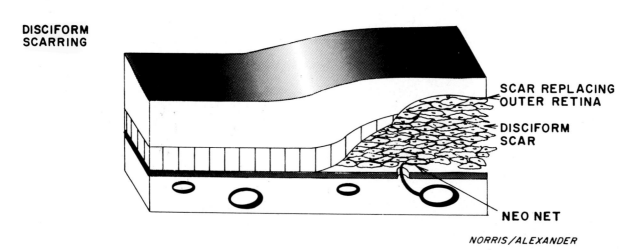

DISCIFORM SCARRING

- SCAR REPLACING OUTER RETINA
- DISCIFORM SCAR
- NEO NET

NORRIS/ALEXANDER

Figure 2–58. The possible consequences of choroidal neovascularization.

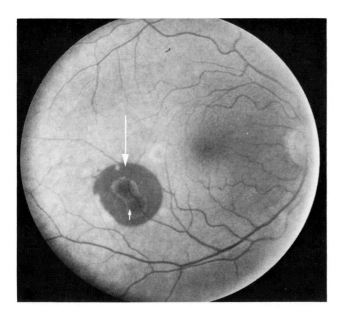

Figure 2–59. The small arrow points to a subretinal pigment epithelial hemorrhage, which is gray-green in color. The overlying subretinal hemorrhage **(long arrow)** is red.

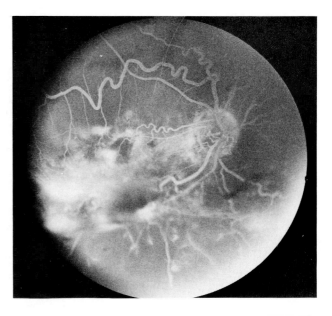

Figure 2–61. Fluorescein angiogram of the resolving vitreous hemorrhage shown in Figure 2–60.

With time, the hemorrhage will settle to the inferior retina. Large clumps of blood remain, with clear zones, whereas in the inferior periphery, large feathery whitish sheets appear. These sheets may persist for years and can create occasional complaints of floaters in an especially syneretic vitreous.

Management of the vitreous hemorrhage consists of first determining the cause and then possible therapeutic intervention once the hemorrhage

has cleared enough to assess the retina. Combined procedures of photocoagulation, vitrectomy, and at times scleral buckling may be necessary to effect a cure. Common causes of vitreous hemorrhage include diabetes, retrolental fibroplasia, sickle cell disease, Eales' disease, hypertension, trauma, and retinal tears.

VITREOUS HEMORRHAGE—PEARLS

- Two forms: retrovitreous and intravitreous
- Usually secondary to rupture of neovascular net or development of a retinal tear
- Often visually devastating
- If long-standing, feathery white sheets into inferior vitreous
- Management
  - Ascertain cause
  - Strongly consider retinology consultation

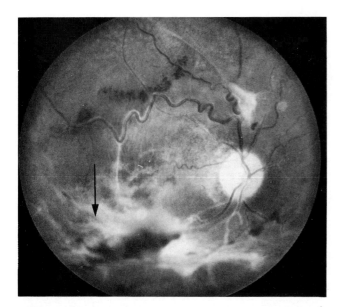

Figure 2–60. Black and white photograph of a resolving vitreous hemorrhage. The arrow points to the gray glial sheaths coursing out into the vitreous cavity.

Retinal Exudates and Cotton Wool Spots

The discussion of retinal exudates is limited to cotton wool spots in the superficial nerve fiber layer and lipid deposition in the deeper retinal layers, known as hard exudates. As with deep hemorrhages, lipid exudates are related to venous congestive retinal diseases. Cotton wool spots are similar to superficial flame-shaped hemorrhages in that they are related to arterial-based retinal diseases.

COTTON WOOL SPOTS

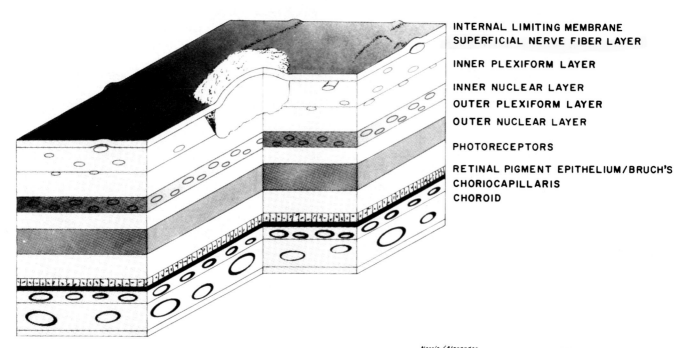

INTERNAL LIMITING MEMBRANE
SUPERFICIAL NERVE FIBER LAYER

INNER PLEXIFORM LAYER

INNER NUCLEAR LAYER
OUTER PLEXIFORM LAYER
OUTER NUCLEAR LAYER

PHOTORECEPTORS

RETINAL PIGMENT EPITHELIUM/BRUCH'S
CHORIOCAPILLARIS
CHOROID

Norris/Alexander

Figure 2–62. Schematic cross section of the retina demonstrating the clinicopathology of cotton wool spots.

Cotton Wool Spots. The retina is a tissue with a very high oxidative capacity and high glycolytic activity. As such, the tissue is very susceptible to hypoxia, which can occur immediately, with arterial occlusive disease such as an embolic branch artery occlusion, or as a sequela to long-standing venous occlusive disease. With venous occlusive disease, hypoxia results when arterial blood supply to a region meets with inflow resistance secondary to edema.

With hypoxia, the retinal capillary endothelium is compromised, leading to edema. The retinal cells destroyed by lack of oxygen lyse, releasing macromolecules that further increase the edema, which ultimately closes down the capillaries. The nuclei and nerve fibers may survive a brief bout with hypoxia, but with long-standing reduction in oxygen, the neurons will be lost and the nerve fibers will degenerate.

Cotton wool spots (Figs. 2–62 and 2–63) are a manifestation of ischemia within the nerve fiber layer. Cotton wool spots are microinfarcts from arteriolar–capillary occlusion. They usually occur in an area of the retina within about 3 disc diameters from the disc except in the foveal avascular zone. This corresponds to an area of the nerve fiber layer richly supplied by the superficial capillary network. The capillaries within the cotton wool spot are usually devoid of blood, with loss of endothelial cells

and intramural pericytes. On resolution of the cotton wool spot, the infarcted area becomes revascularized. In the area of the cotton wool spot, the ganglion cell and nerve fiber layers are swollen by the cytoid body-containing lesion. This swelling and debris accumulation may be the result of interruption in axoplasmic flow. **See color plates 26 and 27.**

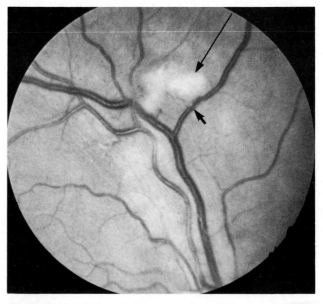

Figure 2–63. Black and white photograph of a very large cotton wool spot.

In the early stages, cotton wool spots appear above the retinal vessels in a fuzzy nondescript shape. If dense enough, they can produce a scotoma at threshold and can minimally block background choroidal fluorescence. The size varies and they are transient, disappearing in 5 to 7 weeks. With resolution, cotton wool spots fade to a gray color and become granular. When they disappear, retinal function resumes in the area with no apparent sequelae.

Many different disease processes can manifest cotton wool spots in the retina. Table 2–8 is a representation of the more common conditions associated with cotton wool spots. It is absolutely imperative that the clinician determine the cause of cotton wool spots, since they are a sign of underlying retinal hypoxia. Any retinal vascular disease that creates low oxygen concentration can manifest cotton wool spots. Retinal hypoxia is the immediate precursor of neovascularization, which occurs to create an alternative oxygen supply to the retina. Control of the underlying systemic disease or internal carotid stenosis should be questioned in retinal vascular disease with cotton wool spots.

COTTON WOOL SPOTS—PEARLS

- Ischemia within nerve fiber layer resulting from arteriolar infarcts
- Usually within 3 disc diameters of optic nerve head
- Edema secondary to interruption of axoplasmic flow
- A definite sign of retinal hypoxia
- Disappear in 5 to 7 weeks
- Management includes ascertaining underlying cause, allowing time for resorption, watching for other signs of hypoxia

---

Lipid (Hard) Exudates. Lipid exudates (Figs. 2–64 and 2–65) represent an excellent sign of retinal vascular compromise, since they are the by-products of breakdown of retinal vessels. They are characteristic of venous-based congestive diseases more often affecting the deeper capillary beds (prevenular). The hard exudates deposit in the outer plexiform layer throughout the retina and Henle's layer in the macular area but may extend from the internal limiting membrane to the outer nuclear layer. Most of the time, hard exudates are confined to the posterior pole except in the case of Coat's disease, when the exudates may be deposited peripherally. It should be noted that in Coat's disease the exudates dominate and can totally occupy the retina, extending into the subretinal space and causing moundlike detachments of the sensory retina.

The genesis of hard exudates is controversial but is thought to be associated with microglial tissue macrophages that are derived from mesodermal tissue or blood monocytes. These macrophages are resistant to hypoxia but are destroyed by anoxia. Macrophages function to remove extravascular blood, exudates, and cellular debris from vascular breakdown. The combination of ingredients of the vascular breakdown forms a lipid soup. The macrophages laden with lipid then remain in the outer plexiform layer. The lipid-laden macrophages along with free lipids migrate to the outer reaches of the diseased edematous retinal area. This "circling of the wagons" serves as a clinicopathologic boundary for identification of intraretinal microvasculopathy. Often, this forms a circle, oval pattern, or partial arcs. This pattern may remain after resolution—either normal or induced by photocoagulation—of the intraretinal disease, much as a ring is left around the bathtub when the water is drained. In the macular area, the pattern may be that of a radiating star because of the absence of an outer plexiform layer, which is replaced by a tightly bound Henle's layer. The absence of hard exudates in retinal ischemic disease, such as branch retinal arterial disease, may be secondary to microglial (macrophage) death from anoxia.

Clinically, hard exudates are dense, with color varying from whitish yellow to gold but most often waxy yellow. Long-standing fatty exudates assume a glittering gold color because of the accumu-

---

TABLE 2–8. CONDITIONS COMMONLY ASSOCIATED WITH COTTON WOOL SPOTS

Hypertension	Purtscher's retinopathy	Papilledema
Diabetes	Anemias	Papillitis
Systemic lupus erythematosus	Leukemias	Papillophlebitis
Blood dyscrasias	Septicemias	Ischemic optic neuropathy
Dermatomyositis	Dysproteinemias	Acquired immunodeficiency syndrome (AIDS)
Scleroderma	Venous occlusive disease	
	Internal carotid stenosis	

HARD EXUDATE FORMATION

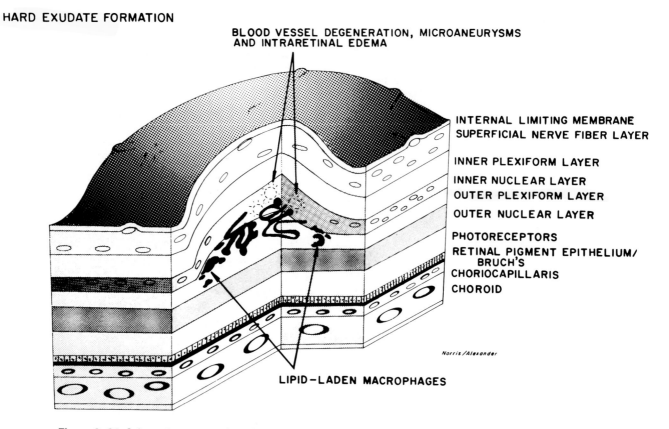

Figure 2–64. Schematic cross section of the retina demonstrating the clinicopathology of hard exudate formation.

lation of cholestrin crystals. The material is space-occupying, pushing aside retinal elements that are already compromised by deep retinal edema and often dot–blot hemorrhages. More often than not, microaneurysms or macroaneurysms can be dem-

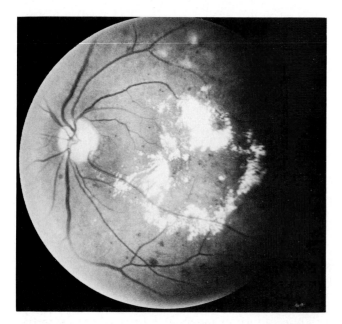

Figure 2–65. Photograph of severe hard exudate formation surrounding the macula in diabetic retinopathy.

onstrated by fluorescein angiography near the hard exudates in the developmental phase. These microaneurysms often are secondary to an obliterated capillary bed. Edema, whether deep in such diseases as diabetes or superficial in such diseases as hypertension, is a necessary precursor to exudate formation.

Exudates are a sign of retinal vasculopathy and in and of themselves require no treatment. It is well known that hard exudates in the fovea are a poor prognostic sign for recovery of vision. This is only because the retina in that area had to be edematous for a long period of time for the development of the exudates. Long-term macular edema creates permanent malfunction of at least some of the tightly packed photoreceptors. When a hard exudate formation is observed, it is a clinicopathologic sign of retinal edema, either present or past, that may be amendable to photocoagulative intervention. If this edema is threatening the macular area, fluorescein angiography is indicated to determine the desirability of photocoagulation. If the exudate pattern is not encroaching on the macula, it is important to determine the underlying cause of the edema, ascertain the control of the systemic disease, and follow the patient on at least a 12-month basis, barring extenuating circumstances. Table 2–9 lists conditions often assoc-

TABLE 2–9. CONDITIONS ASSOCIATED WITH INTRARETINAL HARD EXUDATES

Diabetes: Circular	Retinal macroaneurysms
Hypertension: Star	Leber's miliary
Coat's disease: Dense peripheral	aneurysms
Coat's response in exudative maculopathy	von Hippel-Lindau— angiomatosis retinae
Venous occlusive disease	Papillitis: Macular wing
	Papilledema

iated with intraretinal hard exudates. **See color plate 28.**

LIPID EXUDATES—PEARLS

- Occur in venous stasis diseases in deep retina
- Associated with deep retinal edema
- Usually confined to posterior pole
- Result of macrophages eating a lipid soup within the retina and migrating to the extent of the edema
- Form a ring around intraretinal edema often created by leaking microaneurysms
- Management
  - Ascertain cause
  - If encroaching on or within macula, fluorescein angiography and retinology consultation
  - If away from macula, document, educate, and followup at least every 12 months

---

Retinal Blood Vessel Anomalies and Alterations

Retinal Microaneurysms. Retinal microaneurysms are omnipresent in retinal congestive diseases (Table 2–10). Microaneurysms are 50 to 100 microns in size and, as such, are nonresolvable by direct ophthalmoscopy but become readily apparent on fluorescein angiography. Microaneurysms glow like miniature Christmas tree lights on fluorescein angiography. Larger microaneurysms are visible by ophthalmoscopy, especially when they occur in the

TABLE 2–10. RETINAL DISEASES ASSOCIATED WITH MICROANEURYSM FORMATION

Diabetes	Eales' disease
Venous occlusive disease	Sickle cell disease
Coat's disease	Hypertension (severe)
Blood dyscrasias	Dysproteinemias
Leukemias	Leber's disease
Peripheral retina in aged	

center of active retinal microvasculopathy. Microaneurysms occur in cases of retinal hypoxia when there is associated microcapillary obliteration. They develop most often near the venous side of the deep capillary structure.

Capillary microaneurysms appear as saccules on the wall of the vessel, often in clusters directed toward the areas of capillary obliteration. Within the wall, there is a proliferation of endothelial cells. Initially, these cells leak, but with age the wall, becomes hyalinized sealing the leakage. These may persist 1 to 2 years.

The precise etiopathogenesis of the endothelial proliferation in response to the hypoxia of capillary obliteration is unknown. There are proponents of the theory that the ballooning occurs in response to lipid infiltration of the endothelial walls. Some believe microaneurysms are aborted attempts at neovascularization or revascularization of previously atrophied channels. This theory would gain support with the realization that peripheral retinal microaneurysms are common with aging, since capillary structure normally closes down in the periphery with age. In diabetes alone, there is a selective loss of intramural pericytes that could weaken the capillary wall, allowing for aneurysmal formation. This does not, however, explain the genesis of microaneurysms in other retinal vascular diseases. The only substantiated fact is that microaneurysms occur in areas of hypoxia secondary to capillary obliteration where the endothelium is still viable.

It is important to recognize retinal diseases that may have associated microaneurysms. The microaneurysms leak, creating intraretinal edema with resulting potential acuity or field loss, or both. Although microaneurysms are not routinely observable, there are signs of their presence. Any disease creating stasis microvasculopathy probably will have associated microaneurysms. The signs of these diseases include dot–blot hemorrhages and hard exudates. Any time dot–blot hemorrhages or hard exudates are visible, it is safe to assume that microaneurysms are present or have been present in the recent past. Fluorescein angiography will confirm the presence of microaneurysms.

If microaneurysmal leakage occurs in the macular area, there is a significant threat to vision. The microaneurysms are, however, amendable to photocoagulation to arrest the leakage. It is important to recognize conditions associated with microaneurysms, perform fluorescein angiography to determine their presence, and intervene with photocoagulation when the microaneurysms are a threat to vision. All management must be underscored by the importance of maximal control of the underlying systemic condition.

MICROANEURYSMS—PEARLS

- Usually related to venous stasis
- Often invisible to direct ophthalmoscopy
- Response to a weakening of the capillary wall
- Leak profusely—signs of presence include hard exudates and dot—blot hemorrhage
- Management
  - Ascertain cause
  - If encroaching on or within macula, fluorescein angiography and consider retinology consultation
  - If distant from macula, educate and follow up in at least 12 months

---

Retinal Macroaneurysms. A retinal macroaneurysm is an isolated dilated area of a major retinal arterial branch. The condition is associated with systemic hypertension, arteriosclerosis, and retinal emboli. There is typically not the associated microvasculopathy of capillary obliteration that one finds with microaneurysms, yet there is edema, exudation, and hemorrhage secondary to the macroaneurysm.

Macroaneurysms typically occur in older patients aged 50 to 80 years, with an increased incidence in females. Of these patients, about 50 percent have systemic hypertension and 25 percent demonstrate a high 5-year postdiscovery mortality rate associated with systemic cardiovasculopathy.

Clinical diagnosis is made in the early phase by observation of an isolated ballooning of the vessel usually within the radius of the second branching of the temporal arteries. As the macroaneurysm leaks, retinal edema allows for intraretinal and subretinal hemorrhage and intraretinal and subretinal lipid exudate deposition. Should this process occur in the macular area, there is a definite threat to severe vision loss.

Besides the systemic implications and necessity for a cardiovascular physical examination, it is important to realize that localized ocular treatment may be of benefit. Asymptomatic macroaneurysms need only be observed at 6-month intervals, with the patient monitoring vision at home. These asymptomatic macroaneurysms are characterized by an absence of exudation and hemorrhage. Localized exudation and hemorrhage may be followed at a 3-month interval, with patient self-monitoring if there is no immediate threat to macular vision.

Photocoagulation should be applied if there is a persistence of macular edema or exudate without a spontaneous self-sealing of the macroaneurysm after 3 months of observation. Spread of the effects of the macroaneurysm on serial observations is an-

other indication for photocoagulation. Another indicator for photocoagulative intervention is the observation of pulsation of the macroaneurysmal wall, which suggests a very thin wall that is subject to rupture.

RETINAL MACROANEURYSMS—PEARLS

- Isolated dilatation of major arterial branch usually within radius of second branching
- Associated with hypertension, arteriosclerosis, retinal emboli, and cardiovascular disease
- No microvasculopathy but edema, exudation, and hemorrhage
- Photocoagulation if threat to vision, if lesion pulses, or if lesion spreads
- If asymptomatic, follow up 6 months and home monitoring
- If asymptomatic and localized exudation or hemorrhage, follow up 3 months and home monitoring

---

Parafoveal Retinal Telangiectasia. Parafoveal retinal telangiectasia may be a cause of macular edema and reduced visual acuity. It is a developmental anomaly, with aneurysms of the capillaries involving several retinal areas. The condition is usually unilateral, with males most often affected. Should the leaking telangiectatic vessels occur in the macular area, edema ensues. If severe, intraretinal exudates may occur and even extend into the subretinal spaces, creating a moundlike retinal detachment familiar with Coat's disease.

The clinical picture may be similar to a retinal macroaneurysm, and fluorescein angiography is necessary to make the proper differential diagnosis. Treatment is controversial. Photocoagulation may be useful in reducing the associated edema, but the clinician must remember that there is a high incidence of recurrence associated with parafoveal retinal telangiectasia.

PARAFOVEAL RETINAL TELANGIECTASIAS—PEARLS

- Developmental anomaly
- Series of leaking microaneurysms
- May impact on macular function because of leakage
- Fluorescein angiography indicated, with possible laser intervention, but high incidence of recurrence

---

Retinal Collateralization. Retinal collaterals are blood vessels that develop within the framework of the existing vessel network, usually near or adjacent to areas of nonperfusion of the capillary bed. These areas of collateralization may be contrasted with neovascularization, which occurs in zones of the retina that are normally avascular. Initially, these are capillary in nature but may evolve into vein-to-vein collaterals after venous occlusion, artery-to-artery collaterals after branch arterial occlusion, and occasionally artery-to-vein collaterals after capillary bed obstruction. Artery-to-vein communications without associated capillary bed obstructions are called shunts and may occur isolated as congenital variations or acquired in conditions, such as retinal angiomatosis and Coat's disease.

Collaterals are beneficial to the health of the retina, since they drain venous blood or shunt arterial blood around an area of compromised retinal vascular bed. These channels occur as the blood seeks a new route. The walls of the channels develop, and the lumen of the vessels enlarges to take on more blood. With enlargement, the channels become visible to ophthalmoscopy. These collaterals may be multiple or single and ultimately assume a similar structure to the occluded vessel. Collaterals lie within the retina and do not leak fluorescein. At times, the occluded vessel will become patent and the collateral will recede; other times, the occluded vessel will become sheathed (vein) and the collateral will assume responsibility for the affected retinal area (Fig. 2–66).

A variation of the retinal collateral is the optociliary shunt vessels occurring at the optic nerve head associated with central retinal vein occlusion. These serve to shunt venous blood from the retina to the optic nerve choroidal vasculature, bypassing the occluded central retinal vein.

Collateral formation is an important aspect of resolution of retinal vascular disease. Rapid, extensive collateralization can effectively supply or drain blood to an area of retinal vascular compromise, averting total sensory retinal loss. Identification of collaterals indicates present or past regional retinal vascular disease. It is important to ascertain the underlying systemic cause of this disease and manage it appropriately. Collaterals are never to be photocoagulated. If there is confusion whether the vascular alterations are collaterals or neovascularization, fluorescein angiography will effectively differentiate the two. Collaterals do not leak on fluorescein angiography, but neovascularization does.

Intraretinal microvascular abnormalities (IRMA) describes shunt (collateral) formation and dilated capillaries in areas of nonperfusion in diabetic retinopathy. IRMA looks like intraretinal neovascularization and actually is similar to new vessels in that it is composed of endothelium with only a few intramural pericytes. IRMA does not leak fluorescein in the early phases of development and should not be photocoagulated. It may leak on fluorescein angiography as neovascularization develops in the area. IRMA is considered to be the germination bed for retinal neovascularization, and fluorescein angiography is indicated to determine the stage of development.

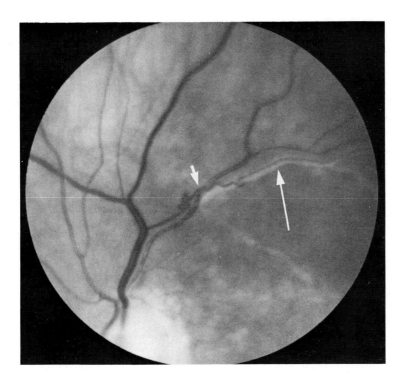

Figure 2–66. The small arrow points to a retinal collateral vessel formed in response to a branch retinal vein occlusion. The large arrow points to the sheathed retinal vein.

Retinal hypoxia
↓
IRMA (Intraretinal Microvascular Abnormalities)
↓
Vasoproliferative stimulus—further hypoxia
↓
Neovascular development through the internal limiting membrane proliferating on the retinal surface—fibrotic scaffolding occurs with additional adherence to the vitreous face if there is no posterior vitreous detachment.

Figure 2–67. Proposed etiology of neovascularization elsewhere in diabetic retinopathy.

RETINAL COLLATERALIZATION—PEARLS

- Develop near zones of capillary nonperfusion
- Develop within the framework of existing vessel network
- Act as a detour to shunt blood around a closed area
- Do not leak, therefore do not photocoagulate
- Optociliary shunt is a sign of past central retinal vein occlusion
- IRMA requires fluorescein angiography to determine stage of development

---

Retinal Neovascularization. Retinal neovascularization is a complex reaction to a simple stimulus—lack of oxygenated blood. Any retinal vascular disease that creates hypoxia can develop neovascularization. Retinal neovascularization typically occurs in avascular zones of the ocular structure to attempt to supply oxygenated blood to a hypoxic retinal area. The attempt is noble, but the new vessels are very fragile and subject to leakage and hemorrhage. The omnipresent fibrotic scaffolding that accompanies neovascularization sets up potential retinal traction, with subsequent detachment. By definition, retinal neovascularization develops from and is contiguous with the preexisting viable retinal vascular bed.

The etiopathogenesis of retinal neovascularization is somewhat controversial, but the effects and proper management are universally accepted. Two theories of genesis of retinal neovascularization are shown in Figures 2–67 and 2–68. It is important to recognize that viable retinal tissue is necessary to support new vessel growth. Anoxic retinal areas will not grow new vessels. Table 2–11 lists some conditions associated with development of peripheral neovascularization.

Retinal neovascularization (Fig. 2–69) is thought to be a proliferation of the endothelium of the capillaries and veins. An arterial association is possible. The lumen is usually larger than a capillary and is differentiated from a capillary also by the profuse leakage of intravascular fluid. All new vessels are accompanied by fibrotic scaffolding, but some may be characterized by a profusion of lacy tortuous vessels, with fibrosis occurring after the network has aged.

As mentioned previously, the new vessels may form on the retinal surface, but they may also emanate from the optic nerve head. When occurring at the optic nerve head, they penetrate easily into the vitreous body because of the lack of a true internal limiting membrane at this location. The possible location for the development of neovascularization in diseases with retinal hypoxia has some predictability. The neovascularization usually will occur within or very near the identified hypoxic zone or on the disc in an area that would face the hypoxic retina. **See color plate 29.**

Retinal neovascularization represents a direct threat to maintenance of vision function. The new vessels can leak, creating edema, can hemorrhage into the vitreous, or can cause retinal traction associated with the fibrotic scaffolding. It is important to ascertain the underlying cause of the neo-

---

Premature infants with immature retinal vascular growth to temporal peripheral retina
↓
Exposure to high oxygen concentrations
↓
Suppression of peripheral retinal vessel development
↓
Return to room air
↓
Peripheral retinal hypoxia
↓
Peripheral retinal vessel proliferation

Figure 2–68. The proposed etiology of neovascularization in retinopathy of prematurity.

TABLE 2–11. DISEASES KNOWN TO BE ASSOCIATED WITH PERIPHERAL NEOVASCULARIZATION

Disease	Age of Onset	Possible Locations	Heredity
Branch retinal vein occlusion	50s–60s	Area of nonperfusion	N/A
Diabetes	Variable usually after 20 years	Entire fundus	N/A
Retinopathy of prematurity	Birth through first year	Temporal periphery	N/A (Prematurity)
Eales' disease	Teens through 30s	Area of involved vein	N/A
Thick blood syndromes	Variable	Periphery	N/A
Sarcoidosis	Variable	Periphery	N/A
Retinal telangiectasia (Coat's disease)	Teens through 30s	Entire fundus	N/A
Familial exudative vitreoretinopathy	Variable	Periphery	Autosomal dominant
von Hippel-Lindau (angiomatosis retinae)	Teens through 40s	Periphery	Autosomal dominant
Hemoglobinopathies, e.g., sickle cell disease	Variable	Temporal periphery	Autosomal
Aortic arch syndrome	After 20 years	Entire fundus	N/A

vascularization. Table 2–12 lists diseases associated with retinal neovascularization. It is important to perform fluorescein angiography to differentiate neovascularization from collaterals. Photocoagulation is indicated to eliminate the hypoxic stimulus and cause regression of the neovascularization. Specific guidelines for intervention are outlined in subsequent sections on diseases associated with new vessel growth. It is important to realize that neovascularization can, at times, regress with re-

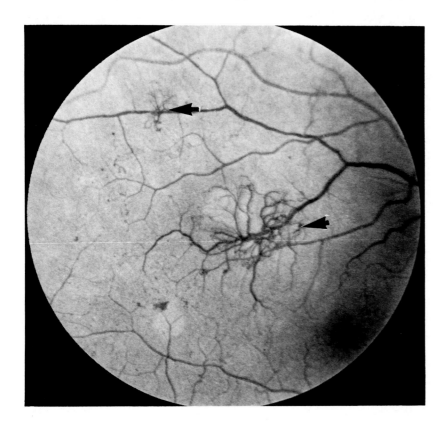

Figure 2–69. Arrows point to neovascularization elsewhere in a case of diabetic retinopathy.

TABLE 2–12. DISEASES COMMONLY ASSOCIATED WITH RETINAL NEOVASCULARIZATION

Diabetic retinopathy	Eales' disease
Branch retinal vein occlusion	Sarcoidosis
Hemicentral retinal vein occlusion	Pulseless disease
Central retinal vein occlusion	Behcet's disease
Sickle cell retinopathy	Hemoglobinopathies
Retinopathy of prematurity	

moval of the hypoxic stimulus, but a conservative approach for all retinal neovascularization would be a retinology consultation.

NEOVASCULARIZATION—PEARLS

- Reaction to hypoxia
- Retinal, disc, and choroidal forms
- Vessels are fragile, leak, and are accompanied by fibrosis
- Develops from viable preexisting vascular bed
- Direct threat to vision
- Management
  Perform fluorescein angiography and determine if amendable to photocoagulation

---

Retinal Vessel Tortuosity. Tortuosity of retinal vessels, specifically veins, can be an important diagnostic sign (Fig. 2–70). Acquired venous tortuosity usually occurs in conditions of retinal hypoxia. The most common vascular tortuosity is, however, congenital. Extreme tortuosity involving all quadrants, tortuosity of the same degree symmetrical in both eyes, or vein tortuosity with associated arterial tortuosity is characteristic of congenital vascular tortuosity. Comparison of both eyes is valuable as a differential diagnostic tool.

Isolated arterial tortuosity is rare. Tortuosity of the veins in just one sector or tortuosity in previously normal channels is of diagnostic significance. There is usually dilatation of the vein and a darkening of the blood column in the affected region. Increased vein tortuosity is indicative of venous stasis, retinal hypoxia in the immediate area, or any form of localized occlusion from blood disease. It is likely that tortuosity in a vein is related to the distensibility of the vein related to increases in internal pressure. The veins do have localized periodic attachments to the retinal tissue. With dilatation, the veins remain attached at certain points, creating a serpentine form. **See color plate 30.**

Retinal vascular tortuosity is important because it is an indicator of blood sludging in the presence of hypoxia. The hypoxia then acts as a neovascular

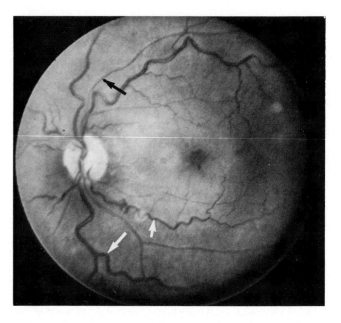

Figure 2–70. The black arrow points to a straight retinal artery; the white arrows point to acquired venous tortuosity.

stimulus. The clinician must attempt to uncover the underlying disease process as well as carefully follow the affected retina for signs of further developments. Tables 2–13 and 2–14 list diseases commonly associated with acquired vascular tortuosity.

RETINAL VESSEL TORTUOSITY—PEARLS

- Congenital
  - Involving all quadrants
  - Symmetrical in both eyes
  - Vein tortuosity associated with arterial tortuosity
- Acquired venous tortuosity
  - Previously documented normalcy
  - Sectoral involvement may occur
  - Associated darkening and thickening of the blood column
  - Indicator of hypoxia
  - Management is to monitor carefully after ascertaining cause

---

Vascular Sheathing. Retinal blood vessel walls usually are invisible by ophthalmoscopic examination. The blood vessel appearance is actually the

TABLE 2–13. DISEASES ASSOCIATED WITH ACQUIRED ARTERY AND VEIN TORTUOSITY

Congenital heart disease
Retinopathy of prematurity
Leber's miliary aneurysms
Coat's disease
Racemose angioma

TABLE 2–14. DISEASES ASSOCIATED WITH ACQUIRED VEIN TORTUOSITY

Ipsilateral internal carotid artery disease
Diabetic retinopathy
Blood dyscrasias
Sickle cell disease
Branch retinal vein occlusion
Central retinal vein occlusion
Hemicentral retinal vein occlusion

visualization of the blood column. Retinal blood vessel walls only become visible when altered by an acquired disease or when congenital sheathing is present. When there is an acquired uniform change of the vessel wall, it is often most visible lateral to the blood column, since the thickness of the viewed wall is greater laterally (Fig. 2–71). Management of all vascular sheathing consists of diagnosis and management of the underlying systemic or retinal disease.

Congenital vascular sheathing is a common occurrence in both retinal arteries and veins. This sheathing is usually continuous with and within 2 disc diameters of the optic nerve head. It usually is densest at the disc, tapering in density toward the periphery. Congenital vascular sheathing is more commonly associated with veins and may be present with persistence of the hyaloid vasculature. It is presumed that there is some connection between congenital vascular sheathing and the residual tissue of the hyaloid vascular network.

Most of the time, *venous sheathing* is a collagenous or lipohyaline thickening of the venous walls, appearing hazy white. Venous sheathing often occurs secondary to long-standing venous obstructive disease. This type of sheathing is uniform and is known as "halo" sheathing. When halo sheathing occurs, the vein may still be patent but may have a slightly reduced lumen.

It is important to note that phagocytized retinal pigment and free fat have an affinity for venous walls. This is most apparent in the condition of pigmented paravenous retinochoroidopathy.

Venous sheathing may occur in 10 to 25 percent of patients with multiple sclerosis (MS). The sheathing in MS usually occurs away from the posterior pole. In the active inflammatory phase, a fuzzy white perivenous cuffing of the vein occurs. This stage is known as periphlebitis (Fig. 2–72) and may come and go with cyclical MS attacks. If prolonged periphlebitis occurs, permanent sheathing of the veins may occur. Periphlebitis can occur with other retinal and systemic diseases, such as Eale's disease, sarcoidosis, toxoplasmosis, acquired retinoschisis, pars plantis, and generalized posterior uveitis. There may be other vascular irregularities, such as hemorrhage associated with vein wall inflammation (periphlebitis) and pigment accumulation with chorioretinal inflammation.

Sheathing of both the arteries and veins may occur near the disc associated with prolonged papillitis, papillophlebitis, and papilledema. This should be easy to differentiate from congenital sheathing by the presence of other signs of nerve head disease.

Arterial sheathing occurs secondary to many systemic conditions that can have a negative impact on arterial wall structure. Early arteriosclerotic

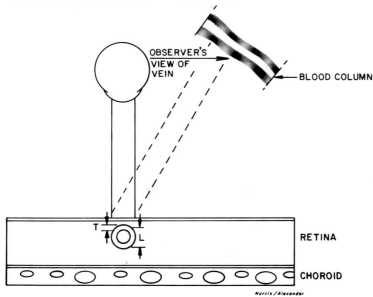

THE TOP VIEW OF A SHEATHED RETINAL VEIN WALL. SECTION L IS THICKER AND MORE VISIBLE THAN SECTION T

Figure 2–71. Top view of a sheathed retinal vein wall. Section L is thicker and more visible than section T.

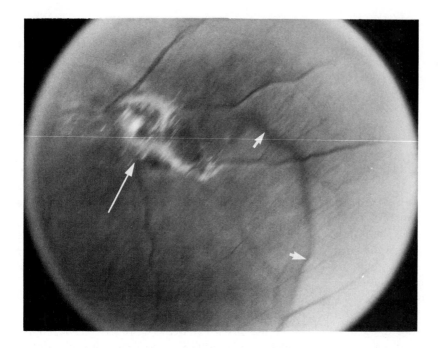

Figure 2–72. The long arrow points to a zone of active periphlebitis. The small arrows demarcate a zone of white without pressure.

changes appear as a broadening of the central white reflex of an artery. This increases to the point where fine white lines may occur along the artery wall. Continued sclerosis of the vessel wall will lead to the classic copper wire appearance of the vessel, which is nothing more than an enhanced reflex. Sclerosis of the arterial wall can lead to artery and vein crossing changes and, ultimately, branch retinal vein occlusions.

With an increase in severity, the sclerosis of vessels may be random but will affect predominantly larger vessels. At the bifurcations of larger arteries, a yellow reflex often develops with crystalline reflections that spread into surrounding areas. There may be associated focal constrictions. Should the patient survive, this sheathing may extend more symmetrically to involve smaller vessels. These severely compromised arteries are still patent but represent a life-threatening underlying systemic disease process.

VASCULAR SHEATHING—PEARLS

- Congenital
  - Continuous with and within 2 disc diameters of optic nerve
  - Most often with veins and may have other hyaloid remnants
- Venous
  - Halo is secondary to venous obstructive disease
  - Phagocytized RPE and fat have an affinity for walls
  - May occur in periphlebitis (MS), Eales' disease, sarcoidosis, toxoplasmosis, retinoschisis, and pars planitis
- Arterial
  - Typical sheathing associated with arteriosclerosis—copper to silver
  - With increasing severity, yellow reflex at bifurcations of large arteries
- Management
  - Ascertain underlying cause and treat accordingly

TABLE 2–15. TRIGLYCERIDE LEVEL IN RELATION TO RETINAL APPEARANCE

Grade of Lipemia Retinalis	Triglyceride Level	Fundus Appearance
I	2500–3500 mg%	Creamy thin peripheral vessels
II	3500–5000 mg%	Creamy thin peripheral vessels, abnormal color in vessels of posterior pole but veins and arteries distinguishable
III	Greater than 5000 mg%	Fundus salmon colored, veins and arteries creamy and difficult to distinguish at disc

Modified and reprinted with permission from Alexander LJ: Ocular signs and symptoms of altered blood lipids. J Am Optom Assoc, 1983; 54:123–126.

Lipemia Retinalis. Lipemia retinalis refers to the ophthalmoscopic picture of the retinal blood vessels assuming a salmon or creamy color secondary to elevated serum triglyceride levels. A grading system for lipemic vessels has been suggested that distinguishes the fundus appearance related to the serum triglyceride levels. Table 2–15 outlines the grading system.

The retinal picture varies with the triglyceride level. The first sign of lipemia retinalis is a creamy appearance to the peripheral retinal vessels (Fig. 2–73). As the triglyceride level increases, the vessels of the posterior pole become affected, ultimately leading to the point where arteries and veins become indistinguishable at the optic nerve head.

Lipemia retinalis is classically recognized as being nonvision-threatening. However, there have been reports of isolated complications, such as macular edema, retinal detachment, and hemorrhages. Other reports have suggested a retinal involvement similar to Coat's disease, with multiple hemorrhages and lipid infiltration. Certainly, the consistency of the blood with such elevated triglyceride levels lends to vaso-occlusive disease.

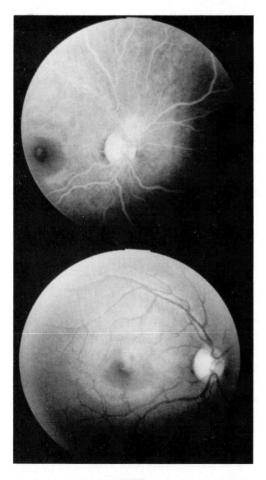

Figure 2–73. Top. Lipemic vessels associated with extremely high triglyceride levels. **Bottom.** Same patient after the triglyceride levels have been controlled.

Of utmost importance in the management of lipemia retinalis is the realization of the impact of the elevated triglyceride levels on the cardiovascular system. The patient should have a complete physical examination with emphasis on differential diagnosis of the hyperlipoproteinemias. Under dietary control and possibly with pharmacologic intervention, the triglyceride level can be controlled, causing total resolution of the lipemic retinal picture. **Table 2–16 summarizes the clinical and ocular signs of hyperlipoproteinemias. See color plate 31.**

Retinal Emboli. Often emboli eroding from remote vascular locations may occur within the retinal vasculature. Theoretically, any foreign substance introduced into the system could travel to the retinal system. The most frequent sites of genesis of retinal emboli are eroding carotid sinus lesions, eroding cardiac vegetations, and self-injected emboli associated with drug usage. Regardless of the source or clinical appearance, there is a strong association of retinal emboli to significant systemic cardiovascular disease.

The clinical picture of retinal emboli varies with the type and extent of the embolus. The embolus may be nothing more than a glowing intravascular plug or may cause vascular occlusion (Fig. 2–74). **Table 2–17 summarizes the characteristics of commonly encountered retinal emboli.** Further discussion of some of the effects of retinal emboli and thrombi are presented in the sections on retinal vaso-occlusive disease. **See color plate 32.**

Preretinal Membrane Formation. Preretinal membrane formation (Figs. 2–75 to 2–78) is discussed in this text because its genesis is often associated with retinal vasculopathy. Preretinal membrane formation is an anatomic alteration that can result from a variety of precipitating factors. The condition often is placed in the category of venous and capillary obstructive diseases because the advanced stages are similar to the retinal reaction seen after the obstruction of a macular draining vein. There also seems to be a relationship between diabetes and preretinal membrane formation, especially in the absence of diabetic retinopathy. Preretinal membrane formation often is associated with surgical procedures for retinal detachment. Preretinal membrane formation has been seen with photocoagulation, trauma, macular holes and inflammation of ocular tissue. Idiopathic preretinal membrane formation occurs also as a separate entity, occurring predominantly in patients over 50 years of age with no demonstrable etiology. It has

TABLE 2–16. THE HYPERLIPOPROTEINEMIAS: CLINICAL LABORATORY AND OCULAR SIGNS

Type of Hyperlipoproteinemia	Clinical Laboratory Signs	Ocular Signs
Type 1 Chylomicronemia	Increased cholesterol Increased chylomicrons (triglycerides)	Lipemia retinalis, palpebral xanthomas, corneal arcus, xanthelasma
Type 2 Hyperbeta-lipoproteinemia	Increased cholesterol Mild to moderately increased triglycerides	Corneal arcus, xanthelasma
Type 3 Abnormal beta-lipoproteins and elevated triglycerides	Variable excesses in cholesterol and triglycerides	Possible corneal arcus, possible xanthelasma, palpebral xanthomas, lipemia retinalis
Type 4 Hyperbeta-lipoproteinemia and elevated triglycerides	Variable excesses in cholesterol and triglycerides	Palpebral xanthomas, lipemia retinalis
Type 5 Hyperchylomicronemia and hyperbeta-lipoproteinemia (type 1 and type 4)	Increased variable cholesterol and increased chylomicrons (triglycerides)	Palpebral xanthomas, lipemia retinalis

Modified and reprinted with permission from Alexander LJ: Ocular signs and symptoms of altered blood lipids. J Am Optom Assoc., 1983; 54:123–126.

been proposed and demonstrated histologically that the glinting reflex of the fundus described in patients with retinitis pigmentosa is the result of preretinal membrane formation.

Preretinal membranes have been classified into three grades according to appearance. Grade 0 is cellophane maculopathy, which appears as a translucent membrane without distortion of the inner retinal surface. Grade 1 occurs as a translucent membrane with the underlying retina gathered into a series of small folds. The underlying vessels may be indistinct, and surrounding small vessels may be slightly tortuous. In grades 0 and 1, visual acuity may be compromised but metamorphopsia is characteristic. Grade 2 appears as a semitranslucent membrane that may obscure the underlying vessels of the retina. Retinal hemorrhages and localized serous detachment may accompany this grade. At this stage, there is evidence of dye leakage with fluorescein angiography. Visual acuity in grade 2 often is compromised.

The etiology of preretinal membrane formation is controversial. Histologic studies support the theory that preretinal membranes occur as the result of proliferation of retinal glial cells on the internal limiting membrane that have escaped through breaks in the internal limiting membrane. This is supported by the appearance of membranes in retinal vascular diseases in which vasculitis contributes to a break in the internal limiting membrane. Trauma and retinal detachment also have the potential to compromise the internal limiting membrane. It should be noted that the membranes often are pigmented in postretinal detachment procedures.

Subjective complaints related to preretinal membrane formation vary according to associated conditions that precipitate the formation. Should the membrane be idiopathic, there may be a visual loss, but more often metamorphopsia is the complaint. Fewer than 5 percent of patients with only preretinal membranes have a visual loss to 20/200 or worse, and fewer than 20 percent have involvement of the fellow eye. More often there are no subjective complaints and preretinal membranes are found on routine examination. The earliest sign is described as a reflex seen on the retinal surface with an ophthalmoscope. This may be accentuated by using the red-free filter. Deviation of retinal vessels also is present. These vessels acquire a corkscrew pattern that is especially enhanced with fluorescein angiography. In approximately 25 percent

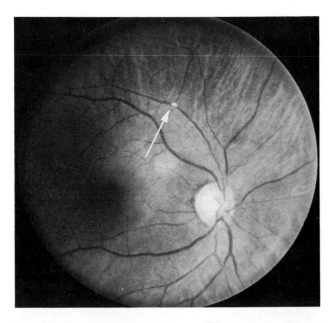

Figure 2–74. The arrow points to a Hollenhorst plaque lodged at an arterial bifurcation.

TABLE 2–17. CHARACTERISTICS OF EMBOLI AND THE RETINAL VASCULAR SYSTEM

Type of Embolus	Color	Location	Source	Retinal Prognosis
Cholesterol	Shiny yellow-orange	Often at bifurcations, may be mobile	Atheromas of carotid and of other vessels	No infarction unless multiple
Calcium	Gray-white	Unbranched arterioles, usually nonmobile	Eroding cardiac atheromas, artificial heart valves	Branch retinal artery occlusion
Platelets	Dull white long plugs	Arterioles but may readily break up	Carotid atheromas and thrombocytopenia	May lead to branch retinal artery occlusion
Fibrin	Not readily observed	Often laminar location, creating occlusion of central retinal artery	Thromboemboli after acute mitral insufficiency	Arterial occlusions
Talc or cornstarch	Shiny red-yellow	Capillaries of posterior pole	Self-injected in drug users	Microinfarcts in capillaries (cotton wool spots)

PRE-RETINAL MEMBRANE FORMATION

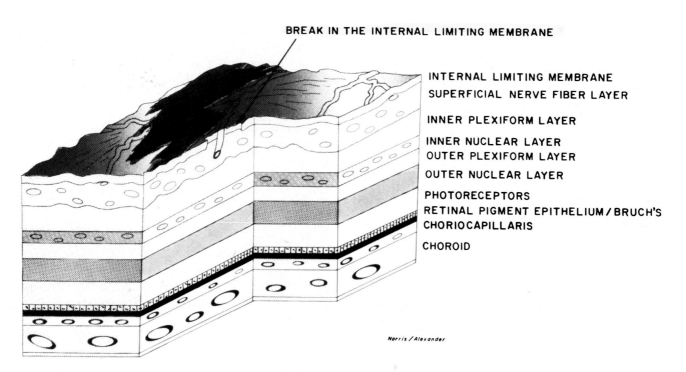

BREAK IN THE INTERNAL LIMITING MEMBRANE

INTERNAL LIMITING MEMBRANE
SUPERFICIAL NERVE FIBER LAYER

INNER PLEXIFORM LAYER

INNER NUCLEAR LAYER
OUTER PLEXIFORM LAYER

OUTER NUCLEAR LAYER

PHOTORECEPTORS
RETINAL PIGMENT EPITHELIUM/BRUCH'S
CHORIOCAPILLARIS

CHOROID

Norris/Alexander

Figure 2–75. Schematic cross section demonstrating the clinicopathology of preretinal membrane formation.

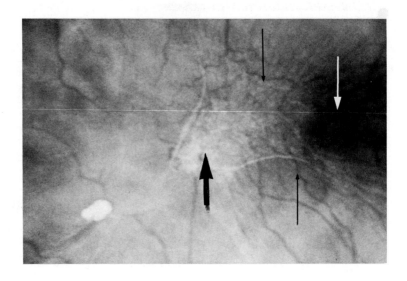

Figure 2–76. Photograph demonstrating a gathered pleat variety of preretinal membrane. The white arrow points to the macula, the large black arrow points to the bulk of the membrane, and the small black arrow points to the tugging of the membrane. (Modified and reprinted with permission from Alexander LJ: Pre-retinal membrane formation. J Am Optom Assoc., 1980; 51:567–572.)

of cases, traction on the retinal vessels from the preretinal membrane will alter vessel physiology, leading to leakage that may cause a further reduction of acuity because of macular edema.

The larger preretinal membranes are visualized more easily with stereoscopic examination techniques and red-free filters. They may become more translucent with age and typically have either a volcano pattern like puckered plastic wrap or a gathered pleat appearance.

In general, preretinal membranes are benign, self-limited processes but may cause significant reduction in vision if they have an impact on the macular area. Should vision be severely compromised or if the membrane is relatively fresh, a retinology consultation is indicated. There has been some success with vitrectomy in fresh cases of preretinal membranes, especially in diabetic retinopathy. There are, however, the potential side effects of long-standing macular edema and anatomically induced aniseikonia in patients who have had vitrectomy. **See color plate 33.**

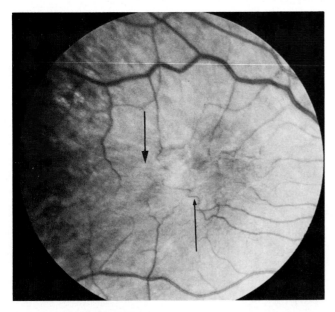

Figure 2–77. A preretinal membrane **(large arrow)** creating vascular tortuosity **(small arrow).**

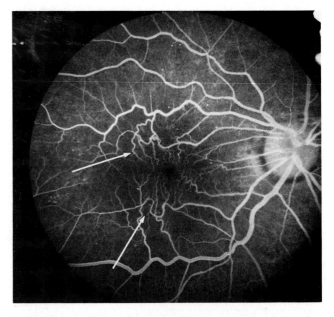

Figure 2–78. Angiogram of the eye shown in Figure 2–77, demonstrating the vascular tortuosity that results from a preretinal membrane.

PRERETINAL MEMBRANE FORMATION—PEARLS

- Associated with a break in the internal limiting membrane
- Volcano and gathered pleat variety
- Create underlying vascular tortuosity
- Create metamorphopsia and vision reduction
- Benign self-limited process but may create macular edema
- Management
  - If vision severely compromised or if fresh, consider retinology consultation
  - If long-standing or removed from macula, educate patient and monitor yearly

---

RETINAL VASO-OCCLUSIVE DISEASE

Retinal vaso-occlusive disease is the second most prevalent retinal vascular disease seen in clinical practice today. It occurs more commonly in the elderly but may occur in younger patients as well. Recent advances and modification of management protocol have, however, brought improvement in the prognosis of these disease processes. All basic principles discussed previously are applied in developing an understanding of the four types of retinal vaso-occlusive disease: branch retinal vein occlusion, central retinal vein occlusion, branch retinal artery occlusion, and central retinal artery occlusion. Brief mention is made of associated systemic ramifications of these diseases. The primary systemic disease process implicated in all retinal vaso-occlusive disease is ipsilateral internal carotid stenosis.

Branch Retinal Vein Occlusion

Branch retinal vein occlusion (BRVO) has been reported to be the second most prevalent of the retinal vascular diseases seen in eye care practice (diabetic retinopathy is first). There is little disagreement about the ophthalmoscopic characteristics of BRVO that assist in the diagnosis. There is, however, considerable controversy surrounding the etiology and management of patients with BRVO. There are also different types of BRVO that occur in clinically different ways, further adding to the confusion.

From an epidemiologic standpoint, the peak incidence of BRVO is in the fifth to sixth decades, with no racial or sexual predilection. There appears to be a 4 to 5 percent incidence of bilaterality.

Although the specific microscopic events surrounding BRVO are somewhat obscure, a few broad statements can be made. Arterial disease plays a part in the process, but it is not possible to state that this is the sole initiating factor in the condition. It can be stated that BRVO has a strong association with systemic-based diseases (57 percent of patients). Hypertension, glucose intolerance, hyperlipidemia, and hypercholesterolemia all have been implicated in BRVO. Recent work implicates platelet coagulation activities in early thrombosis formation in retinal vein occlusion. **Table 2–18 summarizes some of the systemic factors common in BRVO. See color plates 30, 34, and 38.**

The association with systemic disease points to the importance of diagnosis and appropriate management of the underlying systemic vascular condition. Patients with BRVO should have the following minimal screening tests performed: blood pressure, glucose tolerance test, lipid profile, complete blood count (CBC).

Branch retinal vein occlusion can occur as two distinct clinical entities, nonischemic retinopathy and ischemic retinopathy. The ischemic variety implies the possibility of development of neovascularization. The distinction is a clinical impression depending on the degree of superficial hemorrhage, cotton wool spots, and associated arterial changes. The superior temporal veins are affected most often, this being attributed to the fact that there are more arteriovenous crossings in the superior temporal retina than elsewhere.

The clinical picture varies considerably depending on the site of the occlusion, the degree of ischemia created, and the elapsed time since the occlusion (Figs. 2–79 to 2–85). Often a prodromal sign (Bonnet's sign) will occur as small splinter hemorrhages around an area of arteriovenous nicking. Should an occlusion occur either at an arteriovenous crossing or elsewhere, the classic BRVO de-

TABLE 2–18. SYSTEMIC FACTORS COMMON IN BRANCH RETINAL VEIN OCCLUSION

Carotid artery disease	von Hippel–Lindau's disease
Hypertension	Coat's disease
Diabetes	Eales' disease
Hyperlipidemia and hypercholesterolemia	Phlebitis
Altered platelet function	Cavernous sinus thrombosis
Estrogens	Elevated serum immunoglobulins
Chronic lung disease	Elevated intraocular pressure
Trauma	

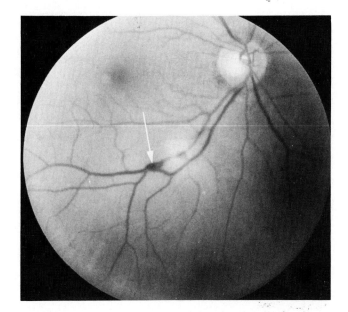

Figure 2–79. A flame-shaped hemorrhage (Bonnet's sign) at an arteriovenous crossing, the sign of a possible impending branch retinal vein occlusion at the site.

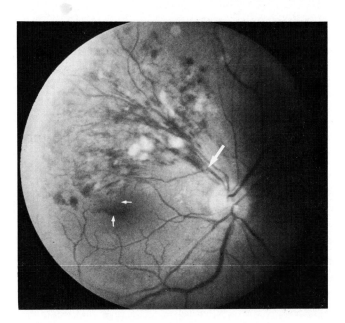

Figure 2–80. A full-blown ischemic branch retinal vein occlusion. The large arrow points to the site of the occlusion; the small arrows outline the ingress of edema into the macular area.

velops. Figure 2–86 demonstrates the factors involved in the genesis of the occlusion. The clinical picture is that of dilated tortuous veins and dot–blot hemorrhages from the site of the obstruction out to the retinal periphery in the sector of the retina normally drained by the affected vein. Microaneurysms also occur in the affected area, leaking and creating retinal edema. As more retinal hypoxia is created, cotton wool spots and flame-shaped hemorrhages are added to the picture.

Lipid infiltrates often occur near the site of the occlusion about 2 months after onset. Figure 2–87 is a schematic representation of the edema and sequelae. If the macular area is not adequately drained, partial or full macular edema (48 to 56 percent of cases) may develop, leading to visual compromise. It is important to understand that edema in the macula is the cause of vision loss in BRVO. As the BRVO progresses, collateral channels open to shunt blood around the occluded zone. The de-

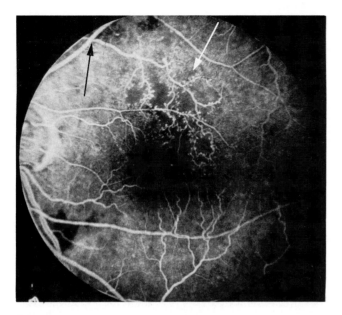

Figure 2–81. Early-phase fluorescein angiogram with the black arrow pointing to the site of the vein occlusion and the white arrow pointing to the area of microaneurysmal formation. These microaneurysms will leak, creating edema in the macula.

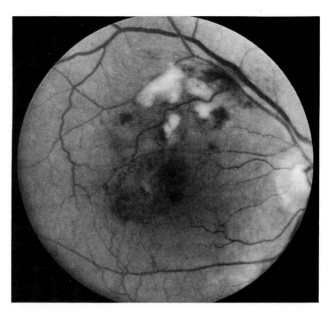

Figure 2–83. Black and white photograph of a branch retinal vein occlusion in the macular area.

velopment of effective collaterals is crucial in the prognosis for recovery. Collaterals observed temporal to the macula crossing the horizontal raphe are pathognomonic of an old BRVO.

Should the affected retinal area not drain properly, increased resistance to incoming oxygenated

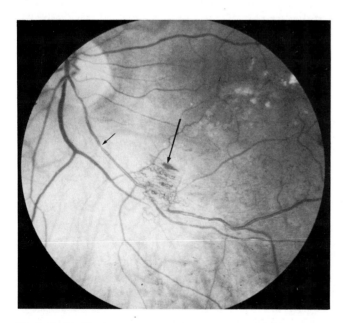

Figure 2–82. Black and white photograph illustrating the aftermath of a branch retinal vein occlusion. The small arrow points to the affected vein, and the large arrow points to a conglomerate of collaterals. (Reprinted with permission from Alexander LJ: The implications and management of retinal vaso-occlusive disease. SJ Optom, 1986; 2:20–34.)

blood occurs. If this oxygenated blood is not allowed sufficient access to the retinal tissue, hypoxia results. If the hypoxia is sufficient, a vasoproliferative stimulus is created, precipitating the development of neovascularization. This neovascularization may occur in the preretinal form, the disc form, and has even been reported at the iris margin. Vitreous hemorrhage or retinal traction may then occur. It appears that neovascularization may occur in approximately 25 to 30 percent of patients with BRVO. Often this neovascularization is hidden by the overlying hemorrhage and becomes apparent only by fluorescein angiography.

When retinal occlusive disease occurs, there appear to be changes in the vitreous overlying the process. When the vitreous is totally attached to the retina in eyes with BRVO, the vitreous adjacent to and overlying the area becomes liquefied. In the early stages, the gel exhibits white degenerative opacities that become larger with resorption of the retinal hemorrhage. Vitreous detachment also has an effect on the development of complications. The status of the vitreous as it relates to complications is summarized in Table 2–19.

Another interesting variety of BRVO can be very visually devastating. Macular branch retinal vein occlusion (MBRVO) results from an occlusion of a small tributary branch near the macula. There is an 85 percent incidence of macular edema associated with MBRVO.

One additional finding that may assist in the diagnosis is the effect of venous occlusive disease

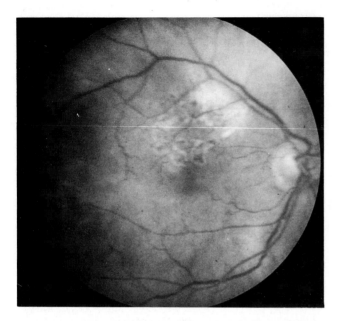

Figure 2–84. Black and white photograph of postphotocoagulation scars of branch retinal vein occlusion shown in Figure 2–83.

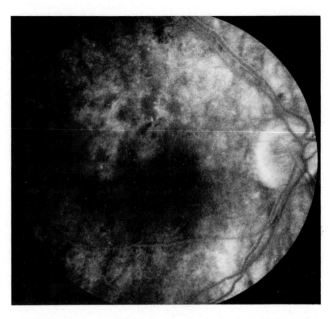

Figure 2–85. Fluorescein angiogram of the eye shown in Figure 2–84, demonstrating total absence of edema after photocoagulation.

on intraocular pressure (IOP). It has been found that 80 percent of patients have a decrease in IOP in the eye with venous occlusive disease. There is a greater decrease in central retinal vein occlusion (CRVO) than BRVO, a greater decrease in ischemic CRVO versus nonischemic CRVO, and a greater decrease in patients with relatively high IOPs in the fellow eye. There appears to be no significant effect in MBRVO. The duration of the hypotensive effect is 3 months in ischemic CRVO, 18 months in nonischemic CRVO, and 24 months in BRVO.

Fluorescein angiographic findings are very important in the diagnostic process of BRVO and can be divided into signs of the acute and chronic phases (Table 2–20).

Much of the controversy surrounding the management of BRVO originates because of the controversy surrounding the natural course of the disease. If untreated, patients often have results very similar to results in patients treated medically or surgically. Certain factors are, however, well documented. In general, studies report visual acuities

BRVO

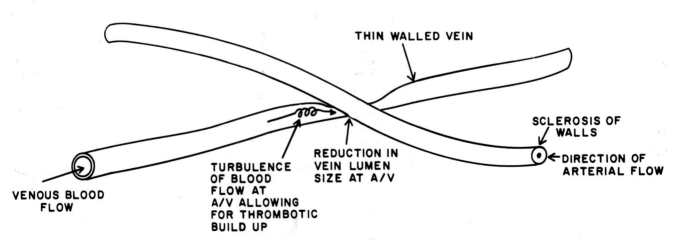

Figure 2–86. Schematic demonstrating the factors involved in the occlusion of a retinal vein. *(Reprinted with permission from Alexander LJ: The implications and management of retinal vaso-occlusive disease. S J Optom, 1986; 2:20–34.)*

BRVO

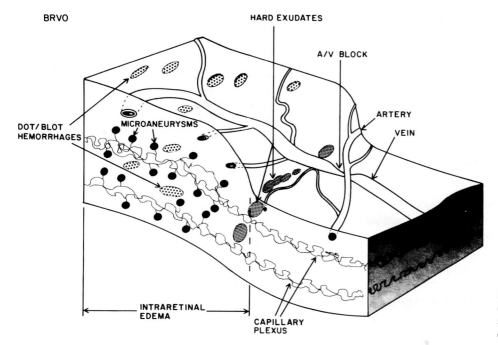

HARD EXUDATES

A/V BLOCK

ARTERY

VEIN

DOT/BLOT
HEMORRHAGES

MICROANEURYSMS

INTRARETINAL
EDEMA

CAPILLARY
PLEXUS

Figure 2–87. Schematic retinal cross section demonstrating the tissue changes secondary to the stasis created by a retinal vein occlusion.

of 6/12 (20/40) or better in 53 to 60 percent of untreated BRVO patients who have been followed for at least 1 year. This neglects, however, the percent who do not improve.

Complications develop, including neovascularization, vitreous hemorrhages, macular edema, macroaneurysms, chronic fibrosis, rhegmatogenous retinal detachment, and possibly neovascular glaucoma. Prognostic indicators are outlined in Table 2–21.

Management of BRVO is the area of greatest controversy, which exists because of the relatively good prognosis associated with the natural course of the disease. One noncontroversial aspect is the need to investigate each patient for the presence of associated systemic diseases. Every patient should have a complete physical examination, including blood pressure determination, blood glucose testing, lipid profile, coagulation profile, CBC with differential and smear, and electrocardiogram with

blood chemistry if hypertension is present.

Several medical management approaches have been advocated for BRVO. Low molecular weight dextran in combination with papaverine hydrochloride, anticoagulants, fibrinolytic agents, antithrombotic agents, steroids, and vasodilators have been tried, but no proof exists as to their efficacy.

Ticlopidine has been evaluated for its action as a platelet aggregation inhibitor in the treatment of BRVO and has been shown to be effective if the occlusion is fresh. Ticlopidine has shown similar results in the treatment of central retinal vein occlusion.

Photocoagulation has a place in the management of BRVO. The rationale for photocoagulation of nonproliferative BRVO is threefold: (1) the scar tissue formed in photocoagulation acts as a barrier to prevent retinal edema from spreading to the fovea, (2) areas of leakage are sealed to prevent further leakage, and (3) destruction of the capillary

TABLE 2–19. EFFECT OF THE STATE OF THE VITREOUS ON VISION-THREATENING FACTORS IN BRANCH RETINAL VEIN OCCLUSION

State of Vitreous	No Vitreous Detachment (%)	Partial Vitreous Detachment (%)	Complete Vitreous Detachment (%)
Neovascularization	16	64	0
Vitreous hemorrhage	12	64	7
Macular edema	54	56	29

Reprinted with permission from Alexander LJ: The implications and management of retinal vaso-occlusive disease. S J Optom, 1986; 2:20–34.

TABLE 2–20. FLUORESCEIN ANGIOGRAPHIC FINDINGS IN STAGES OF BRANCH RETINAL VEIN OCCLUSION

Acute Stage	Chronic Stage
1. Delayed filling of occluded vein, with possible leakage from wall	1. Appearance of collateral channels and shunt vessels
2. Focal hyperfluorescence near spot of occlusion	2. Microaneurysms and macroaneurysms
3. Obscuration of background choroidal fluorescence by hemorrhage	3. Areas of capillary dropout
4. Alterations in the perifoveal capillary net and areas of capillary nonperfusion	4. Macular edema
5. Diffuse intraretinal leakage of fluorescein	5. Neovascularization (disc and elsewhere)
	6. Neurosensory retinal detachment

Reprinted with permission from Alexander LJ: The implications and management of retinal vaso-occlusive disease. S J Optom, 1986; 2:20–34.

bed reduces the input of arterial blood to obstructed areas, which reduces edema and allows the intact bed to drain more effectively.

BRVOs threatening macular vision deserve a consultation with a competent retinologist. BRVO should be photocoagulated according to specific criteria. Argon grid laser application is beneficial for patients who suffer macular edema secondary to BRVO. The fresher the edema, the better the prognosis; however, it is recommended that laser intervention not be applied within the first 3 months postocclusion, since there may be spontaneous regression. If hemorrhage is present in the fovea, laser intervention is of questionable benefit. There is a significantly more favorable prognosis (2:1) in patients treated by these criteria than those left untreated. Regardless of criteria, which may change monthly, a BRVO threatening macular function requires a consultation with a retinologist.

Prophylactic scatter photocoagulation in the involved sector of a BRVO does not seem to be of benefit in the prevention of neovascularization. Scatter photocoagulation in the nonperfused area is, however, of benefit once neovascularization occurs. Regression of neovascularization is important to prevent the possibility of a devastating vitreous hemorrhage.

If photocoagulation is not indicated, patients with BRVOs should be followed very carefully, with routine assessment of visual acuity, Amsler grid (use home Amsler grid), careful dilated fundus examination, and fluorescein angiography when the fundus becomes suspect. It is important not to disregard the fact that there is probably an underlying systemic disease process that deserves careful investigation.

TABLE 2–21. PROGNOSTIC INDICATORS IN BRANCH RETINAL VEIN OCCLUSIONS

Factors	Impact on Prognosis
Location of occlusion	The nearer the disc, the more area involved
	The nearer the macula, the greater the likelihood of macular edema
Caliber of vessel	The larger the caliber (except macular BRVO) the poorer the prognosis
Degree of obstruction	Total obstruction creates poorer prognosis
Intensity and duration of macular edema	86% of patients with macular edema over 6 months and visual acuity of 20/50 or worse fail to improve
Degree of capillary closure: Either fluorescein angiography changes or sheathing of arterioles	The greater the area of capillary closure, the more likely the development of neovascularization
Status of perifoveal capillary net by fluorescein angiography	If perifoveal capillary net unbroken, better resultant vision
Presence of intact venule between obstructed vein and macula	Drainage of macula prevents threat of vision loss secondary to macular edema
Initial visual acuity	If 20/40 or better, excellent prognosis
	If 20/200 or worse, poor prognosis
General systemic health	Blood, vessel, and coagulation status help determine rate of recovery

<table>
<tr><td>

BRANCH RETINAL VEIN OCCLUSION—PEARLS

- Strong association with systemic disease
- Occurs most frequently at arteriovenous crossings
- Nonischemic BRVO characterized by dot—blot hemorrhages and lipid infiltrates in the involved sector
- Ischemic BRVO characterized by dot—blot hemorrhages, lipid infiltrates, cotton wool spots, and flame-shaped hemorrhages
- Collaterals form to drain the affected area
- 25 to 30 percent change of neovascularization of disc or retina
- Management
  - Ascertain underlying systemic disease
  - Fluorescein angiography indicated if threat of edema to macular area
  - Follow carefully for the development of neovascularization
  - When in doubt, a retinology consultation is indicated

</td></tr>
</table>

Central Retinal Vein Occlusion

Central retinal vein occlusion (CRVO) is a very destructive retinal condition with a strong association to systemic diseases or situations that can cause undue pressure on the optic nerve. The pressure within or without can easily compress the thin-walled central retinal vein. CRVO occurs more frequently in men, with the age of onset usually after age 50. Vision invariably is compromised, and in certain instances the eye is totally lost secondary to intractable neovascular glaucoma.

The etiology of CRVO varies considerably but can be categorized as to age of onset. **Table 2–22 summarizes the typical causes by age.** It should be understood that any condition that can create pressure on the central retinal vein has potential to cause closure. Table 2–23 lists some predisposing

TABLE 2–22. SYSTEMIC FACTORS IN CENTRAL RETINAL VEIN OCCLUSION AS RELATED TO AGE OF ONSET

Age	Causes
Under 50 years	Head injuries
	Hyperlipidemia
	Estrogen-containing preparations
Over 50 years	Hypertension
	Abnormal glucose tolerance test
	Hyperlipidemia
	Chronic lung disease
	Elevated serum IgA
All ages	Hyperviscosity syndromes
	Cryofibrinogenemia

Modified from Alexander LJ: Diseases of the retina in Bartlett JD, Jaanus SD (eds): Clinical Ocular Pharmacology, Boston, Butterworth, 1989.

TABLE 2–23. PREDISPOSING FACTORS IN CENTRAL RETINAL VEIN OCCLUSION

Glaucoma
Papilledema
Subdural hematoma
Optic nerve hemorrhage
Drusen of the optic nerve
Cardiovascular and cerebrovascular disease
Diabetes
Hypertension
Leukemia
Thrombocytopenia
Sclerodermatous vascular disease
Reye's syndrome
Systemic lupus erythematosus
Trauma

Reprinted with permission from Alexander LJ: The implications and management of retinal vaso-occlusive disease. S J Optom, 1986; 2:20–34.

factors of CRVO, and Table 2–24 lists reported causes for CRVO. Any condition that allows for a thrombus buildup at the lamina, where the central retinal vein must constrict for passage, can create a potential CRVO. Turbulence occurs at this stricture, allowing debris in the blood to deposit on the wall. Figure 2–88 illustrates this principle. This deposition can lead eventually to a partial (nonischemic) or total (ischemic) closure of the central retinal vein.

As with BRVO, the strong association to systemic diseases, especially carotid artery disease, necessitates a thorough investigation for underlying systemic disease. **See color plate 35.**

CRVO can occur as two distinct clinical entities from an opthalmoscopic standpoint. There is not always, however, a clear distinction, since there may be an in-between variation that is a part of the continuum. The clinical categories are (1) nonischemic retinopathy and (2) ischemic retinopathy. The primary difference involves the presence of significant retinal hypoxia or ischemia created by the totality of blockage. CRVO in either case can occur with the prodromal symptom of transient obscurations (brief blurring of vision associated with postural changes) and the prodromal sign of a yel-

TABLE 2–24. REPORTED CAUSES OF CENTRAL RETINAL VEIN OCCLUSION

Carotid artery disease
Antithrombin deficiency
Secondary to hemodialysis
Increase in platelet aggregability
Elevation of thrombocyte aggregation
Hypercholesterolemia
Hyperlipidemia
Hypertriglyceridemia
Mitral valve prolapse

CRVO

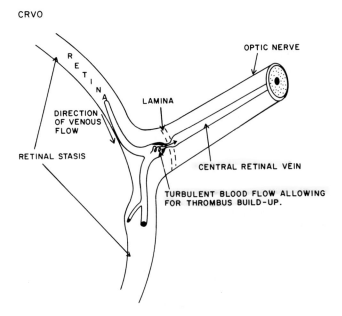

Figure 2–88. Schematic illustrating the turbulent blood flow and buildup of a thrombus at the stricture of the central retinal vein as it passes through the lamina cribrosa. *(Reprinted with permission from Alexander LJ: The implications and management of retinal vaso-occlusive disease. S J Optom, 1986; 2:20–34.)*

lowish hue in the posterior pole when comparing one eye to the other. The prodromata may last months, with the active phase being heralded by dot–blot hemorrhages extending to the periphery, accompanied by intraretinal edema. Evidence of capillary dilatation may occur near the optic disc or temporal vascular arcade as seen by fluorescein angiography. The vision loss that occurs is of rela-

tively sudden onset, since the macular area is very susceptible to intraretinal edema.

The two types of CRVO have specific characteristics, prognoses, and management procedures. Nonischemic CRVO is characterized by dot–blot hemorrhages, intraretinal edema, and various degrees of macular edema (Fig. 2–89). Ischemic CRVO occurs as dot–blot hemorrhages, superficial flame-shaped hemorrhages, cotton wool spots, silver wire or sheathed arteries, and gross intraretinal and macular edema (Fig. 2–90). Another clinical finding that accompanies the acute portion of the occlusion is a lowering of IOP. There is a greater initial reduction of IOP in ischemic CRVO than in nonischemic CRVO, and both of these have a greater reduction than do branch occlusions.

Fluorescein angiographic findings in CRVO vary considerably depending on the types of occlusion as well as the elapsed time. Initially, there is blockage of background choroidal fluorescence by the intraretinal and flame-shaped hemorrhages. The retina will be stained because of intraretinal vascular leakage, and the macula will demonstrate varying degrees of edema. It is possible that neovascularization may develop with its classic fluorescein angiography picture.

The visual prognosis of CRVO is not promising, but one can expect better results in nonischemic CRVO than in ischemic CRVO. Although recovery of visual acuity is variable, it is well established that neovascular glaucoma is an identified complication in 14 to 20 percent of all CRVO cases. Recent work has refined further this expected com-

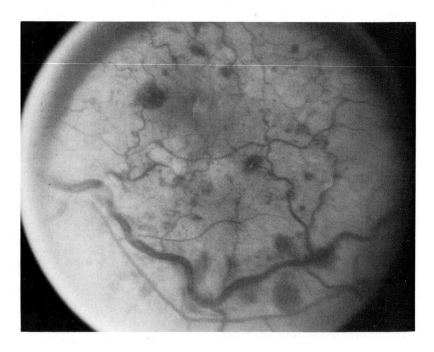

Figure 2–89. Nonischemic central retinal vein occlusion characterized by dot–blot hemorrhages throughout the retina accompanied by reduced visual acuity.

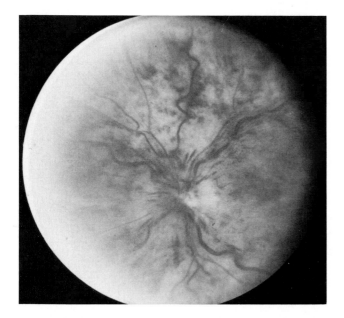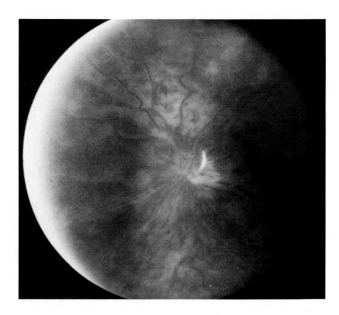

Figure 2–90. Left and Right. Illustration of the progression of severity over a 2-week period of a central retinal vein occlusion. **Right.** Ischemic central retinal vein occlusion.

plication rate, indicating that the risk of neovascular glaucoma is even higher (60 percent) in ischemic CRVO. Neovascularization at the iris occurs secondary to retinal hypoxia, which stimulates neovascularization. However, there is little to no viable retinal germinative capillary tissue in the area of vasostasis. As a result, the stimulus travels through the uveal network in an attempt to find a source for neovascular development. The iris tissue is the only available viable vascularized tissue, and new vessels sprout in this location. This leads to physical blockage of the trabecular meshwork and the development of increased IOP. It is reported that the incidence of chronic open-angle glaucoma in patients with CRVO is increased over the norm. Disc and retinal neovascularization do not represent the same kind of threat in CRVO as in BRVO because of the retinal capillary endothelial death that occurs in CRVO. With capillary death, there is not the germinative tissue necessary for supporting the development of neovascularization.

Of utmost importance are the diagnosis and management of the underlying systemic disease process associated with the CRVO. Management of the acute CRVO process is somewhat controversial. Anticoagulants will not dissolve a thrombus once it has formed, but it is thought that this therapy will limit the propagation of the thrombus. Monitoring of the blood levels is, however, an important aspect of any anticoagulant therapy. It has been suggested that anticoagulation therapy gives slightly better results than no therapy at all and that it lessens the development of neovascular glaucoma. Oral prednisolone therapy has been suggested to minimize the inflammatory component of the disease, but no clinical proof has been presented to substantiate the use of this treatment modality. Recent work has indicated that isovolemic hemodilution improves the visual outcome of patients with CRVO and does offer some hope. As mentioned previously, Ticlopidine (a platelet aggregation inhibitor), may offer some hope in the management of CRVO. Recent work indicates that enzymes, such as streptokinase, may prove valuable.

One indisputable mode of therapy is the use of panretinal photocoagulation to prevent the development of neovascular glaucoma. Visual outcome is not necessarily improved by photocoagulation, but the chance of development of neovascular glaucoma is minimized by elimination of retinal hypoxia. It must be noted that panretinal photocoagulation has little effect in nonischemic CRVO unless it is secondary to ipsilateral carotid artery occlusion, whereas it is of significant benefit in ischemic CRVO. The application of photocoagulation minimizes the vasoproliferative stimulus created by the hypoxic retina, which then reduces the likelihood of iris neovascularization. It should be noted that retinal neovascularization may recur even after panretinal photocoagulation has been applied.

If nonischemic CRVO appears to be progressively worsening and there is associated orbital pain, bypass surgery of the carotid system may produce beneficial results. Patients with neovascular glaucoma but without an obvious precipitating fundus condition should be suspected of having ipsilateral carotid artery disease until proven otherwise.

CENTRAL RETINAL VEIN OCCLUSION—PEARLS

- Strong association with systemic disease
- May be secondary to localized optic nerve compression
- Occlusion occurs at the lamina cribrosa
- Nonischemic variety
    - Dot—blot hemorrhages to the periphery
    - Macular edema
    - Minimal threat to neovascular glaucoma (NVG)
    - Manage by ascertaining cause and possible anticoagulant intervention and follow for potential neovascular glaucoma
- Ischemic variety
    - Dot—blot hemorrhages to the periphery
    - Macular edema
    - Cotton wool and flame-shaped hemorrhages
    - Arterial changes
    - 60 percent chance of NVG
    - Manage by ascertaining cause and consulting with a retinologist

---

Hemicentral Retinal Vein Occlusion

Hemicentral retinal vein occlusion (hemi-CRVO) must be considered as a distinct entity, since it has characteristics of both CRVO and BRVO. The occlusion occurs at the stricture of the vein as it passes through the lamina. The etiopathogenesis is similar to that of a CRVO. The primary difference between the two entities is the anatomic characteristic of the central retinal vein. The central retinal vein in a hemi-CRVO does not become a single vessel until after it passes through the lamina. Figure 2–91 illustrates this principle. Occlusion in one branch creates a picture similar to a BRVO. Since the entire one half of the fundus is nonperfused, there is a strong tendency toward macular edema and hypoxia. Hypoxia in one half of the retina coupled with a viable capillary bed in the other half of the retina lends well to the development of neovascularization. **See color plates 23 and 36.**

The hemi-CRVO can appear either as the ischemic or nonischemic variety (Figs. 2–92 to 2–96). Prognosis depends on the development of macular edema or the development of neovascularization.

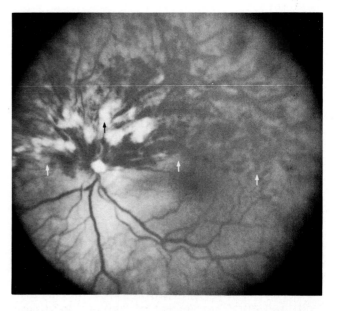

Figure 2–91. Schematic illustrating a hemicentral retinal vein occlusion. Note that the central retinal vein bifurcates retrolaminarly and thus exits the nerve head as two separate branches. This sets up the possibility that only one vein may occlude at the stricture in the lamina cribrosa. *(Reprinted with permission from Alexander LJ: The implications and management of retinal vaso-occlusive disease. SJ Optom, 1986; 2:20–34.)*

Figure 2–92. Black and white photograph of a hemicentral retinal vein occlusion. The white arrows point to the limitations of intraretinal hemorrhage; the black arrow points to a cotton wool spot.

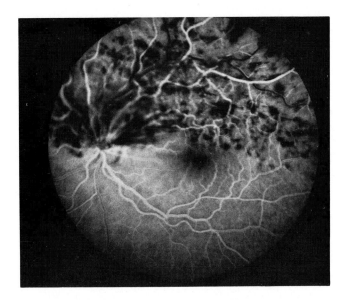

Figure 2–93. An early-stage angiogram of Figure 2–92. The significant amount of intraretinal hemorrhage effectively blocks background choroidal fluorescence.

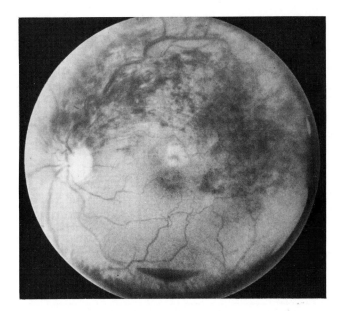

Figure 2–95. Black and white photograph of a superior hemicentral retinal vein occlusion with an inferior preretinal hemorrhage. *(Reprinted with permission from Alexander LJ: The implications and management of retinal vaso-occlusive disease. SJ Optom 1986; 2:20–34.)*

Neovascularization is not expected in the nonischemic variety but may develop in the ischemic variety within 6 months. Neovascularization develops in response to retinal hypoxia.

Management involves the prevention of neovascularization and subsequent neovascular glaucoma. This is accomplished with prophylactic scatter photocoagulation of the affected area in an attempt to eliminate the hypoxic stimulus. Macular edema also may regress in response to photocoagulation. It is important to investigate carefully for the inevitable associated underlying systemic disease.

Table 2–25 summarizes the comparisons of the clinical and pathogenic features of CRVO, hemiCRVO, and BRVO.

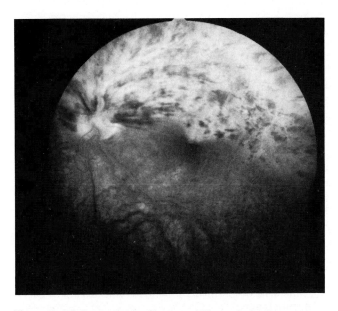

Figure 2–94. Late-stage angiogram of Figure 2–92 demonstrating staining of the intraretinal edema.

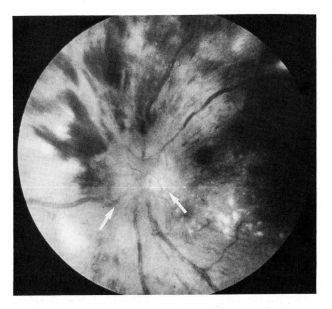

Figure 2–96. Disc neovascularization **(arrows)** secondary to the hypoxia created by a hemicentral retinal vein occlusion.

TABLE 2–25. COMPARISON OF CENTRAL RETINAL VEIN OCCLUSION (CRVO), HEMICENTRAL RETINAL VEIN OCCLUSION (HEMI-CRVO), AND BRANCH RETINAL VEIN OCCLUSION (BRVO)

Features	CRVO	Hemi-CRVO	BRVO
Site of occlusion	In optic nerve at lamina	In optic nerve at lamina	Usually at arteriovenous crossing
Type of retinopathy	Nonischemic 80% Ischemic 20%	Nonischemic 67% Ischemic 33%	Primarily ischemic
Retinal collaterals	Absent	Present	Invariably present
Prognosis	Nonischemic: vision loss Ischemic: vision loss and 60% chance neovascular glaucoma	Vision loss with macular edema, retinal and disc neovascularization possible	Vision loss with macular edema, retinal and disc neovascularization possible

---

HEMICENTRAL RETINAL VEIN OCCLUSION—PEARLS

- Strong association with systemic disease
- Occlusion at lamina cribrosa in one branch of the central retinal vein
- Maximal threat to neovascularization of disc and retina
- Dot–blot hemorrhages and other nonischemic or ischemic signs in the involved sector
- Manage by ascertaining the underlying cause and a retinology consultation

Branch Retinal Artery Occlusion

Both branch retinal artery occlusion (BRAO) and central retinal artery occlusion (CRAO) are the result of emboli dislodged from vasculature elsewhere that travel through the system until they reach a vessel caliber too narrow for passage. With arterial occlusion comes anoxia as the result of an absence of oxygenated blood. This anoxia results in a loss of inner retinal layers, including the nerve fiber layer, ganglion cell layer, inner plexiform layer, and the inner portion of the inner nuclear layer.

BRAO differs from CRAO only because the embolus was small enough to pass through the stricture of the central retinal artery as it traversed the laminar region. The embolus then moved into retinal circulation. The source of the emboli in both cases is essentially identical.

BRAO occurs most frequently in the superior temporal region of the retina and may be produced by multiple emboli. Single cholesterol emboli (Hollenhorst plaques) usually will not create an occlusion but in sufficient numbers will shut the vessel down. Figure 2–97 illustrates the principle of a

BRAO. Visual acuity and visual field loss are dependent on location of the occlusion as well as the extent of blockage. The ophthalmoscopic appearance is dependent on the elapsed time from the occlusion (Fig. 2–98). Initially, the affected arteries narrow and the retina becomes hazy. Over a few hours, the retinal tissue whitens because of the infarct. Segmental optic atrophy may develop in the affected region. The classic field loss associated

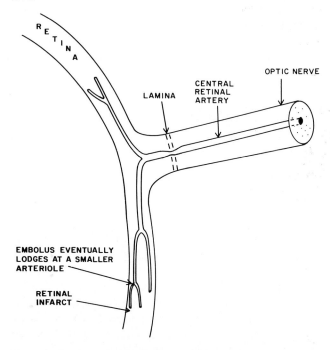

Figure 2–97. Schematic illustrating the etiology of a branch retinal artery occlusion. The embolus is small enough to pass the stricture of the central retinal artery at the lamina but eventually becomes lodged in the smaller-caliber retinal arteries. *(Reprinted with permission from Alexander LJ: The implications and management of retinal vasco-occlusive disease. SJ Optom 1986, 2:20–34.)*

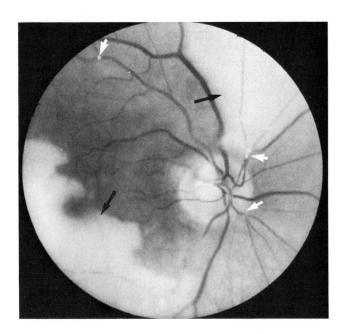

Figure 2–98. A photograph illustrating areas of retinal infarct **(black arrows)** secondary to emboli **(white arrows)** in a branch retinal artery occlusion. *(Photo courtesy of W. Jones.)*

allel that described in the next section on CRAO. Some clinicians advocate pentoxifylline, 300 to 600 mg per day over a 3-month period, to prevent retinal or intravitreal neovascularization caused by retinal ischemia. This mode of prophylaxis is, however, still investigational.

The author has seen BRAOs that are only partial and have been reversed with aggressive therapy. A consultation with a retinologist is indicated in all but long-term BRAO.

BRANCH RETINAL ARTERY OCCLUSION—PEARLS

- Strong association with systemic disease, especially internal carotid and cardiac disease
- Secondary to embolus lodged in retinal artery
- Results in total anoxia of the retina, white retina
- Visual field defect altitudinal respecting the horizontal raphe
- Management
  Attempt to dislodge embolus by physical massage of the eyeball and immediate consultation with a retinologist

---

with BRAO is a sharp-edged defect stopping at the horizontal raphé. The defect occurs because of the termination of retinal arterial supply at the raphe with no crossover of oxygenated blood supply. **See color plates 37 and 38.**

Prognosis depends on rapid institution of therapy. If there is more than a 1 to 2 hour lag, the likelihood of return of vision or visual field is minimal. The initial concern in BRAO is to attempt to reverse the occlusion if it severely affects vision. The next concern is to attempt to diagnose and manage the underlying systemic cause. If vision is severely compromised, aggressive therapy should be instituted immediately. This therapy should par-

Central Retinal Artery Occlusion

The etiology of CRAO is presented in Table 2–26. The emphasis should be placed on the incidence of increased vascular resistance (carotid artery disease) in this disease process. Figure 2–99 illustrates the embolus being lodged at the stricture created in the central retinal artery as it passes through the lamina.

CRAO occurs as a sudden painless loss of vision in an eye that is otherwise disease free. There is often a loss of direct pupillary response associated with the vision loss. If a cilioretinal artery

---

TABLE 2–26. REPORTED ETIOLOGIC FACTORS IN RETINAL ARTERIAL OCCLUSIONS

Emboli from ulcerated atheromatous plaques of the internal carotid artery

Increased vascular resistance (internal carotid disease)

Emboli from cardiac lesions, including atrial myxoma

Mitral valve prolapse

Emboli from artificial cardiac valves

Emboli from subacute bacterial endocarditis

Thrombi secondary to giant cell arteritis, syphilis, fungal sinus infections

Oral contraceptives

Polyarteritis nodosa

Occlusion secondary to methylprednisolone injections of the head and neck soft tissue

Cardiac catherization and other similar diagnostic procedures

Self-injected emboli

Migraine

CRAO

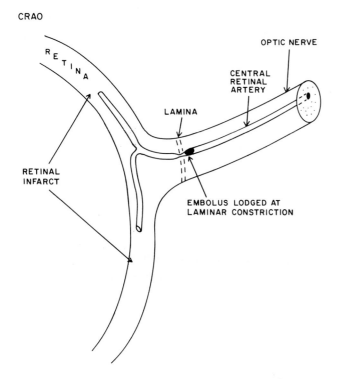

Figure 2–99. Schematic illustrating the etiology of a central retinal artery occlusion. An embolus has broken away from a site in the cardiovascular system, travelled through the ophthalmic artery to the central retinal artery, and lodged at the stricture of the artery as it passes through the lamina. *(Reprinted with permission from Alexander LJ: The implications and management of retinal vaso-occlusive disease. SJ Optom, 1986; 2:20–34.)*

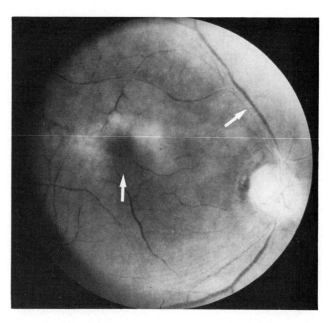

Figure 2–100. Black and white photograph of a central retinal artery occlusion. Arrows point to the macula, which becomes more visible in contrast to the opaque retina and the attenuated retinal arteries. *(Reprinted with permission from Alexander LJ: The implications and management of retinal vaso-occlusive disease. SJ Optom, 1986; 2:20–34.)*

(choroidal vascular origin) is present, a variable island of vision will remain that corresponds to the geography of the vascular supply.

The clinical picture depends on the elapsed time since the occlusion (Fig. 2–100). Early changes involve narrowing of the retinal arteries and a haziness of retinal tissue. Within hours, this haziness of the retina becomes whitish, contrasting with the choroidal macular vascular supply—thus the cherry red spot. The veins then become distended and can exhibit segmentation, which is referred to as "boxcarring." Ultimately, the infarcted retina is replaced by glial tissue, and the arterial tree assumes a more normal appearance except for some irregular narrowing. Optic atrophy can occur, but neovascular glaucoma is rare in CRAO. If neovascular glaucoma should occur associated with CRAO, the patient may have an ocular ischemic syndrome: aqueous flare, rubeosis iridis, midperipheral intraretinal hemorrhages, narrow arteries, cherry red spot, neovascularization of the disc or retina, and common carotid artery obstruction. **See color plate 39.**

Visual prognosis depends on immediate initiation of therapy. Diagnosis and management of the underlying systemic condition are also of immediate concern. Occlusions caused by emboli may be partially reversible if therapy is instituted within 1 to 2 hours. Digital massage of the globe through the eyelid may assist in dislodging the embolus. This coupled with inhalation of carbogen for 15 minutes followed by 15 minutes of room air and repeating the cycle over a 6 to 12 hour period may be of some value. Recent studies, however, show carbogen therapy to be of questionable value.

It seems apparent that attempts at vasodilatation would offer little or no help in managing CRAO. The embolus is lodged at the stricture in the artery as it passes through the lamina. Manipulation of the lamina to facilitate passage of the embolus is a much more logical approach, since the laminar passage will not enlarge with vasodilatation. Paracentesis of the anterior chamber may create enough hypotony to dislodge the embolus. The IOP must then be maintained at a low level for several days by using acetazolamide 250 mg every 6 hours. Retrobulbar injections of acetylcholine, atropine, and 25 mg of tolaxoline also may be beneficial. Papaverine plus heparin via the infraorbital artery has been attempted. Although there is no proof as to the efficacy of any treatment modality, any attempt is worthwhile, since the prognosis is so grim. Again, antiembolic enzymes may offer some promise in the treatment of arterial occlusions.

CENTRAL RETINAL ARTERY OCCLUSION—PEARLS

- Strong association with systemic disease, especially internal carotid and cardiac disease
- Sudden-onset loss of vision
- Embolus lodged at lamina cribrosa
- Narrowing of arteries, haziness of retinal tissue, and boxcar segmentation of veins in the presence of red-brown macula
- If cilioretinal artery present, may have island of healthy retina
- Management
    Ascertain underlying systemic disease and immediate attempts to dislodge embolus while rushing to retinologist

---

Relationship of Retinal Vaso-occlusive Disease to Cerebrovascular Disease

The close relationship of retinal vaso-occlusive disease and cerebrovascular disease deserves brief mention. The patient with retinal vaso-occlusive disease should be a strong suspect for concurrent cerebrovascular disease (Fig. 2–101). There are two basic vascular supply systems to the brain, the internal carotid system and the vertebrobasilar system. Diseases of the internal carotid system are more intimately related to retinal vaso-occlusive disease than are vertebrobasilar occlusions. **Common signs and symptoms of internal carotid stenosis are outlined in Table 2–27. The more common signs and symptoms of vertebrobasilar disease are listed in Table 2–28.** Suggested laboratory tests are listed in Table 2–29.

Awareness of the possible association of retinal vaso-occlusive disease and cerebrovascular disease is a crucial part of management of these patients. The clinician must be well versed in the clinical signs and symptoms of impending stroke syndromes.

DIABETIC RETINOPATHY

Diabetes: The Disease

Glucose is an important nutrient for the human body, being the preferred source of energy for the blood cells and brain. Glucose supplies are pro-

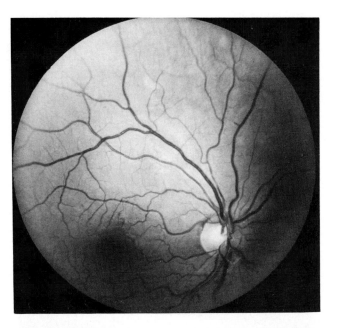

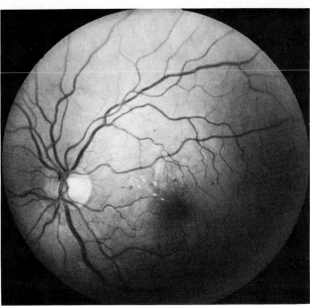

Figure 2–101. Top and Bottom. Black and white photographs illustrating asymmetrical retinopathy. In any patient with asymmetrical hemorrhages, exudates, cotton wool spots, peripheral hemorrhages, or asymmetrical venous tortuosity, internal carotid stenosis should be suspected.

vided through gluconeogenesis, occurring primarily in the liver. The liver is the central organ involved in providing glucose under fasting conditions. Many factors are involved in proper glucose production and use, including glucagon, cortisol, epinephrine, and insulin. Insulin is the primary factor in the control of glucose, and the liver is very sensitive to insulin levels. The peripheral sites of use of glucose are less sensitive to changes in insulin levels.

TABLE 2–27. COMMON SIGNS AND SYMPTOMS OF INTERNAL CAROTID STENOSIS

Sign or Symptom	Description
Transient monocular blindness (amaurosis fugax)	Sudden unilateral blindness that is transient, lasting 15–60 min but returning to normal
Cholesterol, platelet, or calcific emboli lodged in retinal circulation	Cholesterol: Hollenhorst plaque from eroding ipsilateral carotid sinus platelet and calcific (BRAO) from eroding cardiac vegetations
Central retinal artery occlusion	Secondary to eroding emboli lodging at the lamina
Asymmetrical retinal vasculopathy	Caused by relative hypoxic state of one side to the other
Total edema of retina and choroid (no cherry red spot)	Caused by ophthalmic artery obstruction
Unilateral numbness or weakness	Stenosis of blood supply to contralateral cerebral hemisphere
Aphasia	Stenosis of blood supply to dominant cerebral hemisphere
Headache	Frontal that may be associated with other transient ischemic attack symptoms
Unilateral visual loss in bright light	Equivalent of macular photostress recovery due to reduced retinal metabolic activity

Reprinted with permission from Alexander LJ: The implications and management of retinal vaso-occlusive disease. S J Optom, 1986; 2:20–34.

Diabetes is a disease of improper glucose production and use. This may be the result of absence of insulin, reduced supplies of insulin, or inability or reduced ability for receptor sites to use insulin. Insulin-dependent diabetes mellitus (IDDM-type 1) is the result of an absence of insulin. Tables 2–30 and 2–31 outline the common ocular and systemic signs and symptoms of type 1 diabetes. The triggering factors for type 1 diabetes are obscure, but it is known that the afflicted individual has a multigenetic predisposition.

Type 2 diabetes has many names but is classically described as noninsulin-dependent diabetes mellitus (NIDDM). Patients with type 2 diabetes

TABLE 2–28. COMMON SIGNS AND SYMPTOMS OF VERTEBROBASILAR TERRITORY SYNDROME

Bilaterality

Weakness or paralysis of four extremities that may change from side to side in different attacks

Visual field loss that is complete or partial in both homonymous fields, may be altitudinal in nature, may result in tunnel vision

Imbalance or unsteadiness not necessarily associated with vertigo

Numbness, loss of sensation, or parasthesia that often is bilateral but may switch from side to side

Altered hearing that may be unilateral or bilateral

Usual maintenance of consciousness

Occipital–nuchal headaches

Transient confusion, memory problems

Possible drop attacks

Subclavian steal syndrome

Reprinted with permission from Alexander LJ: The implications and management of retinal vaso-occlusive disease. S J Optom, 1986; 2:20–34.

TABLE 2–29. SUGGESTED LABORATORY TESTING IN PATIENTS SUSPECTED OF HAVING RETINAL VASO-OCCLUSIVE DISEASE OR CEREBROVASCULAR DISEASE

Complete blood count with differential and peripheral smear
Fasting blood sugar
Fasting lipid profile
Sedimentation rate
Prothrombin time
Duplex (ultrasonography of carotid system)
Possible digital subraction angiography or more invasive
  arteriography

TABLE 2–31. COMMON OCULAR SIGNS AND SYMPTOMS ASSOCIATED WITH INSULIN-DEPENDENT DIABETES MELLITUS (TYPE 1)

Fluctuating vision
Binocular vision anomalies (double vision)
Corneal epitheliopathy (recurrent corneal erosion)
Neurologic lid and pupil signs
Accommodative insufficiency
Recurrent infections
Early cataract development
Greater prevalence of glaucoma
Kruckenberg spindle
Optic nerve disease
Retinal vasculopathy

may have a relative or partial deficiency of insulin. First phase insulin secretion is markedly reduced in type 2 diabetes. Type 2 diabetes also may be the result of resistance to insulin action. This may be the result of an intracellular defect or alteration of insulin receptors. Type 2 diabetes usually develops in the following manner: (1) obesity creates insulin resistance and decreased insulin production, and (2) postreceptor defects occur, leading to glucose intolerance. Table 2–32 lists the common systemic and ocular signs and symptoms of type 2 diabetes.

Emergency situations associated with diabetes mellitus include ketoacidosis and hyperosmolar coma. Characteristics of ketoacidosis include (1) lack of insulin, with blood glucose in the 300 to 600 mg percent range, (2) vomiting, (3) abdominal pain from sodium and potassium loss, (4) labored breathing, and (5) dehydration. Characteristics of hyperosmolar coma include (1) lack of insulin and electrolyte imbalance in an older diabetic with acute illness, (2) severe dehydration, (3) mild ketone elevation, (4) shock, (5) tachycardia, (6) hyperventilation, and (7) possible seizures.

Proper management of types 1 and 2 diabetes includes a combination of diet modification by a nutritionist, education by a nurse educator, proper timing and proper levels if insulin injection, control of hepatic glucose production, increasing peripheral uptake and oxidation of glucose by potentiating insulin action, increasing peripheral uptake and

oxidation of glucose by insulin, and careful follow-up of the patient, assessing for the complications of diabetes to ensure timely therapeutic intervention.

Diabetes mellitus is easily diagnosed by laboratory and office tests. Probably the most common office screening test for diabetes is the fasting blood glucose test. This is performed by asking the patient to fast after 10 PM the night before. The patient then reports to the office early in the morning. A fingerprick often is sufficient to generate a fasting glucose level. Diabetes is suspect in the 100 to 120 mg percent range and is likely above the 120 mg percent range. This along with a random blood sample is often useful in patients who profess to be under control but in whom the clinician finds such signs as ketone breath or severe retinopathy that would cause questioning of the degree of control. Never assume that your patients are under good control. If a suspect or abnormal screening level is present or if you suspect hypoglycemia, a glucose tolerance test (GTT) should be ordered. The GTT is an uncomfortable test and should not be ordered in a cavalier fashion but certainly is diagnostic. Another useful test to ascertain compliance over a prolonged period is hemoglobin A_1C. Hemoglobin A_1C is a measure of glycosolated hemoglobin that is the most abundant component of hemoglobin in normal red blood cells. Hemoglobin A_1C can be elevated as a much as three times in diabetes. It is particularly sensitive to the degree of glucose control over the preceding 2 to 3 months.

TABLE 2–30. COMMON SYSTEMIC SIGNS AND SYMPTOMS ASSOCIATED WITH INSULIN-DEPENDENT DIABETES MELLITUS (TYPE 1)

Fatigue[a]	Cardiovascular disease
Excessive thirst[a]	Neurologic disease
Excessive hunger[a]	Impotence
Excessive urination[a]	Ketoacidosis
Weight loss	Hyperosmolar coma
Recurrent infections (vaginitis)[a]	Oral disease, periodontal
Ketone (fruity) breath	Podiatric disease
Nephropathy, responsible for death in 40%	

[a]Early.

TABLE 2–32. SYSTEMIC AND OCULAR SIGNS AND SYMPTOMS OF NONINSULIN-DEPENDENT DIABETES MELLITUS (TYPE 2)

Often unaware of disease
Refractive changes
Mild weight loss, fatigue, weakness
Perhaps polyuria, polydipsia, polyphagia
Infection

Another important consideration in patients with diabetes is the level of blood lipids. Often lipid levels are elevated in diabetic patients because of the need to catabolize lipid for energy. Should triglyceride, cholesterol, and phospholipids be elevated, retinal vascular complications may occur. Lipid levels should be ordered in patients with diabetes at intervals to ensure the health of the vascular system. Several excellent office testing systems are available for glucose and lipid screening. Proper management of diabetic patients includes routine blood work. Never assume proper control of the patient with diabetes.

From an epidemiologic standpoint, diabetes is a severe problem in today's society. Figure 2–102 shows estimates of the occurrence of diabetes in the general population as of 1980. Data from the 1982 National Health Interview Survey estimated that there were approximately 5.8 million persons in the civilian noninstitutionalized population of the United States with known diabetes, with the South having the highest rate. Other studies estimate that 5 percent of the population have diabetes, with only 50 percent of the cases actually having been diagnosed. There are over 600,000 new cases diagnosed per year, with an estimate that the numbers will double every 15 years. The numbers are there. Diabetes is a major national health problem.

The American Diabetes Association states that "Diabetic eye disease is the number one cause of new blindness in people between ages 20–74 in this country, and each year over 5000 Americans lost their sight because of diabetes." Diabetic ocular changes are responsible for 12 percent of the blind population of the United States. Statistics of incidence of diabetic retinopathy in the diabetic population are clouded by definitions. It can be said, however, that the development of diabetic retinop-

athy increases in incidence with age and is somewhat related to degree of control in the early phases of the systemic process. Over time, at least 50 percent of diabetics develop some form of diabetic retinopathy.

Blindness from diabetes peaks in incidence between ages 30 and 50 and is race and sex related. Nonwhite females have a 3.8 times risk of blindness, nonwhite males a 1.3 times risk of blindness, white females a 1.3 times risk of blindness, and white males a 1.0 times risk factor. Diabetics as compared to nondiabetics are 25 times more prone to blindness, 17 times more prone to renal disease, 20 times more prone to gangrene, and 2 times more prone to myocardial infarct or stroke. **The prevalence of diabetic retinopathy is presented as a summary of several studies in Table 2–33.**

Diabetic Retinopathy: Genesis

The genesis of diabetic retinopathy is certainly controversial but seems to be secondary to changes in the capillary basement membrane or capillary walls combined with sticky blood, resulting in nonperfusion in the capillary bed. This nonperfusion results in hypoxia. The combination of hypoxia and altered vascular wall structure (selective loss of intramural pericytes) unfolds into diabetic retinopathy. A great deal of research is now being done in the area of the conversion of glucose to sorbitol by aldose reductase because of the implication that accumulation of sorbitol is a possible trigger in the genesis of diabetic retinopathy. Figure 2–103 is a simplification of the role of sorbitol in the complications of diabetes. It is thought that if the conversion to sorbitol can be blocked by an aldose reductase inhibitor, diabetic retinopathy may be avoided. Figure 2–104 summarizes some of the current theory regarding the genesis of diabetic microvasculopathy.

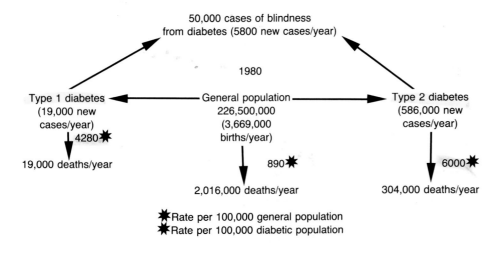

Figure 2–102. Prevalence of diabetes in the general population of the United States.

TABLE 2-33. PREVALENCE OF DIABETIC RETINOPATHY

	Mitchel 1985	Klein et al 1984	Dwyer et al 1985	Grey et al 1986	Klein et al 1985	Klein 1985	Klein et al 1984	Jerneld and Algvere 1984
Type 1 diabetes	Total in types 1 and 2, 49%	Total in types 1 & 2, DX over 30 yrs. a. Duration less than 5 yrs. 28.8% DR 2.0% PDR b. Duration over 15 yrs. 78.8% DR 15.5% PDR	Cumulative 70% 3 times incidence of retinopathy	43.4% DR[a] 13.3% VTR	Under age 13 years, 9% — Over age 13 DX after 13 34%	DX under age 30 70% DR — Duration 15 years, 18% MAC — Duration 20 years, 50% PDR — DX over age 30, 60% DR — Duration 15 years, 20% MAC — Duration 20 years, 25% PDR	DX under age 3 — Duration under 5 years, 17% DR — Duration under 10 years, 1.2% PDR — Duration over 15 years, 97.5% DR — Duration over 20 years, 29% MAC — Duration over 35 years, 67% PDR	DX under age 4 — Duration under 5 years, 11% DR — 6–10 years, 42% DR — 11–15 years, 84% DR — 16–30 years, 90% DR — Over 30 years, 100 DR
	With 13% VTR							
Type 2 diabetes			Obese cumulative, 30% — Nonobese cumulative 36% 4 times total retinopathy	20.1% DR 4.3% VTR		General incidence, 36% DR — Duration 15 years, 12% MAC	DX under age 30 — Duration under 5 years, 3% MAC — Duration over 20 years, 28% MAC	

[a]DR, diabetic retinopathy; MAC, diabetic maculopathy; PDR, proliferative diabetic retinopathy; VTR, vision-threatening retinopathy; DX, diagnosis.

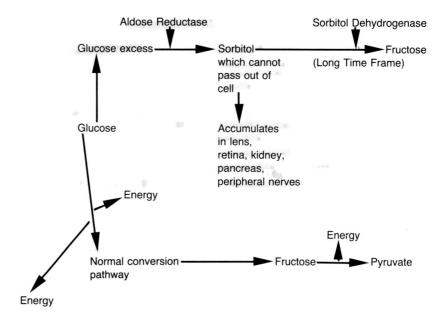

Figure 2–103. The proposed role of sorbitol in the genesis of the complications of diabetes.

Once the basic microvasculopathy is established, a number of retinal vascular changes can occur. Figures 2–105 to 2–107 illustrate potential retinal vascular changes associated with diabetes. It should be noted that large vessel disease (atherosclerosis) also increases in patients with diabetes. Patients with diabetes have 2 times the risk of stroke, 5 times the risk of myocardial infarction, and 8 times the risk of peripheral vasculopathy.

Background Diabetic Retinopathy

Broad statements about background diabetic retinopathy (BDR) being relatively benign can be very misleading. Certain components of BDR can have a negative impact on vision when located in the macular area. The retinal vasculopathy components commonly attributed to BDR are microaneu-

rysms, dot–blot (deep) retinal hemorrhages, and hard exudate formation. The specifics of each of these components are discussed in detail in the section on the clinicopathologic basis of retinal vasculopathy.

Microaneurysms are balloonlike structures along weakened capillary walls. These microaneurysms usually are not visible by ophthalmoscopy but become readily apparent with fluorescein angiography. Microaneurysms leak into the retina, creating edema. Should this edema spread into the macula, visual acuity may become compromised. If there is demonstrable leakage into the macular area, fluorescein angiography is indicated to determine the advisability of photocoagulative intervention. Should the microaneurysms become hyalinized, they will be visible because of the white

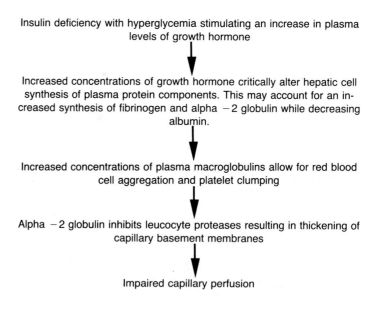

Figure 2–104. Summary of the theory regarding the etiopathogenesis of the microvasculopathy of diabetic retinopathy.

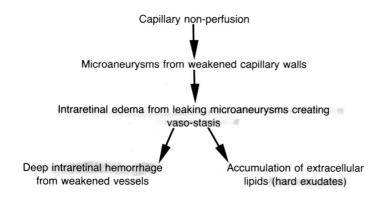

Capillary non-perfusion

Microaneurysms from weakened capillary walls

Intraretinal edema from leaking microaneurysms creating vaso-stasis

Deep intraretinal hemorrhage from weakened vessels

Accumulation of extracellular lipids (hard exudates)

Figure 2–105. The basics of the genesis of background diabetic retinopathy. The primary feature is intraretinal edema.

sheath. If there is evidence of microaneurysmal formation away from the macular area, it is safe to follow this patient in 1 year. Always instruct diabetic patients to use some method of monocular home monitoring of vision. It is important to question degree of control of the diabetes whenever there are all signs of diabetic retinopathy.

Dot–blot or deep retinal hemorrhages represent ruptures in weakened capillary walls. Once the hemorrhage occurs, the condition is static, but hemorrhages indicate the presence of deep intraretinal edema. A dot–blot hemorrhage in the macular area indicates edema encroaching into the foveal avascular zone (FAZ) and an immediate threat to vision. Dot–blot hemorrhages are not treatable, since they resolve of their own accord. Dot–blot hemorrhages do, however, offer a sign of diabetic microvasculopathy and intraretinal edema. If dot–blot hemorrhages are not in the macular area, they may be followed in 12 months using some method of home monitoring. However, if dot–blot hemorrhages are present in the macular area, fluorescein angiography is indicated to determine the advisability of photocoagulative intervention. A preponderance of widespread dot–blot hemorrhages indi-

cates the need for investigation for either an evolving CRVO or ocular ischemia.

Hard exudates represent areas of lipid deposits that are a sign of chronic retinal edema secondary to leaking microaneurysms or a choroidal neovascular net. The exudates in and of themselves are benign but indicate long-standing edema. Most often, the exudates will circle the area of leakage and, if they are around the macula, are known collectively as circinate maculopathy. The hard exudates indicate the boundary of the intraretinal edema and often remain for a time after resolution of the edema. They are the ring around an area of nonperfused retinal microvasculopathy. Since exudates are a sign of long-standing edema, their presence around the macular area or in the FAZ indicates relatively poor prognosis for return of good vision because the macular retinal tissue has been compromised for a prolonged period. If the hard exudates are remote to the macular region, it is safe to follow the patient in 6 to 12 months after establishing a system of monitoring the monocular vision at home. Should diabetic maculopathy—macular edema with hard exudates in the macula, encroaching on the macula or surrounding the macula—be

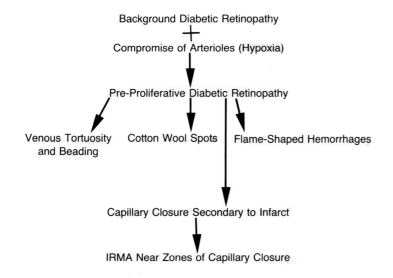

Background Diabetic Retinopathy
+
Compromise of Arterioles (Hypoxia)

Pre-Proliferative Diabetic Retinopathy

Venous Tortuosity and Beading   Cotton Wool Spots   Flame-Shaped Hemorrhages

Capillary Closure Secondary to Infarct

IRMA Near Zones of Capillary Closure

Figure 2–106. The basics of the genesis of preproliferative diabetic retinopathy. The primary features are the retinal signs of hypoxia.

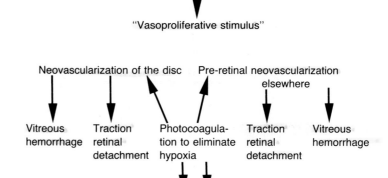

Figure 2–107. The basics of the genesis of proliferative diabetic retinopathy. The primary feature is the vasoproliferative stimulus.

present, fluorescein angiography is indicated to assess the desirability of photocoagulative intervention. Prognosis for treatment in diabetic maculopathy is shown in Table 2–34. The advent of grid photocoagulation has improved the prognosis for cases of diabetic maculopathy that were previously thought unmanageable. When in doubt, a competent retinologist should be consulted. **See color plates 25 and 28.**

BACKGROUND DIABETIC RETINOPATHY—PEARLS

- Dot—blot hemorrhages to be followed every 12 months if away from macula plus home monitoring of vision
- Microaneurysms to be followed every 12 months if away from the macula plus home monitoring of vision
- Hard exudates to be followed every 6 months if away from the macula plus home monitoring of vision
- If evidence of any of these components is in the macula, fluorescein angiography is indicated to determine if amendable to photocoagulation
- Communicate findings to patient's diabetologist

Preproliferative Diabetic Retinopathy

Recognition of the signs of preproliferative diabetic retinopathy (PPDR) is absolutely crucial in the management of the patient with diabetes. All of the retinal signs of PPDR are indicators of retinal hypoxia, which is the immediate precursor to the vasoproliferative stimulus that stimulates retinal neovascularization. The components of PPDR include cotton wool spots, intraretinal microvascular abnormalities (IRMA), venous tortuosity and beading, arteriolar abnormalities such as flame-shaped hemorrhages, and areas of capillary closure. The specif-

ics of each of these components other than capillary closure are discussed in detail in the section on the clinicopathologic basis of retinal vasculopathy. As with BDR, PPDR should cause concern about the degree of control of the underlying diabetic condition.

Cotton wool spots are the result of microinfarcts of arterioles in the nerve fiber layer. The cotton is the result of axoplasmic stasis, with resultant deposition of debris. The cotton wool spots never occur in the macular area and usually are confined to a distribution pattern within 3 disc diameters of the disc. The spots may cause small scotomas at threshold but are essentially benign and nontreatable. Cotton wool spots serve as an indicator of retinal hypoxia. Eyes with cotton wool spots should be monitored at 3 to 4 month intervals.

IRMA (Figs. 2–108 to 2–110) represents an intraretinal shunting system associated with tortuous capillaries in an area of severe capillary nonperfusion. IRMA forms to attempt to drain an area of stasis and is no threat to vision, since the vessels do not leak on fluorescein angiography. In fact, in the performance of photocoagulation, IRMA should be avoided. IRMA is an indicator of stasis severe enough to create retinal hypoxia and is thought to be the germination bed of neovascularization. Eyes with IRMA should be followed at 3 to 4 month intervals after performance of fluorescein angiography.

TABLE 2–34. PROGNOSIS IN DIABETIC MACULOPATHY

Poor Prognosis	Good Prognosis
Hard exudates in fovea	Exudates away from a foveal avascular zone
Poor initial acuity	
Long-term maculopathy	Good initial acuity
Diffuse nonidentifiable leakage	Short-term maculopathy
Break in perifoveal capillary net	Focal identifiable leakage
	Healthy perifoveal capillary net

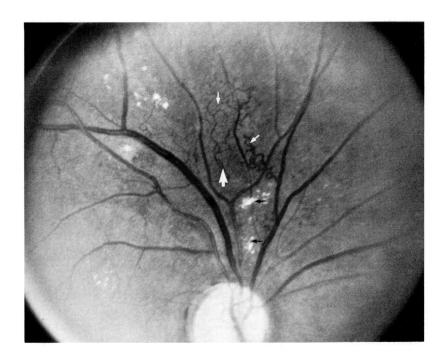

Figure 2–108. The white arrows point to zones of intraretinal microvascular abnormalities, and the black arrows point to hard exudates.

Venous tortuosity or beading is the result of sludging or slowing of venous blood, causing localized areas of venus dilatation. Again, tortuosity is of no threat to vision but represents stasis to the point that retinal hypoxia exists. Venous tortuosity is a sign that retinal hypoxia exists; the patient should return in 3 to 4 months.

Arteriolar abnormalities occur as superficial flame-shaped hemorrhages or areas of focal arteriolar narrowing. The flame-shaped hemorrhages are the result of compromised arterioles in the nerve fiber layer. The flames usually stay within the area of radial peripapillary distribution. Any arteriolar compromise results in localized hypoxia. With the presence of flame-shaped hemorrhages, the patient with diabetes should be followed in 3 to 4 months. **See color plates 24, 26, 40.**

Areas of capillary closure are evident only on high-resolution fluorescein angiography, appearing as dark spots in the normally lighted-with-fluores-

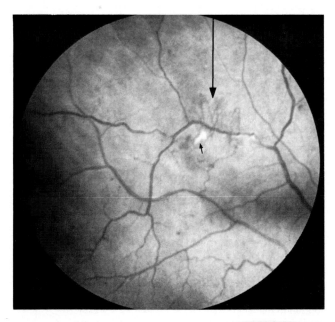

Figure 2–109. The long arrow points to a zone of intraretinal microvascular abnormalities, and the small arrow points to a cotton wool spot.

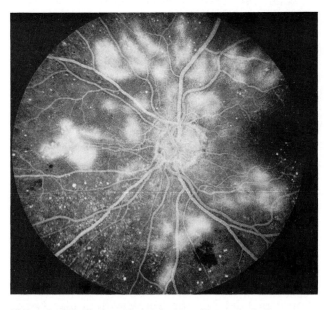

Figure 2–110. Fluorescein angiogram of intraretinal microvascular abnormalities evolving into severe neovascularization elsewhere as evidenced by the leaking hyperfluorescence. Note the glowing microaneurysms spread throughout the posterior pole.

cein capillary bed. This area of capillary closure represents an area of localized infarct (multiple) of the capillary bed. This infarct will cause relative hypoxia in the area of capillary distribution. Areas of capillary closure indicate the need to recall the patient in 3 to 4 months.

The Diabetic Retinopathy Study found that approximately 50 percent of eyes with at least three preproliferative signs progress to proliferative diabetic retinopathy within 2 years. Fluorescein angiography is indicated if there are three or more signs of PPDR.

■ Clinical Note

Any diabetic retinopathy (BDR or PPDR) that occurs in an asymmetrical fashion should be considered secondary to unilateral internal carotid or ophthalmic artery stenosis until proven otherwise. In these cases, always at least palpate the internal carotid area for asymmetrical pulsation and auscultate for carotid sinus bruits. Should internal carotid stenosis be suspected, consultation with a neurovascular surgeon should be arranged.

PREPROLIFERATIVE DIABETIC RETINOPATHY—PEARLS

- Indicates hypoxia
- Cotton wool spots, flame-shaped hemorrhages, venous beading and tortuosity, arteriolar narrowing, and IRMA are all signs of hypoxia and should be followed at 3- to 4-month intervals
- Areas of capillary closure are visible only on fluorescein angiography
- IRMA is the germination bed for neovascularization elsewhere
- Management
  - Fluorescein angiography indicated if three or more signs of preproliferative retinopathy
  - Fluorescein angiography indicated with IRMA
  - Communicate findings to patient's diabetologist

Proliferative Diabetic Retinopathy

Proliferative diabetic retinopathy (PDR) was devastating before the development of laser photocoagulation. Patients with PDR had an extremely poor visual prognosis with radical intervention, such as pituitary ablation, as their only hope. Every component of PDR has the potential to create blindness. The components of PDR include neovascularization of the disc, neovascularization elsewhere, fibrotic proliferation accompanying the neovascu-

larization, traction retinal detachment, and vitreous hemorrhages (Figs. 2–111 to 2–117). The specifics of these components are discussed in detail in the section on the clinicopathologic basis of retinal vasculopathy. Effective care of the diabetic patient with proper monitoring should avert development of PDR in most patients. If, however, the components of PDR are present, laser photocoagulation and vitrectomy offer some hope. There is approximately a 50 percent risk of blindness in an eye with PDR within 5 years after the onset of neovascularization if laser intervention is not applied.

Neovascularization of the disc (NVD) occurs in approximately 25 percent of the patients that develop PDR. This neovascularization occurs as a response to hypoxia in the retinal tissue. NVD and neovascularization elsewhere (NVE) both seem to progress more rapidly in young patients with diabetes than in older patients with diabetes. NVD and NVE both usually appear after a minimum of 15 years of diabetes. NVD initially occurs as a very fine network arising from the disc capillaries, which soon establishes connections with larger retinal veins in the immediate area. This early neovascularization grows slowly but is not restricted by an internal limiting membrane at the disc. All new vessels leak, and the clinician may notice a hazy appearance to the disc borders and fine vessels of the disc as the result of this leakage. These exposed vessels are subject to trauma and posterior vitreous detachment that may lead to intravitreous or retrovitreous hemorrhage.

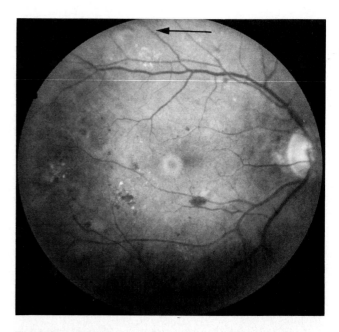

Figure 2–111. Black and white photograph of apparent background diabetic retinopathy. The arrow points to a zone that proved to be neovascularization.

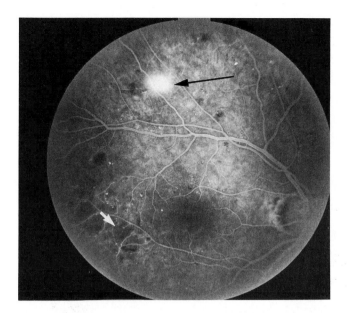

Figure 2–112. Early-stage angiogram of Figure 2–111, demonstrating the neovascularization **(black arrow)** and an area of capillary dropout **(white arrow).**

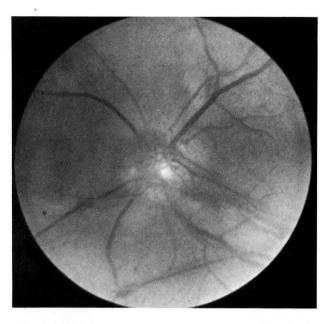

Figure 2–114. Black and white photograph demonstrating fragile neovascularization of the disc. Note the haze over the disc created by the leaking neovascularization.

Should the NVD progress unchecked, a fibrotic scaffolding will become more prominent. The addition of fibrotic scaffolding increases the likelihood of the future development of traction retinal detachment. As the net expands, there is a greater chance of vitreal hemorrhage. The hypoxia may be severe enough at this stage to initiate iris neovascularization, complicating the eye with neovascular glaucoma.

Eventually, hypoxia will be severe enough to actually create retinal death, which reduces the hypoxic stimulus. With a reduction of oxygenated blood, the new vessels may regress, leaving the fibrotic scaffolding to do its damage through traction retinal detachment.

NVE takes a similar course to NVD albeit more insidious. The new vessels are thought to sprout from areas of IRMA in the capillary bed. The new

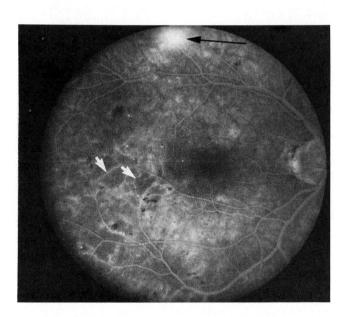

Figure 2–113. Late-stage angiogram of Figure 2–111.

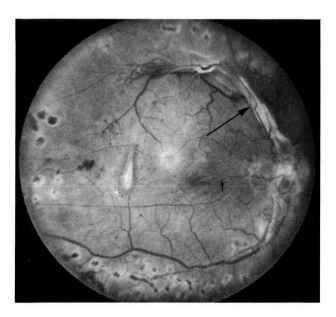

Figure 2–115. An example of proliferative diabetic retinopathy. The long arrow points to fibrotic scaffolding, and the short arrow points to the traction created by the proliferation.

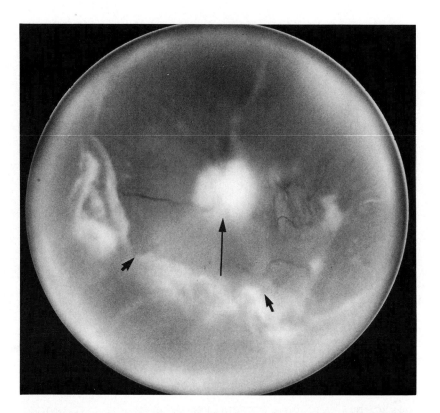

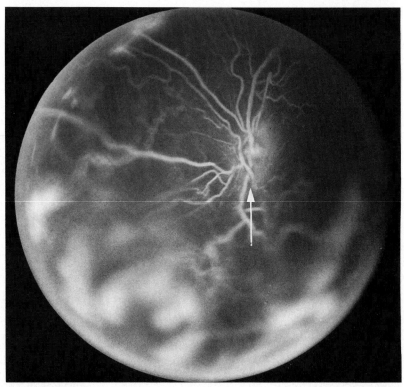

Figure 2–116. A traction retinal detachment associated with proliferative diabetic retinopathy. The small arrows **(Top)** point to the forward detachment of the retina. **Bottom.** Fluorescein angiograms of the detachment.

vessels eventually may perforate the internal limiting membrane to proliferate along the retinal surface. These vessels adhere to the vitreal hyaloid membrane and grow rapidly. They may later regress, but the accompanying fibrotic scaffolding remains adherent to the membrane. With vitreous syneresis and collapse, there is potential for both vitreous hemorrhage and retinal detachment. The vitreous detachment in the patient with diabetes is more insidious than in the nondiabetic, creating

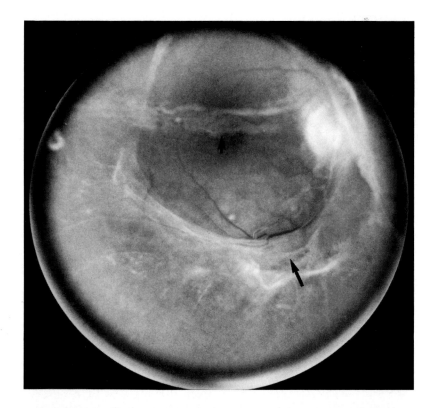

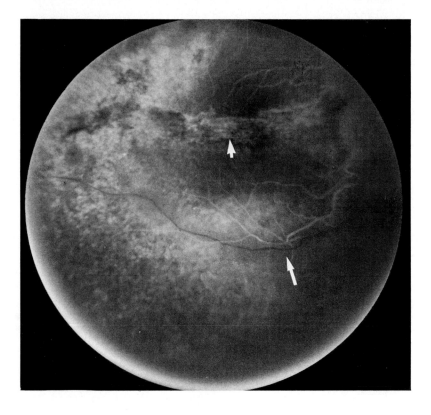

Figure 2–117. This is the fellow eye to that in Figure 2–116, also with a detachment. A band of traction coarses directly through the macula of the photograph **(Top)** and the angiogram **(Bottom).**

pockets of detachment. These pockets may create isolated retrovitreous hemorrhage or isolated areas of retinal detachment. NVE may regress to the point where no treatment is necessary (15 percent). **See color plates 29 and 41.**

The Diabetic Retinopathy Study Group established the standard of care in the case of NVD and NVE. This study demonstrated that the risk of severe vision loss—visual acuity at less than 5/200 at two consecutive 4-month follow-up visits—was much greater without photocoagulation than with photocoagulation.

Although many theories exist about the most effective method of application of panretinal photocoagulation (PRP) and when to photocoagulate, the statistics support the efficacy of photocoagulation in PDR. Photocoagulation actually destroys retina, eliminating the need for oxygen and short-circuiting the vasoproliferative stimulus. Elimination of hypoxia results in regression of new vessel growth. Remember, however, that the fibrotic scaffolding remains. Management of NVD or NVE is fluorescein angiography to assess the potential for photocoagulative intervention. There are complications to PRP or panretinal ablation. The common complications are listed in Table 2–35. A skilled retinologist is the consultant of choice to minimize complication rates.

Fibrotic proliferation is the response of retinal glial cells to provide a support scaffold for new vessel growth. The presence of the vitreous is necessary to support this scaffolding. Elimination of the vitreous by vitrectomy effectively prevents future scaffolding for neovascularization. Vitrectomy also cuts and eliminates existing scaffolding. The attachment of the scaffolding between the retina and vitreous face is the point of genesis of a traction retinal detachment when vitreous degeneration occurs. Again, vitrectomy may be used to cut the abnormal adhesions and allow the relief of retinal traction. Fibrotic scaffolding does not directly alter vision, but its presence opens the potential of traction retinal detachment even resulting in retinal tears and rhegmatogenous retinal detachment. The fibrotic scaffolding will remain even with regression of neovascularization. Fibrotic scaffolding resulting in areas of potential retinal traction should be seen by a retinologist to determine if vitrectomy would be of benefit.

Hemorrhage into the vitreous may result in a broad range of reduced acuities. If the hemorrhage is only partial, it may be possible to ascertain the site of the bleeding and intervene with photocoagulation. Should intravitreal blood totally block the view of the retina, the retinologist

TABLE 2–35. COMMON COMPLICATIONS ASSOCIATED WITH PANRETINAL PHOTOCOAGULATION

Constriction of visual fields
Mobility problems especially at night
Transient cystoid macular edema
Choroidal neovascularization in scars
Retinal–choroidal detachments
Flattened anterior chamber
Transient retinal hemorrhage

TABLE 2–36. POTENTIAL COMPLICATIONS ASSOCIATED WITH VITRECTOMY

Corneal folds
Corneal edema
Iris damage with hemorrhage
Neovascularization of the Iris
Cataract formation
Intraocular hemorrhage
Retinal breaks
Retinal detachment
Fibrinoid syndrome (cornea decomposition + vitreous strands → retinal detachment)
Endophthalmitis

has the option of waiting to allow blood to clear (6 to 12 months) before performing photocoagulation or vitrectomy or clearing some of the hemorrhage by pars plana vitrectomy, then performing endo-photocoagulation. With further clearing of blood, addition of photocoagulation or vitrectomy may be necessary.

Vitrectomy is not without risk. There is about a 25 percent complication rate with vitrectomy (Table 2–36). Any of the signs of PDR deserve a consultation with a highly competent retinologist.

PROLIFERATIVE DIABETIC RETINOPATHY—PEARLS

- Neovascularization of the disc, neovascularization elsewhere, fibrotic scaffolding, traction retinal detachment, and vitreous hemorrhage
- All signs are vision threatening and deserve fluorescein angiography and a retinology consultation
- Photocoagulation has positive effect on arresting NVD and NVE
- Vitrectomy of some benefit but also carries some risk
- Communicate findings to diabetologist

Patients with diabetes must be evaluated carefully for signs of diabetic retinopathy. The signs become more prevalent with an increase in the duration of diabetes. All patients with diabetes without signs of retinopathy should have annual dilated fundus examinations. The etiology of all of the signs of diabetic retinopathy is initiated in the deep capillary bed, with edema and hypoxia being the culprits in the visually destructive phases of retinopathy. Edema spreading into the macula as evidenced by hard exudates and dot–blot hemorrhages in the macula is a threat to vision. Likewise, the components of PDR threaten vision. All attempts at therapeutic intervention are directed toward elimination of hypoxia or severing of fibrotic proliferative strands. In addition, vitreous blood is at times removed by vitrectomy.

TABLE 2–37. RECOMMENDED STANDARDS OF CARE FOR THE OCULAR COMPLICATIONS OF DIABETES

Condition	Management[a]	
Background diabetic retinopathy	Encroaching on or within macula	Distant from macula
Dot–blot hemorrhages	Fluorescein angiography (FA)	Educate and follow 1 year
Hard exudates		Educate and follow 1 year
Microaneurysms		Educate and follow 1 year
Preproliferative diabetic retinopathy		
Cotton wool spots	→ Educate and follow 3 months	
Venous tortuosity	→ Educate and follow 3 months	
Capillary closure	→ Educate and follow 3 months	
Arteriolar abnormalities	→ Educate and follow 3 months	
IRMA[b]	→ FA, educate and follow 3 months	
Note: If three or more signs	→ FA	
Note: If asymmetry	→ Probable internal carotid artery stenosis	
Proliferative diabetic retinopathy		
NVD	→ Educate and FA + retinology consultation	
NVE	→ Educate and FA + retinology consultation	
Fibrotic proliferation	→ Educate and retinology consultation	
Traction detachment	→ Retinology consultation	
Vitreous hemorrhage	→ Retinology consultation	

[a]In all cases, communicate findings to patient's diabetologist.
[b]IRMA, intraretinal microvascular abnormalities; NVD, neovascularization of the disc; NVE, neovascularization elsewhere.

The accepted standards of care for patients with ocular complications of diabetes are summarized in Table 2–37.

EALES' DISEASE (RETINAL PERIPHLEBITIS)

The classic form of Eales' disease occurs in otherwise healthy young men in their 20 to 30s. It appears as a bilateral perivasculitis most often affecting the veins. If unilateral, the left eye is involved most often. There may be an associated anterior uveitis. The cause is obscure, most often being attributed to a nonspecific inflammatory reaction to antigens (tubercular).

Signs and Symptoms. The signs and symptoms vary depending on the severity of the disease. Early in the disease, acuity is usually unaffected, with complaints associated with floaters. In the periphery, there is perivascular sheathing sometimes with associated hemorrhages that emanate into the vitreous. Vitritis naturally occurs overlying the inflammatory locus. Vision eventually may be compromised secondary to vitreous blood, retinal traction, or macular edema. The venous stasis may spread to the posterior pole, resulting in considerable manifestations of retinal edema.

Management. The patient presumed to have Eales' disease should have a complete medical evaluation, including a PPD and chest x-ray, to rule out tuberculosis. The vitreous hemorrhage may be allowed to clear on its own, or vitrectomy may be used. Areas of leakage and neovascularization in the retina should be assessed by fluorescein angiography (Fig. 2–118). Should there be active leakage or neovascularization, photocoagulation may be attempted. Intervention as early as possible will improve the chances of retention of retinal function. A patient suspected of having Eales' disease must have fluorescein angiography to determine if a retinology consultation is necessary.

EALES' DISEASE—PEARLS

- Healthy young (20–30) men
- Perivasculitis with occasional anterior uveitis
- Vitritis and occasional vitreous hemorrhage
- If unilateral, most often affects left eye
- May be associated neovascularization
- Management
  - Rule out tuberculosis, and fluorescein angiography if neovascularization suspected, a retinology consultation should be considered

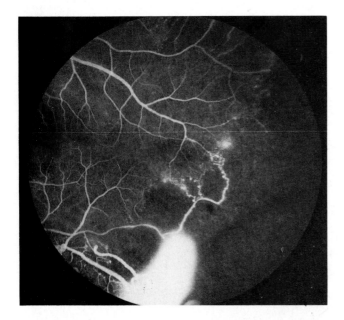

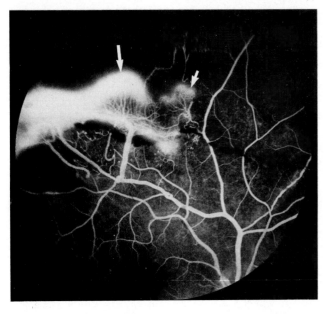

Figure 2–118. Top and Bottom. Fluorescein angiograms demonstrating neovascularization in a case of Eales' disease.

SICKLE CELL RETINOPATHY

Sickle cell retinopathy is the result of compromise of normal retinal circulation by abnormal hemoglobin. The result is retinal hypoxia, which then stimulates abnormal vascular growth. The majority of activity occurs pre-equatorial because of vascular narrowing in the periphery, lending to closure by sickled red blood cells combined with inherently reduced oxygenation in the periphery.

The normal population has only hemoglobin A, whereas sickle cell patients have an abnormal hemoglobin because of an inherited substitution of amino acid valine for glutamic acid (hemoglobin S) or lysine for glutamic acid (hemoglobin C) in the beta chain. Of American blacks, approximately 10 percent have a variety of hemoglobinopathy. About 80 percent of those have the trait (SA), 10 percent have sickle thalessemia (S-thal), 4 percent have sickle cell anemia (SS), and 1 to 2 percent have SC hemoglobinopathy. The SC and S-thal patients have higher hematocrit levels, leading to increased viscosity. This increased viscosity, combined with sickling and hypoxia, creates a higher incidence of proliferative retinopathy than the other hemoglobinopathies. Sickled hemoglobin has the potential to have a lower oxygen-carrying ability as well as developing unusual shapes that block vessels. This blockage usually occurs near the arteriole–capillary zone.

Signs and Symptoms. Intraretinal hemorrhages appearing salmon in color and a black sunburst spot representing reactive RPE hyperplasia occur near the site of obstruction in the arteries. Venous tortuosity may also occur in these patients. There may be shining retinal crystals that represent residue of hemorrhage. Angioid streaks occur in 6 to 8 percent of the patients (Fig. 2–119). Proliferative retinopathy may occur as the result of the hypoxia. The neovascularization grows near the occluded area and spreads out in a fan shape from a single vessel. This neovascularization carries the same risk to vision as does neovascularization in any other retinal vasculopathy process. Figure 2–120 illustrates the sequence of development of proliferative retinopathy. Some patients with sickle cell disease also have areas of retinal dark without pressure in the posterior pole.

Management. Management of sickle cell retinopathy with photocoagulation is definitely indicated when neovascularization appears. Treatment at earlier stages is controversial, and that decision should be made by a competent retinologist. Often sickle cell retinopathy will occur in patients who are unaware of the systemic disease. These patients need a consultation with a hematologist or internal medicine specialist knowledgeable in the manifestations of sickle cell disease.

The complication of vitreous hemorrhage often is allowed to clear on its own. Should a retinal tear occur, it is usually at the base of the lesion and often creates a rhegmatogenous retinal detachment. Surgical intervention, often with scleral buckling, is necessary. The risk of anterior segment necrosis secondary to buckling is very high (70 percent) in patients with sickle cell retinopathy as compared to

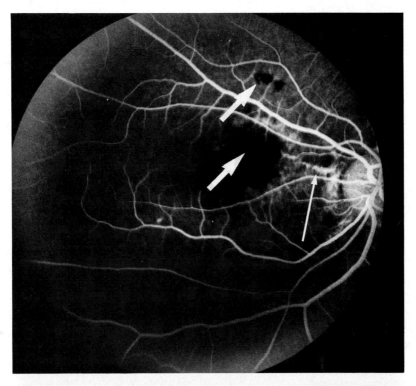

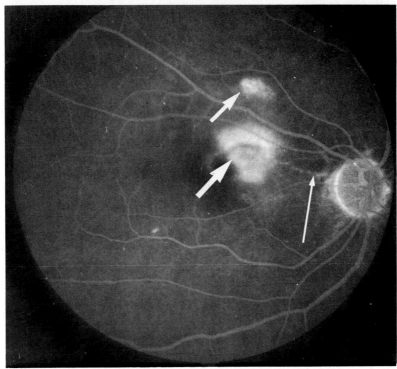

Figure 2–119. Early-stage **(top)** and late-stage **(bottom)** angiograms of choroidal neovascularization **(large arrows)** secondary to angioid streaks **(small arrows)** in a case of sickle cell disease.

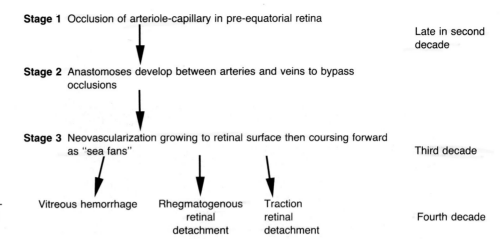

Stage 1 Occlusion of arteriole-capillary in pre-equatorial retina

Late in second decade

Stage 2 Anastomoses develop between arteries and veins to bypass occlusions

Stage 3 Neovascularization growing to retinal surface then coursing forward as "sea fans"

Third decade

Vitreous hemorrhage   Rhegmatogenous retinal detachment   Traction retinal detachment

Fourth decade

Figure 2–120. The sequence of development of proliferative sickle cell retinopathy.

under 5 percent in nonsickle cell patients. A skilled surgeon is of utmost importance for these patients.

SICKLE CELL RETINOPATHY—PEARLS

- Result of closure of retinal circulation and hypoxia by sickled hemoglobin
- Usually manifests in pre-equatorial retina as hemorrhage, black sunburst spot, and seafan neovascularization
- If allowed to progress will result in vitreous hemorrhage or retinal detachment
- Management includes:
    - Consultation with hematologist if not previously diagnosed
    - Consultation with retinologist for possible photocoagulation or vitrectomy

---

RETINOPATHY OF PREMATURITY (RETROLENTAL FIBROPLASIA)

Retinopathy of prematurity (ROP) has once again surfaced as a severe problem as the result of improved technology in neonatology.

As discussed previously, retinal vascularization to the oral region is just barely complete at full gestation in the human. The last area of the retina to be vascularized is the temporal periphery. If birth occurs before full gestation, this peripheral retinal region is susceptible to altered vasculopathy because of incomplete maturation. Retinopathy of prematurity has three distinctive stages: (1) vaso-obliterative, (2) proliferative, and (3) cicatricial.

Signs and Symptoms. The vaso-obliterative phase is related to the rise in available oxygen when the premature infant is placed in oxygen-rich incubation. The excessive oxygen stunts the normal maturation of vessels (vaso-obliteration). Once the child is returned to room air, there is a sudden deficiency in oxygen, creating a demand that cannot be met by the child's existing vessels. Vasoproliferation then ensues to satisfy the demand. As one would expect, this activity occurs most frequently in the temporal periphery, appearing first as endothelial nodules in the inner retina followed by proliferation of intraretinal capillaries. This neovascularization breaks through the internal limiting membrane to proliferate on the retinal surface and may then spread into the vitreous in the form of hemorrhage, fibrotic proliferation, and retinal traction. Traction can cause retinal detachment as well as mild forms of retinal dragging that may result in heterotopic macula. The extent of proliferation is determined by several factors, including the elapsed time of the oxygen therapy. Spontaneous recovery from vasoproliferative ROP occurs in a very high percentage of patients, resulting in mild temporal periphery changes that are typically static.

The cicatricial phase is considered the regressive phase and is identified by pigment irregularities, vitreoretinal membranes, pale optic nerve head with temporally dragged vessels, retinal folds, and a retrolental mass in the pupillary area (Fig. 2–121). The development of ROP is summarized in Figure 2–122. Most of the time, the retinal vasculopathy is bilateral, but the author has observed unilateral cases.

Management. The importance of recognition and management of ROP results from the severe visually debilitating results of progression. Recognition and diagnostic difficulties are compounded by the difficulty of examining the peripheral retina of the infant. Maximal dilation (0.5 percent cyclopentolate + 0.5 percent tropicamide + 2.5 percent phenyle-

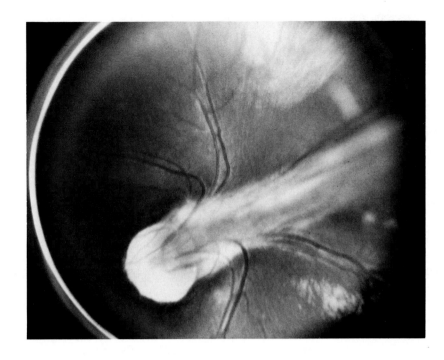

Figure 2–121. The dragged disc characteristic of severe stages of retinopathy of prematurity.

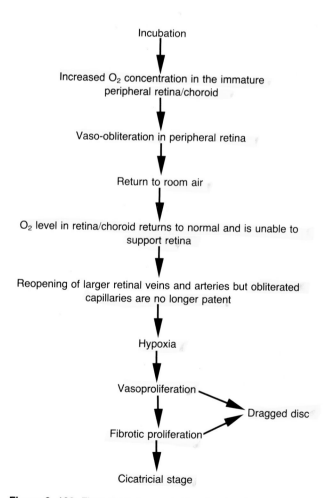

Incubation

↓

Increased O₂ concentration in the immature peripheral retina/choroid

↓

Vaso-obliteration in peripheral retina

↓

Return to room air

↓

O₂ level in retina/choroid returns to normal and is unable to support retina

↓

Reopening of larger retinal veins and arteries but obliterated capillaries are no longer patent

↓

Hypoxia

↓

Vasoproliferation → Dragged disc

↓

Fibrotic proliferation → Dragged disc

↓

Cicatricial stage

Figure 2–122. Flow chart demonstrating the development of retinopathy of prematurity.

phrine), in addition to mild anesthesia, is preferable for complete examination. This should be performed before age 10 weeks and every month thereafter for 6 months. Should an active phase—vasoproliferative component—be diagnosed, a retinal consultation is indicated for possible photocoagulative or cryopexy intervention. Vitrectomy in skilled hands also may be beneficial. Should the patient have cicatricial components of ROP and such potential complications as retinoschisis and retinal detachment, the individual complication must be managed by proper surgical protocol. It is also important to watch for other complications such as glaucoma.

The best method of management of retinopathy of prematurity is prevention. Although strides constantly are being made in monitoring of blood gases and improved neonatologic techniques, some cases are unavoidable. Recent work has indicated that prophylactic cryopexy of low birth weight infants may delay or eliminate the development of ROP. The increased success in neonatology also results in more potential candidates for ROP. Research in this area is aggressive, but recent setbacks, such as the vitamin E experience, indicate that retinopathy of prematurity is a difficult problem in eye care.

BECHET'S DISEASE

Bechet's disease is systemic and thought to be a vaso-occlusive immune complex disease. It is characterized by recurrent iridocyclitis, mucous membrane ulcers of the mouth and genitals, and central nervous system and joint disorders (acute polyarthritis). Bechet's disease affects young (18 to 40 years) adults (male/female 2:1) and is more common in Japan (20 to 30 percent of iridocyclitis) and the Mediterranean area. Iridocyclitis with hypopyon is the most prevalent ocular feature, but vaso-occlusive manifestations may occur as peripheral retinal vasculitis (26 percent of patients).

In the retina, the small peripheral veins are affected most often. With this, there is retinal edema, exudates deep in the retina, sheathing, and large vessel occlusion. This is a necrotizing vasculitis and, as such, is irreversible. The ophthalmoscopic view often is hampered by the almost omnipresent cells of the accompanying iridocyclitis. Treatment is the systemic use of chlorambucil.

RETINAL VASCULAR TUMORS

Several different tumors arise from the vascular tissues of the retina and optic nerve, some of which may threaten vision. In addition to ocular signs, there may be associated lesions in other systems of the body, including the skin, central nervous system, and visceral tissues. When retinal vascular tumors are associated with remote changes in other systems, the complex is sometimes grouped under the term "phakomatoses" or "systemic hamartomatoses."

Cavernous Hemangioma of the Retina

Cavernous hemangioma of the retina is a relatively rare condition that occurs at an average age of 23 years. In the past, however, it was often misdiagnosed as one of the other retinal vascular tumors or abnormalities. The majority of the patients reported in the literature are white. Cavernous hemangioma usually is unilateral with no preference for laterality. There is increasing evidence in the literature that cavernous hemangioma of the retina is inherited in an autosomal dominant pattern, with highly variable penetrance and expressivity.

Signs and Symptoms. Cavernous hemangioma of the retina appears ophthalmoscopically as dark red saccular clusters projecting from the inner retinal layers (Fig. 2–123). There is usually an associated overlying white epiretinal membrane. The saccular clusters rarely demonstrate change over time, but the epiretinal membrane may increase in size and density. Exudation and hemorrhage are extremely rare, which contrasts with Coat's disease (retinal telangiectasia) and capillary hemangioma of the retina. When a cavernous hemangioma occurs on the disc, the ophthalmoscopic appearance is similar.

The patient with a cavernous hemangioma is usually asymptomatic and has good visual acuity if the epiretinal membrane does not tug on the macula. The visual fields may show a scotoma corresponding to the site of the lesion if assessed at threshold. Vision may become compromised if a rare vitreous hemorrhage occurs. There may be an associated extraocular muscle palsy if the central nervous system is the peripheral site of a similar tumor.

The most important diagnostic test in all retinal vascular tumors is fluorescein angiography, which produces results that are very characteristic, if not pathognomonic, of cavernous hemangioma of the retina. The epiretinal membrane may produce a mild autofluorescence. The prearterial (cho-

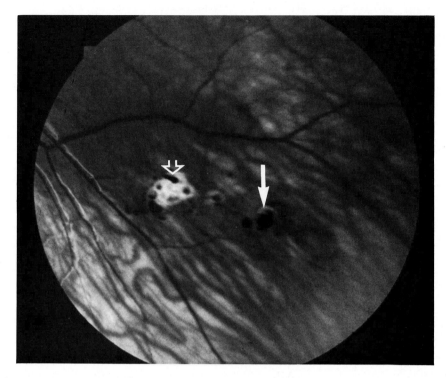

Figure 2–123. Black and white photograph of a retinal cavernous hemangioma. The solid arrow points to the saccular dilatations, and the open arrow points to a preretinal membrane.

roidal flush) phase of fluorescein angiography demonstrates hypofluorescence of the area of the lesion, whereas the surrounding retina is normal. The hypofluorescence remains throughout the arterial phase. During the later parts of the venous phase, fluorescein begins slowly to enter the clusters of the hemangioma. The fluorescein pools in the plasma in the superior portion of each vascular space, whereas the blood collects in the inferior portion of the ballooning of the vessel. This plasma–erythrocyte sedimentation pattern is pathognomonic of cavernous hemangioma. There is usually no leakage of dye into the surrounding tissue. The fluorescein angiography findings may be summarized as slowed venous drainage, no arteriovenous shunting, no leakage into or under surrounding retinal tissue, and the classic plasma–erythrocyte sedimentation.

Cavernous hemangiomas of the retina and optic nerve are composed of multiple isolated saccular dilatations of blood vessels that replace the normal tissue of the inner half of the retina and optic nerve head (Fig. 2–124). The saccular dilatations are lined with a continuous layer of nonfenestrated endothelial cells. Electron microscopic studies have shown normal anatomic features for retinal vessels within a cavernous hemangioma. Within the hemangioma, the vessels often abut one another with lumen connected by small orifices. The saccular dilatations are relatively independent of the remainder of the retinal vascular system. The endothelial lining is responsible for the fact that leakage is not a

factor in a cavernous hemangioma as contrasted to some of the other vascular tumors with fenestrated vessel walls.

In addition to the saccular dilatations, the internal limiting membrane overlying these tumors is altered. In places, the internal limiting membrane is thin to absent, allowing for communication between the inner retina and the vitreous face. Migration of retinal glial cells up through these focal breaks allows for proliferation of the glial tissue on the surface of the internal limiting membrane. The proliferation and subsequent contraction of these glial cells produce the epiretinal membrane often associated with cavernous hemangioma.

Management. Emphasis should be placed on ruling out associated central nervous system dysfunction and symptoms. The patient should be questioned carefully about cutaneous vascular anomalies. Cutaneous vascular lesions may occur in a variety of ways and may even give an appearance similar to the fundus lesion. The classic skin lesion is a cherry hemangioma. The clinician must always consider the possibility of an associated vascular tumor elsewhere in the body. A number of conditions associated with cavernous hemangioma of the retina has been reported (Table 2–38).

Probably the most important clinical association is the triad of cavernous hemangioma of the retina, intracranial vascular lesions, and cutaneous angiomas. Pedigree analysis of the neuro–oculocutaneous presentation supports an autosomal domi-

RETINAL CAVERNOUS HEMANGIOMA

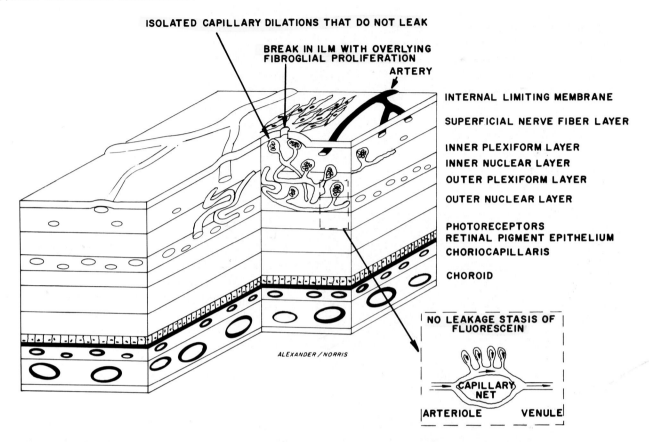

Figure 2–124. Schematic retinal cross section demonstrating the development of a retinal cavernous hemangioma. *(Reprinted with permission from Alexander LJ, Moates KN: Cavernous hemangioma of the retina. J Am Optom, Assoc 1988; 59:539–548.)*

nant inheritance pattern with variable penetrance and expressivity. A few cases have been presented in which the entire neuro–oculocutaneous syndrome has been transmitted. Any history of seizure, cranial nerve palsies, paresthesias, convulsions, visual field variations, strokes, and neurologic seizure in a patient with a cavernous hemangioma of the retina may be indicative of central nervous system involvement. The clinician should refer all questionable signs and symptoms in patients for computed tomography (CT) or magnetic resonance imaging (MRI). The lesions in the brain are often amendable to surgical intervention.

TABLE 2–38. SYSTEMIC ANOMALIES ASSOCIATED WITH CAVERNOUS HEMANGIOMA OF THE RETINA

Neuro–oculocutaneous syndrome
Congenital cardiovascular anomalies
Hypogammaglobulinemia
Cranial nerve palsies
Angioma serpiginosum
Agenesis of the internal carotid system
Blue rubber bleb syndrome

CAVERNOUS HEMANGIOMA OF THE RETINA—PEARLS

- Congenital malformation characterized by clusters of vascular abnormalities
- Usually unilateral, intraretinal, and often covered by a preretinal membrane
- No demonstrable vision-threatening consequences
- Possible associated hemangiomas in the central nervous system
- Management includes:
  - Ruling out neurologic signs and routine eye examinations

Angiomatosis Retinae

Angiomatosis retinae (capillary hemangiomas) is a benign retinal angioma that usually occurs within the first two decades of life. The lesion is inherited in an autosomal dominant manner, with incomplete penetrance and variable expressivity. Capillary hemangioma may appear at the optic nerve head (Fig. 2–125) or within the retina. When the ocular lesion is associated with an intracranial or spinal cord hemangioblastoma, the syndrome is referred to as von Hippel-Lindau disease. Association with systemic tumors occurs in about 25 percent of the cases, and the presentation is bilateral in approximately 50 percent of the cases.

Signs and Symptoms. Angiomatosis retinae usually occurs as an ophthalmoscopically observable lesion in the 20 to 40-year-old patient. The temporal periphery is the most common location of the

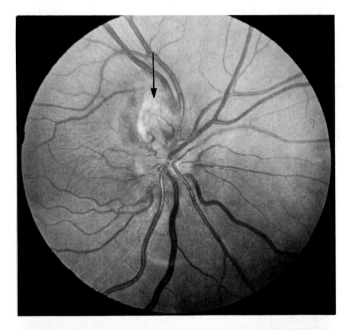

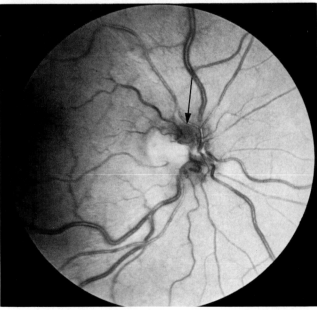

Figure 2–125. Top and Bottom. Two cases of capillary hemangioma of the optic nerve head.

hemangioma, which originates as a proliferation of endothelial cells between arterioles and venules in the capillary bed. At this stage, the lesion is small, with a red-gray color. As the hemangioma enlarges to occupy the sensory retina, arteriovenous communications develop, with further growth of the capillaries surrounding the hemangioma. The lesion then assumes a pink balloon pattern. The capillary growth exists to supply and drain the tumor. These capillary channels eventually develop into a large fistular single arteriole and venous channel. As the blood is shunted to the tumor from the surrounding retina, microvasculopathy occurs in the capillary bed. This nonperfused area may then develop intraretinal edema, hemorrhages, and exudation (Fig. 2–126). The intraretinal edema may lead to cystoid maculopathy. If allowed to progress unchecked, the hemangioma decompensates, allowing for intraretinal and subretinal exudation with the potential for retinal detachment. Figure 2–127 summarizes the sequence in the development of angiomatosis retinae. The exudation has a strong propensity for the posterior role, resulting in reduced acuity (Fig. 2–128). Fluorescein angiography will demonstrate the tumor and the leakage from the site.

Management. Since it is most likely that the angioma will progress, it is important to intervene surgically as soon as possible. The exception to this is the case of the optic nerve hemangioma. The earlier the angioma is treated, the better the prognosis. Cryopexy and photocoagulation are both effective methods of treatment when in experienced hands. Genetic counseling is indicated in cases of angiomatosis retinae, as is a neurologic consultation to rule out intracranial and spinal hemangioblastomas and the possibility of pheochromocytomas.

ANGIOMATOSIS RETINAE—PEARLS

- Retinal angioma transmitted as autosomal dominant
- May have intracranial or spinal cord hemangioblastoma (25 percent) and possibly pheochromocytomas
- Most often in the 20s to 30s in temporal periphery
- Develops to a pink balloon with a single feeder artery and draining vein
- The lesion leaks, creating hemorrhage, exudate, and retinal detachment
- Management includes:
  - Genetic counseling
  - Neurologic consultation
  - Retinology consultation for possible photocoagulation

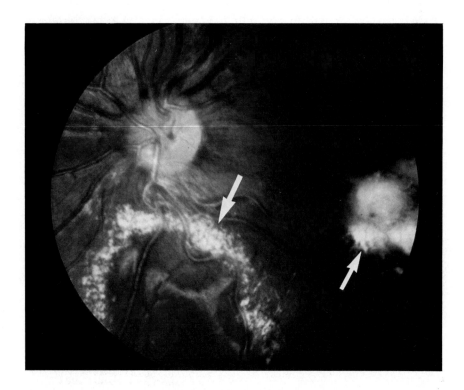

Figure 2–126. The exudative response associated with a retinal capillary hemangioma.

Retinal Telangiectasia

Retinal telangiectasia often is confused with cavernous hemangioma. Coats' disease is a variety of exudative retinopathy resulting from telangiectasias of the retinal vessels. Leber's miliary aneurysms are similar telangiectatic vessels without the presence of extensive exudation. Coats' disease usually occurs unilaterally in the first to second decades. Coats' disease is about four times more common in males than females and usually is discovered in the first to

second decades in spite of the fact that the telangiectasias are actually congenital.

Signs and Symptoms. The congenital vascular anomalies are altered over time, leading to leakage, degeneration, and development of hard exudates. It has been proposed that the conversion of benign congenital telangiectasias is stimulated by a growth hormone. Figure 2–129 illustrates the clinicopathology of retinal telangiectasias.

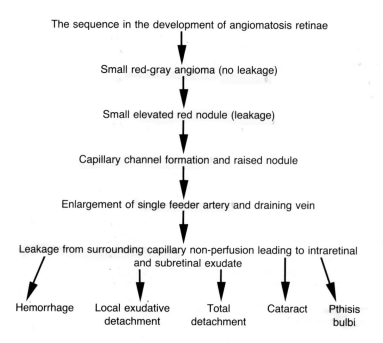

Figure 2–127. The sequence in the development of angiomatosis retinae. (Reprinted with permission from Alexander LJ, Moates KN: Cavernous hemangioma of the retina. J Am Optom Assoc. 1988; 59:539–548.)

The sequence in the development of angiomatosis retinae

↓

Small red-gray angioma (no leakage)

↓

Small elevated red nodule (leakage)

↓

Capillary channel formation and raised nodule

↓

Enlargement of single feeder artery and draining vein

↓

Leakage from surrounding capillary non-perfusion leading to intraretinal and subretinal exudate

Hemorrhage   Local exudative detachment   Total detachment   Cataract   Pthisis bulbi

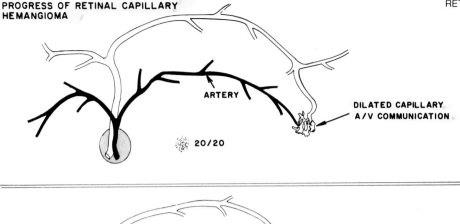

ARTERY

DILATED CAPILLARY
A/V COMMUNICATION

20/20

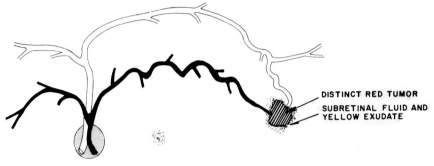

DISTINCT RED TUMOR
SUBRETINAL FLUID AND
YELLOW EXUDATE

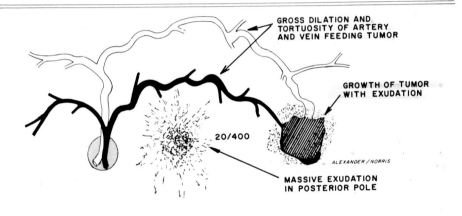

GROSS DILATION AND
TORTUOSITY OF ARTERY
AND VEIN FEEDING TUMOR

GROWTH OF TUMOR
WITH EXUDATION

20/400

ALEXANDER/NORRIS

MASSIVE EXUDATION
IN POSTERIOR POLE

Figure 2–128. Schematic illustrating the progression of a retinal capillary hemangioma. (Reprinted with permission from Alexander LJ, Moates KN: Cavernous hemangioma of the retina. J Am Optom Assoc. 1988; 59:539–548.)

The breakdown in the blood–retinal barrier results in an accumulation of lipid-rich soup under the retina. The macrophages pick up the lipids and migrate, resulting in intraretinal and subretinal exudation (Fig. 2–130). In addition to exudation creating vision loss, the intraretinal edema may spread to the posterior pole, creating cystoid macular edema. Ischemic foci may develop within the capillary bed near the telangiectasias. Retinal hemorrhage, neovascularization, and subsequent vitreous hemorrhage may occur in these areas of hypoxia. As the exudative process evolves and becomes more chronic, cholesterol crystals accumulate, and tortuous vessels develop in the periphery with the potential toward arteriovenous shunting. Ghost cells characteristic of Coats' disease appear and are thought to originate from retinal histocytes, retinal pigment epithelial cells, or lipid-laden macrophages. Table 2–39 outlines the stages of development of Coats' disease, with recommended therapeutic intervention.

Fluorescein angiography in telangiectasia demonstrates that the lesions are in the mainstream of the vascular tree and that arteriovenous collateral channels are present. Leakage of fluorescein dominates the picture.

Management. The patient suspected of having Coats' disease should have fluorescein angiography performed to determine if the lesions are amendable to photocoagulation. The earlier the disease is detected with application of therapy, the better the prognosis. The end result of Coats' disease, if allowed to progress unchecked, is retinal detachment. **Table 2–40 compares cavernous hemangioma, retinal telangiectasia, and capillary hemangioma.**

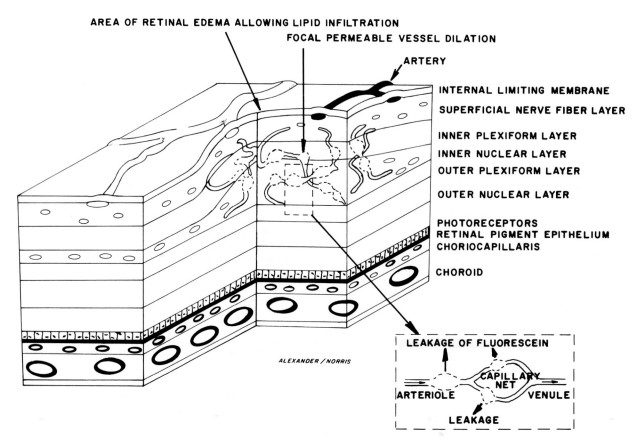

AREA OF RETINAL EDEMA ALLOWING LIPID INFILTRATION
FOCAL PERMEABLE VESSEL DILATION
ARTERY
INTERNAL LIMITING MEMBRANE
SUPERFICIAL NERVE FIBER LAYER
INNER PLEXIFORM LAYER
INNER NUCLEAR LAYER
OUTER PLEXIFORM LAYER
OUTER NUCLEAR LAYER
PHOTORECEPTORS
RETINAL PIGMENT EPITHELIUM
CHORIOCAPILLARIS
CHOROID
ALEXANDER / NORRIS
LEAKAGE OF FLUORESCEIN
CAPILLARY NET
ARTERIOLE
VENULE
LEAKAGE

Figure 2–129. Schematic illustrating the clinicopathology of retinal telangiectasia. *(Reprinted with permission from Alexander LJ, Moates KN: Cavernous hemangioma of the retina. J Am Optom Assoc. 1988; 59:539–548.)*

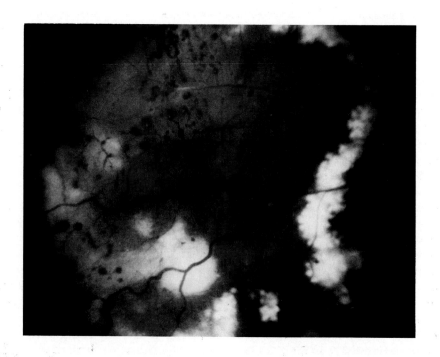

Figure 2–130. An example of the severe exudation occurring secondary to the leakage associated with telangiectasia.

TABLE 2–39. CLINICAL STAGES OF COATS' DISEASE WITH RECOMMENDATIONS REGARDING THERAPEUTIC INTERVENTION

Clinical Stage of Coat s' Disease	Recommendations Regarding Therapeutic Intervention after Fluorescein Angiography
I. Retinal vessel telangiectasia (dilated tortuosity, edema, minor exudates)	I. Xenon (children) or argon photocoagulation to areas of telangiectasia A. Thermal necrosis of telangiectasia B. Possible cryopexy
II. Localized intraretinal exudates (obscuration of telangiectasia by exudate)	II. Higher energy photocoagulation or cryopexy
III. Localized (partial) retinal detachment (sensory RD by subsensory exudate)	III. A. Photocoagulation to affected area (often repeated) B. Drainage of subretinal exudate C. Cryopexy
IV. Total retinal detachment (massive exudation and subretinal membrane)	IV. Same as stage III with addition of scleral buckle
V. Uveitis, phthisis bulbi, glaucoma, cataract, massive subretinal membrane	V. Symptomatic relief of pain

TABLE 2–40. COMPARISON OF CAPILLARY HEMANGIOMA, RETINAL TELANGIECTASIA, AND CAVERNOUS HEMANGIOMA

Characteristic	Capillary Hemangioma	Retinal Telangiectasia	Cavernous Hemangioma
Age of onset	1st–2nd decade	1st–2nd decade	1st and 2nd decade
Laterality	Bilateral 50%	Unilateral	Unilateral
Sex	No pattern	Male	Female
Genetics	Autosomal dominant with variable penetrance and expressivity	None	Possible autosomal dominance with variable expressivity and penetrance
Progression	Common	Common	Only epiretinal membrane
Ophthalmoscopic appearance	1. Distinct red tumor with large feeder 2. Arteriovenous shunt 3. Massive intraretinal and subretinal exudation 4. Surrounding retina involved	1. No distinct tumor 2. Arteriovenous collaterals 3. Intraretinal and subretinal exudation 4. Surrounding retina involved	1. Dilatations isolated from vascular tree 2. No collaterals 3. No exudation 4. No involvement of surrounding retina 5. Preretinal membrane
Histology	Abnormal blood–retinal barrier	Abnormal blood–retinal barrier	Intact blood–retinal barrier
Fluorescein angiography	Dye leakage	Dye leakage	No dye leakage but classic sedimentation
Complications	Hemorrhage Retinal detachment Glaucoma	Retinal detachment Hemorrhage	Rare hemorrhage
Associated systemic conditions	25% with CNS involvement	Usually no association	Possible Neuro–oculocutaneous syndrome
Treatment	Photocoagulation Cryopexy Scleral buckle Genetic counseling Neurologic consultation	Photocoagulation Cryopexy Scleral buckle	Not indicated Possible Neurologic consultation

Modified from Alexander LJ, Moates KN: Cavernous Hemangioma of the retina J Am Optom Assoc. 1988, 59:539–548.

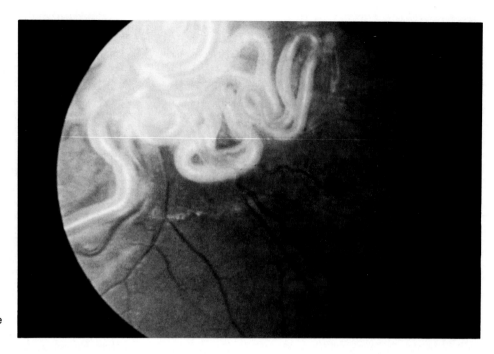

Figure 2–131. An example of a racemose hemangioma emanating from and returning to the optic nerve head. *(Photo courtesy of J. Potter.)*

Parafoveal and perifoveal retinal telangiectasia also may occur as an isolated entity not associated directly with Coats' disease or Leber's miliary aneurysms. Parafoveal retinal telangiectasia occurs as capillary malformation at the edge of the foveal avascular zone. This condition usually occurs as vision reduction in the third to fifth decades of life and has a possible relationship to diabetes. Treatment by photocoagulation is controversial, since results sometimes are poor.

RETINAL TELANGIECTASIA—PEARLS

- Occurs unilaterally in first two decades
- Most often in males
- Progresses to intraretinal and subretinal exudate accumulation
- A retinology consultation is indicated

Racemose Hemangioma

Racemose hemangioma (Fig. 2–131) usually occurs unilaterally as extremely dilated, tortuous arteriovenous communications associated with reduced acuities. There usually are no other ocular anomalies. With fluorescein angiography, it appears as if there is no capillary bed between the arteriovenous communication.

Racemose hemangioma does not progress and does not have any tendencies toward leakage. There is some concern that racemose hemangioma

may be associated with similar aberrant vasculature within the optic nerve and intracranial cavity. These associations are referred to as the Wyburn–Mason syndrome. A neurologic consultation is, therefore, necessary in cases of racemose hemangioma.

RACEMOSE HEMANGIOMA—PEARLS

- Extremely dilated tortuous arteriovenous communications
- Reduced acuities
- No particular retinal complications
- Possible intracranial associations necessitating a neurologic consultation

---

REFERENCES

Alexander LJ: How to perform and interpret fluorescein angiography. *Rev Optom* 1988;125:72–82.

Alexander LJ: Retinal vein occlusion. A literature update. J Am Optom Assoc 1986;57:557–560.

Alexander LJ: Implications of retinal vaso-occlusive disease. *S J Optom* 1986;4:20–34.

Alexander LJ, Jones W, Potter JW: *Retina, Retina, Retina. Primary Care.* Philadelphia, 1985.

Alexander LJ: The prevalence of corneal arcus senilis in known insulin dependent diabetic patients. *J Am Optom Assoc* 1985;56:556–559.

Alexander LJ: Ocular signs and symptoms of altered blood lipids. *J Am Optom Assoc* 1983;54:123–126.

Alexander LJ: Pre-stroke signs and symptoms. *Rev Optom* 1980;117:58–73.

Alexander LJ: Pre-retinal membrane formation. *J Am Optom Assoc* 1980;51:567–572.

Alexander LJ: Optometric detection of pre-stroke signs and symptoms. *Rev Optom* 1979;116:45–53.

Alexander LJ: Diseases of the retina, in Bartlett JD, Jaanus SD (eds): *Clinical Ocular Pharmacology*. Boston, Butterworths, 1984.

Alexander LJ, Moates KN: Cavernous hemangioma of the retina. *J Am Optom Assoc* 1988;59:539–548.

Balogh VJ: The use of oral fluorescein angiography in idiopathic central serous chorioretinopathy. *J Am Optom Assoc* 1986;57:909–913.

Barnett AH, Armstrong S, Wakelin K, et al: Specific thromboxane synthetase inhibition and retinopathy in insulin-dependent diabetics. *Diabetes Res* 1986;3:131–134.

Blankenship GW: Diabetic macular edema and argon laser photocoagulation: A prospective randomized study. *Ophthalmology* 1979;86:69–75.

Branch Vein Occlusion Study Group: Argon laser scatter photocoagulation for prevention of neovascularization and vitreous hemorrhage in branch vein occlusion. *Arch Ophthalmol* 1986;104:34–41.

Branch Vein Occlusion Study Group: Argon laser photocoagulation for macular edema in branch vein occlusion. *Am J Ophthalmol* 1984;98:271–282.

Brown GC, Magargal LE, Schachat A, Shah H: Neovascular glaucoma. Etiologic considerations. *Ophthalmology* 1984;91:315–320.

Brown GC, Magargal LE, Simeone FA, et al: Arterial obstruction and ocular neovascularization. *Ophthalmology* 1982;89:139–146.

Brown GC, Shah HG, Magargal LE, Savino PJ: Central retinal vein obstruction and carotid artery disease. *Ophthalmology* 1984;91:1627–1633.

Brown RE, Sabates R, Drew SJ: Metochlopramide as prophylaxis for nausea and vomiting induced by fluorescein. *Arch Ophthalmol* 1987;105:658–659.

Brunette I, Boghen D: Central retinal vein occlusion complicating spontaneous carotid cavernous fistula. Case report. *Arch Ophthalmol* 1987; 105:464–465.

Butner RW, McPherson AR: Adverse reactions in intravenous fluorescein angiography. *Ann Ophthalmol* 1983;15:1084–1086.

Buzney SM, Frank RN, Varma SD, et al: Aldose reductase in retinal mural cells. *Invest Ophthalmol Vis Sci* 1977;16:392–396.

Caird FT: Control of diabetes and diabetic retinopathy, in Goldberg MF, Fine SL (eds): *Symposium on the Treatment of Diabetic Retinopathy*. US Public Health Service Publication No. 1890. Washington, DC, US Government Printing Office, 1969, pp 115–118.

Carter JE: Panretinal photocoagulation for progressive ocular neovascularization secondary to occlusion of the common carotid artery. *Ann Ophthalmol* 1984;16:572–576.

Chopdar A: Dual trunk central retinal vein incidence in clinical practice. *Arch Ophthalmol* 1984;102:85–87.

Christensen JE, Varnek L, Gregersen G: The effect of an aldose reductase inhibitor (sorbinil) on diabetic neuropathy and neural function of the retina: A double-blind study. *Acta Neurol Scand* 1985;71:164–167.

Cogan DG (moderator): Aldose reductase and complications of diabetes. *Ann Intern Med* 1984;101:82–91.

Cunha-Vaz JG, Mota CC, Leite EC, Abreu JR, Ruas MA: Effect of sorbinil on blood–retinal barrier in early diabetic retinopathy. *Diabetes* 1986;35:574–578.

Deutsch TA, Read JS, Ernest JT, Goldstick TK: Effects of oxygen and carbon dioxide on the retinal vasculature in humans. *Arch Ophthalmol* 1983;101:1278–1280.

Diabetic Retinopathy Study Research Group: Preliminary report on effects of photocoagulation therapy. *Am J Ophthalmol* 1976;81:388–396.

Diabetic Retinopathy Study Research Group: Photocoagulation therapy of proliferative diabetic retinopathy: The second report of diabetic retinopathy study findings. *Ophthalmology* 1978;85:82–106.

Diabetic Retinopathy Study Research Group: Four risk factors for severe visual loss in diabetic retinopathy. The third report from the diabetic retinopathy study. *Arch Ophthalmol* 1979;97:654–655.

Diabetic Retinopathy Study Research Group: A modification of the Airlie House classification of diabetic retinopathy. Report number 7. *Invest Ophthalmol Vis Sci* 1981;21:210–226.

Diabetic Retinopathy Study Research Group: Design, methods and baseline results. Report number 6. *Invest Ophthalmol Vis Sci* 1981;21:149–209.

Diabetic Retinopathy Study Research Group: Indications for photocoagulation treatment of diabetic retinopathy. Report number 14. *Int Ophthalmol Clin* 1987;28:239–253.

Dodson PM, Galton DJ, Hamilton JM, Blach RK: Retinal vein occlusion and the prevalence of lipoprotein abnormalities. *Br J Ophthalmol* 1982;66:161–164.

Doft BH, Kingsley LA, Orchard TJ, et al: The association between long-term diabetic control and early retinopathy.*Ophthalmology* 1984;91:1796–1806.

Drury TF, Powell AL: Prevalence, impact, and demography of known diabetes in the United States. *NCHS Advance Data* 1986;114:1–14.

DRVS Research Group: Two-year course of visual acuity in severe proliferative diabetic retinopathy with conventional management. *Ophthalmology* 1985;92:492–501.

Dvornik D, Porte D: *Aldose Reductase Inhibition—An Approach to the Prevention of Diabetic Complications*. New York, Biomedical Information Corporation, 1987.

Dwyer MS, Melton LJ, Ballard DJ, et al: Incidence of diabetic retinopathy and blindness: A population-based study in Rochester, Minnesota. *Diabetes Care* 1985;8:316–322.

Early Treatment Diabetic Retinopathy Study Research Group: Photocoagulation for diabetic macular edema. Report number 1. *Arch Ophthalmol* 1985;103:1796–1806.

Early Treatment Diabetic Retinopathy Study Research Group: Treatment techniques and guidelines for photocoagulation of diabetic macular edema. Report number 2. *Ophthalmology* 1987;94:761–774.

Ellis PP, Schoenberger M, Rendi MA: Antihistamines as prophylaxis against side reactions to intravenous fluorescein. *Trans Am Ophthalmol Soc* 1980;78:190–205.

Ferris FL, Podgor MH, Davis MD: (DRSRG). Macular edema in diabetic retinopathy study patients. Diabetic retinopathy study report number 12. *Ophthalmology* 1987;94:754–760.

Flynn JT, Bancalari E, Bachynski BN, et al: Retinopathy of prematurity. Diagnosis, severity and natural history. *Ophthalmology* 1987;94:620–629.

Friberg TR, Rosenstock J, Sanborn G, et al: The effect of long-term near normal glycemic control on mild diabetic retinopathy. *Ophthalmology* 1985;92:1051–1058.

Frucht J, Shapiro A, Merin S: Intraocular pressure in retinal vein occlusion. *Br J Ophthalmol* 1984;68:26–28.

Gass JD, Tiedeman J, Thomas MA: Idiopathic recurrent branch retinal arterial occlusion. *Ophthalmology* 1986;93:1148–1157.

Gonder JR, Magargal LE, Walsh PN, Raok, Denenberg BE: Central retinal vein obstruction associated with mitral valve prolapse. *Can J Ophthalmol* 1983;18:220–222.

Grey RH, Malcolm N, O'Reilly D, Morris A: Ophthalmic survey of a diabetic clinic. I: Ocular findings. *Br J Ophthalmol* 1986;70:797–803.

Gutman FA: Discussion of macular branch vein occlusion. *Ophthalmology* 1980;87(2):98–104.

Gutman FA, Zegarra H, Rauer A, Zakov N: Photocoagulation in retinal branch vein occlusion. *Ann Ophthalmol* 1981;13:1359–1363.

Gutman FA, Zegarra H: Macular edema secondary to occlusion of the retinal veins. *Surv Ophthalmol* 1984;18(suppl):462–470.

Hansen LL, Daniseyski P, Arntz HR, Ovener G, Wiederholt M: A randomized prospective study on treatment of central retinal vein occlusion by isovolemic hemodilution and photocoagulation. *Br J Ophthalmol* 1985;69:108–116.

Hayreh SS, Hayreh MS: Hemi-central retinal vein occlusion. Pathogeneses, clincial features, and natural history. *Arch Ophthalmol* 1980;98:1600–1609.

Hayreh SS, March W, Phelps CD: Ocular hypotony following retinal vein occlusion. *Arch Ophthalmol* 1978;96:827–833.

Hedges TR Jr, Giliberti OL, Magargal LE: Intravenous digital subtraction angiography and its role in ocular vascular disease. *Arch Ophthalmol* 1985;103:666–669.

Herman WH, Sinnock P, Brenner E, et al: An epidemiologic model for diabetes mellitus: Incidence, prevalence and mortality. *Diabetes Care* 1984;7:367–371.

Hunter JE: Oral fluorography in retinal pigment epithelial detachment. *Am J Optom Physiol Opt* 1982;59:926–928.

Hunter JE: Oral fluorography in papilledema. *Am J Optom Physiol Opt* 1983;60:908–910.

Jalkh AE, Avila MP, Zakka KA, Trempe CL, Schepens CL: Chronic macular edema in retinal branch vein occlusion: Role of laser photocoagulation. *Ann Ophthalmol* 1984;16:526–529, 532–533.

Jerneld B, Algvere P: The prevalence of retinopathy in insulin-dependent juvenile-onset diabetes mellitus—A fluorescein angiographic study. *Acta Ophthalmol (Copenh)* 1984;62:617–630.

Joffe L, Goldberg RE, Magaragal LE, Annesley WH: Macular branch vein occlusion. *Ophthalmology* 1980;87:91–97.

Kahn HA, Moorehead HB: Statistics on blindness in the model reporting area 1969 to 1970. U.S. Department of Health, Education and Welfare Publication No. (NIH) Washington, DC, 73-427.

Kinoshita JH: Aldose reductase in the diabetic eye. *Am J Ophthalmol* 1986;102:685–692.

Klein R, Davis MD, Moss SE, Klein BE, DeMets DL: The Wisconsin epidemiological study of diabetic retinopathy. *Adv Exp Med Biol* 1985;189:321–335.

Klein R, Klein BE, Moss SE, Davis MD, DeMets DL: Retinopathy in young-onset diabetic patients. *Diabetes Care* 1985;8:311–315.

Kraushar MF, Brown GC: Retinal neovascularization after branch retinal artery occlusion. *Am J Ophthalmol* 1987;104:294–296.

Liggett PE, Lean JS, Barlow WE, Ryan SJ: Intraoperative argon endophotocoagulation for recurrent vitreous hemorrhage after vitrectomy for diabetic retinopathy. *Am J Ophthalmol* 1987;103:146–149.

Lipson LG: Diabetes in the elderly: Diagnosis, pathogenesis, and therapy. *Am J Med* 1986;80:10–21.

Little HL: Pathogenesis, in L'Espérance FA, James WA (eds): *Diabetic Retinopathy: Clinical Evaluation and Management.* St. Louis, Mosby, 1981, pp 58–88.

Magargal LE, Brown GC, Augsburger JJ, Parrish RK: Neovascular glaucoma following central retinal vein obstruction. *Ophthalmology* 1981;88:1095–1101.

Mason G: Iris neovascular tufts. *Ann Ophthalmol* 1980;12:420–422.

Mazze RS, Sinnock P, Deeb L, et al: An epidemiological model for diabetes mellitus in the United States: Five major complications. *Diabetes Res Clin Pract* 1985;1:185–91.

McDonald HR, Verre WP, Aaberg TN: Surgical management of idiopathic epiretinal membranes. *Ophthalmology* 1986;93:978–983.

McGrath MA, Wechsler F, Hunyor ABL, Penney R: Systemic factors contributory to retinal vein occlusion. *Arch Intern Med* 1978;138:216–220.

Mitchell P: Development and progression of diabetic eye disease in Newcastle (1977–1984): Rates and risk factors. *Aust NZ J Ophthalmol* 1985;13:39–44.

Minturn J, Brown GC: Progression of nonischemic central retinal vein obstruction to the ischemic variant. *Ophthalmology* 1986;93:1158–1162.

Morgan KS, Franklin RM: Oral fluorescein angioscopy in aphakic children. *J Pediatr Ophthalmol Strabismus* 1984;21:33–36.

Noble MH, Cheng H, Jacobs PM: Oral fluorescein and cystoid macular edema: Detection in aphakic and pseudophakic eyes. *Br J Ophthalmol* 1984;68:221–224.

Novotny HR, Alvis DL: A method of photographing fluorescein in circulating blood in the human retina. *Circulation* 1961;24:82–86.

Olk RJ: Modified grid argon (blue–green) laser photocoagulation for diffuse diabetic macular edema. *Ophthalmology* 1986;93:938–950.

Oral Fluorescein Study Group: Oral fluorography. *J Am Optom Assoc* 1985;10:784–792.

Pacurariu RI: Low incidence of side effects following fluorescein angiography. *Ann Ophthalmol* 1982;14:32–36.

Patz A, Fine SL: *Interpretation of the Fluorescein Angiogram.* International Ophthalmology Clinics, Boston, Little, Brown, 1977.

Patz A, Schatz H, Berkow JW, Gittelson AM, Ticho U: Macular edema: An overlooked complication of diabetic retinopathy. *Trans Am Acad Ophthalmol Otolaryngol* 1973;77:34–42.

Pfiefer MA: Clinical trials of sorbinil on nerve function. *Metabolism* 1986;35(suppl 1):78–82.

Pitts NE, Vreeland F, Shaw GL, et al: Clinical experience with sorbinil—An aldose reductase inhibitor. *Metabolism* 1986;35(suppl 1):96–100.

Ramsay RC, Knobloch WH, Cantrill HL: Timing of vitrectomy for active proliferative diabetic retinopathy. *Ophthalmology* 1986;93:283–289.

Rosenstock J, Friberg T, Raskin P: Effect of glycemic control on microvascular complications in patients with type I diabetes mellitus. *Am J Med* 1986;81:1012–1018.

Sanborn GE, Magargal LE: Characteristics of the hemispheric retinal vein occlusion. *Ophthalmology* 1984;91:1616–1626.

Schatz H: *Interpretation of Fundus Fluorescein Angiography.* St. Louis, Mosby, 1978.

Sheng FC, Quinones-Baldrich W, Machleder HI, et al: Relationship of extracranial carotid occlusive disease and central retinal artery occlusion. *Am J Surg* 1986;152:175–178.

Shilling JS, Jones CA: Retinal branch vein occlusion: A study of argon laser photocoagulation in the treatment of macular edema. *Br J Ophthalmol* 1984;68:196–198.

Smith RJ: Rubeotic glaucoma. *Br J Ophthalmol* 1981;65:606–609.

Solerte SB, Ferrari E: Diabetic retinal vascular complications and erythrocyte filtrability: Results of a 2-year follow-up study with pentoxifylline. *Pharmatherapeutica* 1985;4:341–350.

Starup K, Larsen HW, Enk B, Vestermark S: Fluorescein angiography in diabetic children. *Acta Ophthalmol* 1980;58:347–354.

Tasman W, Magargal LE, Augsburger JJ: Effects of argon laser photocoagulation on rubeosis iridis and angle neovascularization.

Thompson JT, de Bustros S, Michels R, Rice TA: Results and prognostic factors in vitrectomy for diabetic traction detachment of the macula. *Arch Ophthalmol* 1987;105:497–502.

Thompson JT, de Bustros S, Michels R, Rice TA, Glaser BM: Results of vitrectomy for proliferative diabetic retinopathy. *Ophthalmology* 1986;93:1571–1574.

Trempe CL, Takahashi M, Topilow HW: Vitreous changes in retinal branch vein occlusion. *Ophthalmology* 1981;88:681–687.

Vision Research Center: A national plan: 1978–1982. National Advisory Eye Council 1977. U.S. Department of Health, Education and Welfare Publication (NIH) No. 78–1258.

Wilson PM, Anderson KM, Kannel WB: Epidemiology of diabetes mellitus in the elderly. The Framingham Study. *Am J Med* 1986;80:3–9.

Yamana Y, Ohnishi Y, Taniguchi Y, Ikeda M: Early signs of diabetic retinopathy by fluorescein angiography. *Jpn J Ophthalmol* 1983; 27:218–227.

Zegarra H, Gutman FA, Conforto J: The natural course of central retinal vein occlusion. *Ophthalmology* 1979;86:1931–1942.

Zegarra H, Gutman FA, Zakov N, Carim M: Partial occlusion of the central retinal vein. *Am J Ophthalmol* 1983;96:330–357.

3

Exudative and Nonexudative Macular Disorders

INTRODUCTION

The clinician is well aware of the importance of maintenance of integrity of the macular area of the retina. The concentration of photoreceptors in this area requires an exquisite vascular supply for proper function. This complex and active vascular supply makes the macular area particularly susceptible to compromise. Often this compromise can be predicted, and with proper and timely intervention, severe loss of vision can be averted. Prevalence of the various macular disorders is on the rise because of the relationship of macular disease to age, coupled with the increasing age of the world population. To understand diagnosis and management of macular disease, the clinician must first have a working knowledge of the clinicopathology of the macular region of the retina.

RETINAL ANATOMY RELEVANT TO THE MACULOPATHIES

Grossly, the central posterior portion of the eye is clinically known as the posterior pole. The area is usually considered to be demarcated by the major vascular arcades. The diagrammatic representation is shown in Figure 3–1. The macula is about 1.5 mm centered around the 0.35-mm fovea. The macular region is brownish yellow as compared to the remainder of the retina. The yellow coloration is due to xanthophyll pigment and is more apparent in darkly pigmented individuals. This yellow pigment combined with high-density retinal pigment epithelium (RPE) creates blockage of background choroidal fluorescence in all phases. The area devoid of retinal capillaries surrounding the fovea is known as the foveal avascular zone and is 0.5 to 0.6 mm in diameter. This portion of the retina receives nutrition from the choriocapillaris.

Sensory Retina

The sensory retina is comprised of nine specific layers. From the vitreous toward the RPE the retina consists of the (1) internal limiting membrane, (2) nerve fiber layer, (3) ganglion cell layer, (4) inner plexiform layer, (5) inner nuclear layer, (6) outer plexiform layer, (7) outer nuclear layer, (8) external limiting membrane, and (9) rod and cone inner and outer portions. For this clinical discussion these nine layers will be referred to as the sensory retina. The retinal pigment epithelium binds loosely to the sensory retina; then Bruch's membrane binds more solidly to the RPE. Underneath Bruch's membrane is the swamplike choroid/choriocapillaries. The sclera envelopes the entire package.

The retinal structure is markedly different in the macular zone. In the central fovea the only layer present is the photoreceptor layer. The majority of cells in this area are cones. As the fovea unfolds up the clivus, the retina accumulates additional layers from the outer retina inward. Very near the fovea,

THE CLINICAL POSTERIOR RETINA

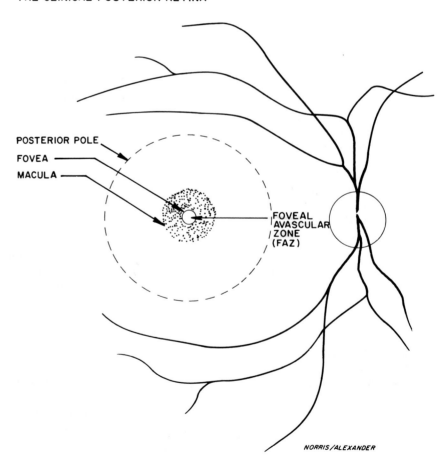

Figure 3–1. A schematic representation of the clinical posterior retina.

NORRIS/ALEXANDER

the outer plexiform layer forms the thickened Henle's layer. This variation of structure in the macular zone lends to the characteristic patterns that develop in many disease processes, such as cystoid macular edema.

RPE

The RPE is a uniform single layer of cells that is situated between the sensory retina and Bruch's membrane. The cells of the RPE are cuboidal, are usually heavily pigmented (melanin granules in cytoplasm), and are hexagonal in shape. The cells have a reasonably tight junction to one another. The RPE functions to hold structures together, provides a barrier to the swamplike choroid, processes metabolites, and absorbs light.

Bruch's Membrane

Bruch's membrane functions with the RPE to provide a barrier and supportive system to the retina. Bruch's membrane is considered to consist of five layers: (1) the basement membrane of the RPE, (2) the inner collagenous zone, (3) the elastic layer, (4) the outer collagenous zone, and (5) the basement membrane of the choriocapillaris.

Choroid/Choriocapillaris

The choriocapillaris layer is the capillary structure adjacent to Bruch's membrane. The short posterior ciliary arteries, the recurrent branches of the long ciliary arteries, and the branches of the anterior ciliary arteries provide the arterial blood supply to this area. This area drains into the vortex veins. The vessels in the choriocapillaris are fenestrated, allowing for a free exchange of fluids with surrounding tissues. The choriocapillaris is densest beneath the macula. The density at the macula allows for the necessarily high hemodynamic activity and creates the potential for multitudes of vascular-related disease conditions.

The choroidal stroma lies external to the choriocapillaris. The choroid is comprised of blood vessels, nerves, immune cells, fibroblasts, collagenous supportive tissue, and melanocytes. The larger choroidal vessels seen by ophthalmoscopy are usually veins. The presence of immunological cells in the choroid speaks to the relationship of choroidal disease to some of the systemic immunological diseases. The suprachoroid lies between the choroid and the sclera. The choroid is responsible for the nutritional (vascular) supply to the RPE and the outer one third of the sensory retina.

Sclera

The entire ocular structure is surrounded by the predominantly acellular sclera, which functions to maintain the shape and integrity of the intraocular contents. The sclera does not actively participate in ocular metabolism.

THE ISSUE OF DRUSEN

Retinal drusen have been put in a big clinical diagnostic pot, have been stirred up by many clinicians, and have yielded a totally confusing diagnostic soup. The drusen may take on multiple clinical presentation, and the only for-sure thing about drusen is that if you see them in one eye, you should see a mirror image in the fellow eye. If you do not, you may be seeing something other than drusen.

While neither the true pathogenesis nor the total implications of drusen are entirely understood, it is known that drusen do represent an altered state of the metabolically healthy retinal complex. If multiple extramacular drusen are present, there is an over 80 percent chance of macular degenerative abnormalities as compared to only a 2 percent chance in the population without drusen.

Drusen have been described as hyaline deposits lying underneath the retinal pigment epithelium. Drusen are associated with retinal pathology, Bruch's membrane disease, choriocapillaris and choroidal disease, retinal pigment epithelial disease, systemic diseases such as diabetes, and space-occupying lesions of the choroid such as benign choroidal melanomas.

The retinal pigment epithelium/Bruch's membrane complex is the area of activity in the genesis of drusen. The RPE is derived from the neuroectoderm and acts to maintain the health of the outer retinal layers. The RPE forms an outer blood-retina barrier, is integral in vitamin A metabolism, works in the transport of metabolites between the choriocapillaris/choroid complex and the retina, manufactures extracellular mucopolysaccharides, functions to eliminate damaged and discarded photoreceptor outer segments, and also works to envelop and negate the effects of developing choroidal neovascular nets. There is a strong juncture between RPE cells known as the zonula occludens that prevents significant fluid seepage between the choriocapillaris and the retina. The metabolism of the RPE is intimately related to the health of the choriocapillaris. It is also important to note that the RPE is tightly adherent to Bruch's membrane and very loosely adherent to the overlying retina.

When RPE cells are not functioning properly, they elaborate an extracellular material such as collagen and basement membrane material that is deposited or "spit out" onto Bruch's membrane. The resulting excrescences are called drusen and are composed of mucopolysaccharides and lipids. The triggering mechanism is unknown but is thought to be related directly to choriocapillaris disease.

When considering drusen in the macular area, the health of the choriocapillaris has an intimate relationship. The choriocapillaris supply to the macular area is derived primarily from arterioles coming from the short posterior ciliary arteries. These arterioles terminate in small compartments. In the eyes of patients with age-related macular disease (ARM), there is a narrowing of the capillary lumen, foci of atrophy of the capillaries, and a loss of cellularity of the capillaries. This situation may create a condition of "zone hypoxia" such as that which occurs overlying a benign choroidal melanoma (choroidal nevus). This "zone hypoxia" results in a "sick" RPE area that creates the deposition of drusen. The concept of local or "zone hypoxia" is supported by the occurrence of drusen with systemic vascular diseases such as cardiovascular disease, hypertension, and diabetes.

Drusen may then progress to further changes that can impact on the health and architectural integrity of the overlying retina. The drusen are, however, observable in well over 70 percent of the population over the age of 50 years but do not negatively affect all of those eyes. As the deposition of the drusen increases with age, the RPE cells undergo further thinning and loss of function. In addition, there are fibrovascular changes within the drusen. There can be a variable color presentation that is associated with lipofuscin accumulation. These zones of drusen may progress on toward cal-

cification (Fig. 3–2) and the development of rifts in Bruch's. The final aging change that occurs related to drusen is the accumulation of granular deposits near the drusen lying between the RPE and Bruch's. These areas of deposition seem to be the actual sites of ingress of choroidal neovascularization. It is well recognized that small, discrete drusen are less likely to be associated with choroidal neovascularization than larger soft "drusen." What in fact may be occurring is the deposition of drusen in the classical sense with nearby granular deposits in a larger area giving the appearance of soft confluent drusen. These soft confluent drusen may be localized zones of RPE detachment.

Drusen are then signs of RPE abnormalities that are not necessarily an assurance that atrophy of the overlying retina will occur or that choroidal neovascularization will occur, leading to exudative maculopathy. The only "for-sure" is that the appearance of large, soft, fuzzy-white "drusen" indicates an ill RPE that may be conducive to exudative maculopathy. These fuzzy-white drusen may be referred to as choroidal infiltrates.

One last point to be made is that the risk of choroidal neovascularization and exudative maculopathy decreases as RPE atrophy progresses. Further progression of RPE atrophy indicates poor choroidal vascular perfusion. If the vessels are dying, it is impossible to support new vessel growth. Therefore, when significant RPE loss occurs or if drusen calcify with cholestrin crystal deposition, the possibility of growth of neovascularization is reduced. **See color plates 42 and 43.**

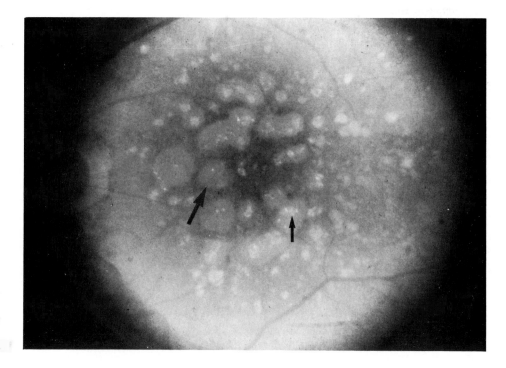

Figure 3–2. A photograph demonstrating "drusen" variations. The large arrow points to a large "soft drusen." The small arrow points to areas of calcification within drusen.

THE ISSUE OF CHOROIDAL NEOVASCULARIZATION AND RPE DETACHMENT

Once an alteration of Bruch's membrane occurs, there is the possibility of choroidal neovascular growth and infiltration under the retinal pigment epithelium or sensory retina or both (Figs. 3–3 through 3–9). There is also the possibility that seepage through the alterations may occur, creating a localized RPE detachment. The primary area of concern within the retina is the macular zone, as the hemodynamic activity is very high in this area and small changes in oxygenated blood flow can create dramatic changes in function and structure.

Detachment of the RPE without choroidal neovascularization can occur. This usually occurs associated with other signs of RPE dysfunction such as drusen. In over 90 percent of cases of RPE detachment, an associated sensory detachment occurs as well. The diagnosis of the RPE detachment requires a combination of stereoscopic observation and fluorescein angiography. When the detachment occurs without hemorrhage, the appearance is a dome with turbid intralesional fluid that may have accompanying hard exudate deposition. On fluorescein angiography, the lesion glows early and evenly and remains stained late into the process. The presence of an RPE detachment does not necessarily guarantee the presence of a choroidal neo-

vascular net. It is possible to have spontaneous RPE detachment remission or progression toward further retinal destruction. Choroidal neovascularization can occur in many ocular disease processes. A number of these are listed in Table 3–1.

There are several routes of retinal destruction associated with choroidal neovascularization. All routes of destruction start with the growth of a neovascular net up through an area of compromise in the RPE/Bruch's complex. This neovascular net initially appears as a gray-green area. This appearance occurs as the result of fibrosis accompanying the new vessels. As the fibrosis progresses, the color becomes yellowish. With the development of the net there is RPE hyperplasia and leakage, causing RPE or sensory retinal elevation or both. This elevation creates metamorphopsia or vision reduction or both. This fluid accumulation of the sensory retinal detachment is to be contrasted with that of idiopathic central serous choroidopathy (ICSC). The fluid in ICSC is clear, and that associated with choroidal neovascularization creating a sensory retinal detachment is turbid due to protein extravasation. The RPE detachment associated with choroidal neovascularization is often indistinguishable from a leak-induced RPE detachment until fluorescein angiography is performed. In all cases of choroidal neovascularization, fluorescein angiography will demonstrate an early-onset, hot-spot–spoked wheel that spreads to include the entire area of leakage.

Evolution of Choroidal Neovascular Nets

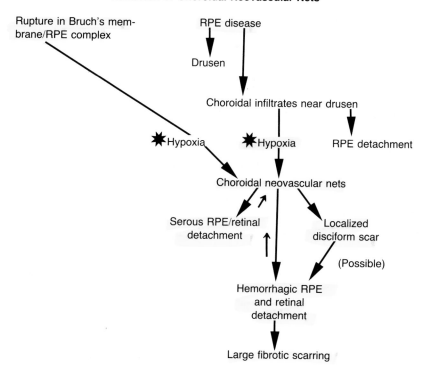

Figure 3–3. A flow chart demonstrating the stages in the evolution of choroidal neovascular nets.

THE BREAKDOWN OF BRUCH'S MEMBRANE

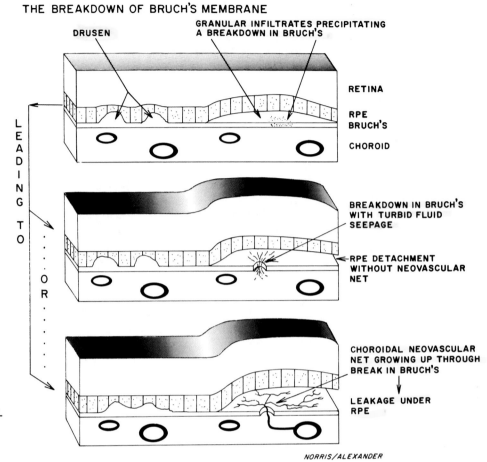

Figure 3–4. This figure illustrates alterations of Bruch's membrane in the form of drusen and granular infiltration. The granular infiltration allows for choroidal neovascular net development.

The neovascular net may regress if enveloped by RPE, or it may progress to hemorrhage or disciform scarring. When the net hemorrhages, blood first accumulates between Bruch's and the retinal pigment epithelium. The hemorrhage at this phase is gray green. Should the hemorrhage spread through the RPE into the subretinal space, it will assume a reddish coloration. This type of hemorrhage has also been known to break through into the vitreous cavity. In all stages, subretinal and intraretinal exudate is possible and is classically known as Coat's response. In fact, hard exudate formation in the absence of ophthalmoscopically visible retinal vascular disease is a very strong indicator of choroidal neovascular disease.

During the involutional stage, the hemorrhage can organize with accompanying fibrotic scarring, resulting in severe, widespread retinal destruction and a resultant extensive central scotoma.

The neovascular net may also pursue a more insidious course of development. The net may grow, being somewhat retarded by disciform scarring and RPE hyperplasia. The development of the disciform scar complex will initially limit the totality of retinal destruction and limit the size of the central scotoma. This scar may, however, reactivate, leading to a more destructive hemorrhagic scar. **See color plates 44 through 50.**

AGE-RELATED MACULAR DEGENERATION

Age-related macular degeneration (ARM) is the number one cause of legal blindness in the United States in persons over 60 years of age. The Framingham Eye Study reports rates of up to 7 percent of the aged population.

There are two distinct forms of ARM, with variations within these categories. The more common form of ARM is dry ARM, or geographic retinal pigment epithelial atrophy. This is present in about 15 percent of eyes by the age of 80 years. Of the patients with ARM who are not legally blind, about 90 percent have dry ARM. The less common form of ARM is wet ARM. Wet ARM can be of several forms: (1) choroidal neovascularization, (2) exudative degeneration, (3) hemorrhagic degeneration

THE POSSIBLE CONSEQUENCES OF CHOROIDAL NEOVASCULARIZATION

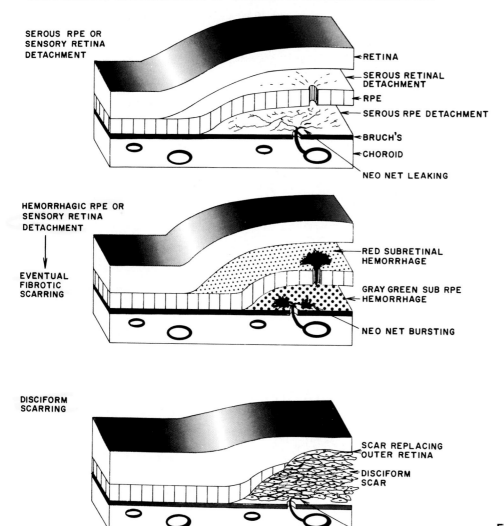

Figure 3–5. The possible consequences of the development of choroidal neovascularization.

NORRIS/ALEXANDER

leading to fibrotic scarring, and (4) disciform macular degeneration. Of the patients who are legally blind from ARM, about 90 percent have the wet variety. In both cases, the presence of RPE/Bruch's disease seems to be the precursor.

While etiology and predisposing factors are uncertain, some reports suggest a familial tendency in the development of ARM. One interesting finding is that the more lightly pigmented the iris is in a patient, the more likely the patient is to develop ARM at an earlier age.

The distinction between wet and dry ARM is crucial, as the severe vision loss of wet ARM may be delayed or prevented by timely photocoagulative intervention. The more benign dry ARM will now be differentiated from the potentially vision-threatening wet ARM.

Dry ARM

Appearance and Layers Involved. Discussion of dry ARM is a direct extension of the previous section on RPE/Bruch's membrane abnormalities. Patients with macular drusen are at an increased risk to develop ARM both dry and wet. Both an increase in the incidence of drusen and dry ARM occur in patients over 60 years of age.

From an ophthalmoscopic view, there is initially an observable alteration of the RPE in dry ARM (Fig. 3–10). This is bilateral and eventually symmetrical. There are areas of depigmentation, areas of granular clumping of RPE, and areas of RPE hyperplasia. Patterns are unpredictable. With time these areas of "RPE change" may coalesce into geographical patterns.

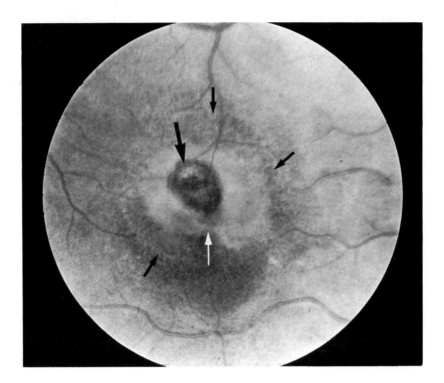

Figure 3-6. A photograph of a neovascular net **(large black arrow)** creating a sensory retinal elevation, the limits of which are indicated by the small black arrows. The white arrow indicates the notch in the sensory elevation at the fovea that occurs because of the anatomic resistance in this area.

From a clinicopathologic standpoint it appears that there is initially a change noted in the RPE cells that may be the result of isolated poor vascular supply from the choriocapillaris. The RPE cells eventually undergo complete degeneration resulting in photoreceptor loss. This creates a situation where the inner nuclear layer actually comes in contact with Bruch's membrane. The outer retinal layers then degenerate. In the past it was thought that the underlying choriocapillaris was also lost, but recent work implies that it is kept intact. **See color plate 43.**

Signs and Symptoms. Dry ARM creates a variable degree of loss of central vision that invariably becomes bilateral. Because of loss of cone function, color vision may also be compromised. It is well known that "wet forms" of degeneration may coexist with the dry forms, and therefore other symptoms such as metamorphopsia may present.

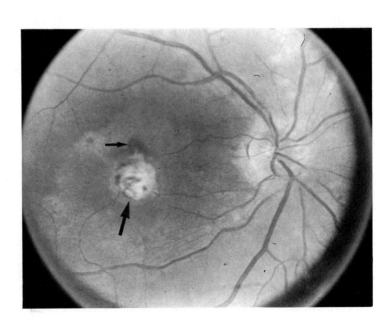

Figure 3-7. This photograph illustrates a "golf-ball" disciform sear **(large arrow)** and subretinal hemorrhage **(small arrow)** secondary to a choroidal neovascular net.

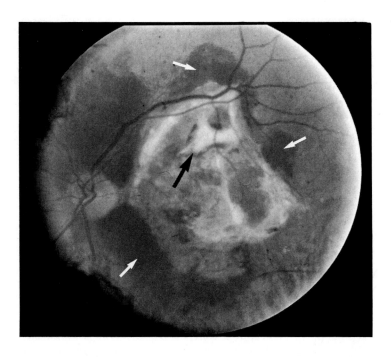

Figure 3–8. An example of a hemorrhagic retinal detachment secondary to a ruptured neovascular net. The small white arrows point to residual hemorrhage, while the large black arrow points to scarring.

Prognosis and Management. Visual acuity is rarely reduced to legal blindness in dry ARM. The primary goal in management of the patient with dry ARM is education and maximizing usable vision. The patient must be educated regarding the potential of progression of dry ARM to wet ARM. These individuals must be on some form of home monitoring and must be followed on routine intervals (every 3 to 12 months). Should signs of "soft drusen" or other exudative signs develop (hard exudates or intraretinal hemorrhages), fluorescein angiography must be performed. At this point in time it is difficult to accurately predict which, if any, of the patients with dry ARM will convert to wet ARM. It has been suggested that as drusen calcify and as RPE disappears, the risk of progression to wet ARM in that area is virtually nonexistent. My conservative approach is to assume the worst, to cover for the possibility, and to be ecstatic when nothing occurs.

To maximize usable vision, the doctor must provide the best prescription, low-vision devices, and patient education regarding eccentric viewing.

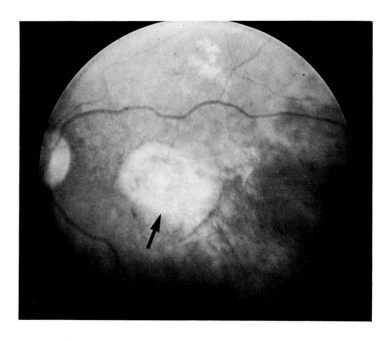

Figure 3–9. An example of a large disciform scar associated with wet age-related maculopathy.

TABLE 3–1. CONDITIONS ASSOCIATED WITH CHOROIDAL NEOVASCULAR DEVELOPMENT

Wet age-related maculopathy

Presumed ocular histoplasmosis

Inflammatory chorioretinal diseases

Postphotocoagulative scarring

Angioid streaks

Degenerative myopia

Choroidal rupture

Dominant drusen

Vitelliform dystrophy

Optic nerve head drusen—even at a very young age

Benign choroidal melanoma

Rubella retinopathy

Harada's disease

APMPPE

Osseous choroidoma

Geographical helicoid peripapillary choroidopathy

Retinal hamartomas

Cryosurgery

Behçet's disease

Chronic uveitis

Idiopathic

DRY ARM—PEARLS

- Usually over age 60 years
- Granular disorganization of the RPE in macula/RPE hyperplasia
- Degeneration of outer retinal layers
- Variable bilateral loss of central vision, color vision compromise
- Rare severe loss of central vision
- Management
  - Patient education and home monitoring of vision
  - Maximize visual correction
  - Follow patient at 3 to 12-month intervals
  - Fluorescein angiography and retinology consult if threat of "wet" arm

Wet ARM

Appearance and Layers Involved. It has long been regarded that drusen are the visible precursors of wet ARM even though the neovascular growth actually occurs away from visible drusen in areas of RPE/Bruch's breakdown. If a patient has bilateral macular drusen, it appears that about 10 percent develop exudative maculopathy over a 4.3 year period. It is suspected that extramacular drusen and macular degeneration have similar pathogenic mechanisms.

As suggested previously, wet ARM may assume four patterns: (1) choroidal neovascularization, (2) exudative degeneration, (3) hemorrhagic degeneration, and/or (4) disciform degeneration (Fig. 3–11).

Choroidal neovascularization occurs as the result of disruption in the RPE/Bruch's barrier. New ves-

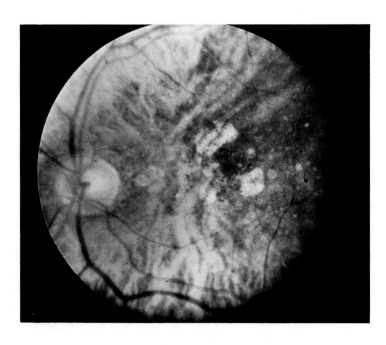

Figure 3–10. This photograph illustrates an example of dry ARM. The ophthalmoscopic picture of this disease presents in many ways but usually has drusen, RPE clumping, and areas of RPE atrophy.

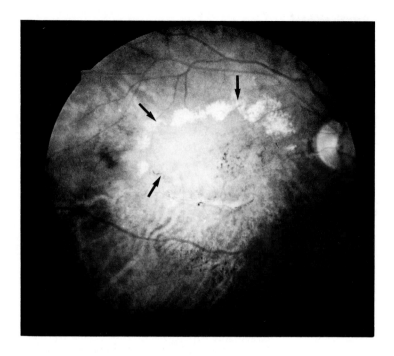

Figure 3–11. An example of hard exudates (Coat's response) surrounding an area of sensory retinal elevation created by a leaking choroidal neovascular net. Note the RPE clumping and loss of choroidal detail. One of the many presentations of wet ARM.

sels from the choriocapillaris grow up through the disruption in Bruch's in response to a hypoxic stimulus. The neovascularization may then (1) leak, creating an RPE detachment or a sensory retinal detachment; (2) hemorrhage, creating a sub-RPE or subretinal hemorrhage; or (3) form a disciform scar. Whichever option is pursued, the results are visually devastating. The section on choroidal neovascularization outlines all options in detail. **See color plate 51.**

Signs and Symptoms. Often the only complaint of a patient with evolving wet ARM is reduced vision, distorted vision, or color distortion. Unfortunately a lot of patients come into the office after irreversible damage has already occurred. When this occurs the best option is to guard against involvement of the fellow eye. **See color plates 49 and 50.**

Prognosis and Management. Untreated, prognosis for usable vision in wet ARM is poor. Functional vision, such as reading large print, currency discrimination, and color recognition, is known to be significantly better with better Snellen acuity. It is best to attempt some sort of intervention within reasonable guidelines rather than tempt fate relying on natural progression. The goal is maintenance of the best possible vision.

Primary care practitioners must recognize the early signs of the evolution of wet ARM. All elderly patients with macular drusen should be placed on

home monitoring systems to be used daily and should be followed at least at yearly intervals. All elderly patients with unexplained vision reduction or distortion should be suspected of having choroidal neovascularization or retinal pigment epithelial detachments until proven otherwise. The appearance of soft drusen—really choroidal infiltrates or RPE detachments—should heighten the practitioner's suspicion. All hard exudates or hemorrhages in the macular area in the absence of documented retinal vascular disease should alert the practitioner to the possibility of choroidal neovascular nets. All gray-green areas in the macular area should be assumed to be choroidal neovascular nets until disproven by fluorescein angiography. Any unusual appearance in the macular area in an elderly patient that cannot be explained should have a fluorescein angiography evaluation. Should the evolution progress to hemorrhage or disciform scarring, intervention will be of little value.

It is well proven that expertly placed laser photocoagulation applied in a timely manner reduces the risk of severe vision loss for patients with extrafoveal wet ARM degeneration. The elapsed time of choroidal neovascular development is crucial. It has been estimated that at least 75 percent of patients with wet ARM degeneration secondary to choroidal neovascularization pass through a potentially treatable stage. At the same time it has been suggested that only 20 percent of patients with symptoms secondary to choroidal neovascularization will be treatable after eight weeks and only 15 percent after four months. Up to 80 percent of patients with visual symptoms for less than 2 weeks and over 50 percent with symptoms less than 4 weeks will be treatable. There is a small window for success; therefore early detection and rapid intervention are crucial. It should be noted that once the eye is treated, proper follow-up is mandatory, as there is up to a 25-percent recurrence rate, and 12 percent of fellow eyes develop wet ARM.

The type of laser (argon, Krypton, dye) used is at the discretion of the retinal specialist. The theory behind use of the Krypton is that it allows treatment closer to the fovea than argon because of Krypton's specificity for choroidal layers. The same theory applies to dye lasers. Studies of patients with choroidal neovascularization within the foveal avascular zone treated with Krypton laser demonstrated that improvement of stabilization may occur. In addition to these findings, there is a strong argument that the resultant scar created by the Krypton laser will create a smaller scotoma than had the neovascular net progressed naturally. The smaller scar and resultant scotoma create improved functional vision for the patient.

Photocoagulation of retinal pigment epithelial detachments by argon and Krypton laser has also demonstrated some encouraging results. The photocoagulation can actually collapse the detachment, and good results may be achieved if the detachment is away from the fovea.

In all, early recognition and expeditious consultation with a highly competent retinologist is indicated, as the visual prognosis for the forms of wet ARM untreated is very grim.

WET ARM—PEARLS

- In aged patients with drusen/choroidal infiltrates as precursors
- May present as:
  - Choroidal neovascularization—gray-green net
  - Exudative degeneration—hard exudates
  - Hemorrhagic degeneration
  - Disciform degeneration
- Reduced vision or metamorphopsia
- Elderly patients with metamorphopsia or reduced vision should be suspected of neovascular nets and should have fluorescein angiography
- Management
  - If one eye has a disciform scar, assume the other eye will develop vision loss, and monitor appropriately.
  - If there is suspicion of development of a net, ask for a retinology consult.
  - Watch soft choroidal infiltrates carefully, or ask for a retinology consult.

CHOROIDAL NEOVASCULARIZATION RELATED TO CHORIORETINAL SCARRING

The initiating factor in the development of choroidal neovascularization is the disruption in the RPE/Bruch's membrane barrier. Certainly degenerative changes such as ARM can create the situation for the development of alterations in the barrier. There is also the possibility that physical damage to the eye can create the possibility for a disruption in the membranes, leading to neovascular development. There are many possibilities for this disruption, including trauma, postuveitic scarring, postcryopexy scarring, postphotocoagulation scarring, and neovascularization arising from a drainage site after scleral buckling procedures.

Choroidal Ruptures
Choroidal ruptures (Fig 3–12) in the posterior pole are fairly common complications of contusion injuries to the eye. The ruptures are the result of contrecoup shock waves. The ruptures are usually crescentric in nature with the concavity toward the disc. Depending on the severity of the blow, there may be hemorrhages of the following types: intrachoroidal, subretinal pigment epithelium, subretinal, intraretinal, and vitreous. As the hemorrhage resorbs and the retinal and choroidal edema disappear, a scar forms with migration and hyperplasia of the overlying RPE. Despite the damage, the overlying retina and retinal vessels often remain intact.

Vision loss or visual field defects vary considerably, depending upon the severity, the particular area involved, and the extent of retinal edema. The field defect may be larger than that expected because of inherent damage to the nerve-fiber layer. There is no particularly effective management for the acute phase of choroidal rupture.

One of the concerns regarding choroidal rupture is the possibility of delayed onset of complications. It is possible that choroidal neovascularization can occur within the scar up to 5 years after the original trauma. This choroidal neovascularization has the potential toward leakage, hemorrhage, or disciform scarring. Photocoagulation of the developing neovascular net may create variable results, as the RPE/Bruch's membrane barrier is already very fragile from the trauma.

The management of the patient with choroidal rupture in the posterior pole consists of education, monitoring on a yearly interval, home monitoring of vision, and provision of protective eyewear in eye hazard situations. **See color plate 52.**

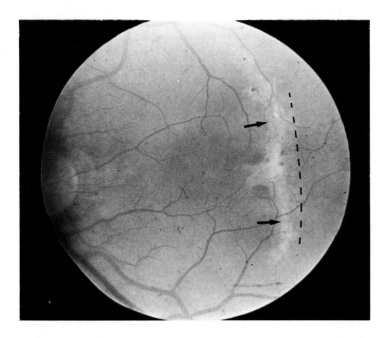

Figure 3–12. An example of a choroidal rupture **(small arrows).** The contour is indicated by the dotted line and follows the contour of the disc.

CHOROIDAL RUPTURES—PEARLS

- Result of blunt trauma
- Crescentic, following contours of the disc
- An active rupture may bleed, then scar
- Vision and visual field loss is variable
- Possibility of development of choroidal neovascularization in zone of scar up to five years later
- Management
  - Patient education and yearly monitoring
  - Home monitoring of vision
  - Protective eyewear

Postphotocoagulative and Postcryopexy Scarring

Photocoagulation and cryopexy have provided the ophthalmic surgeon with effective tools to combat blindness. Unfortunately the scar created by these processes represents a destruction of tissue that may support choroidal neovascular growth when a situation of hypoxia occurs. The first reported cases of choroidal neovascular net development within photocoagulative scars were in association with Eales's disease. Other reports have associated choroidal neovascular net development in sickle cell proliferative retinopathy, sarcoidosis, and diabetic retinopathy. Over 60 percent of photocoagulated proliferative retinopathy has been shown to develop neovascular nets in the scars. It has also been shown that there may be up to a 6-year delay in the development of nets within the scars. **See color plate 53.**

New approaches to photocoagulation have been undertaken to minimize the likelihood of the choroidal neovascularization. The type of photocoagulative procedure that is *most likely* to create a situation conducive to neovascular growth is a combination of small spot size, short exposure durations, high peak power, and retreatment.

Once a neovascular net develops within a scar, it is recommended that no treatment be applied unless there is active hemorrhage. It appears that outcome is better with no intervention.

POSTPHOTOCOAGULATIVE AND POSTCRYOPEXY SCARRING—PEARLS

- Choroidal neovascularization may develop in photocoagulation or cryopexy scars—it may be delayed by six years
- Occurs in Eales' disease, sickle cell proliferative retinopathy, sarcoid retinopathy, and diabetic retinopathy
- Management is prevention by proper photocoagulation and cryopexy. If the net occurs, it appears that the best results occur with no intervention.

DEGENERATIVE OR PATHOLOGICAL MYOPIA

Introduction

Degenerative or pathological myopia differs significantly from the more prevalent refractive myopias in that there is a true alteration of structure of the globe that is progressive and often leads to blindness. True degenerative myopia has a prevalence of only about 2 percent in the United States and seems to have an ethnic predilection for Chinese, Japanese, Arabians, and Jews. While low in prevalence, pathological myopia is the seventh leading cause of blindness in the United States. Associated diseases are listed in Table 3–2.

The clinician cannot rely on refractive error as the sole predictor of pathological myopia, as many highly myopic patients will never progress toward pathological alteration of ocular structure. The diagnosis of degenerative myopia is based primarily on ophthalmoscopically observable signs.

Myopia has been categorized into three easily clinically definable conditions. Stationary myopia typically develops during periods of rapid body growth and rarely exceeds 6 to 9 diopters. While there is an increased incidence of retinal detachment in these individuals, the pathological changes found in degenerative myopia are usually absent. Late myopia begins after bodily growth ceases and is often associated with work conditions. This can best be characterized by the myopia a first-year law student develops associated with an inordinate amount of reading. Degenerative myopia typically develops in youth and progresses through stages as the patient ages. Some individuals are, however, born with staphylomas of the globe that are usually associated with the later stages of development of degenerative myopia. Whether congenital or developmental, the ocular structure changes associated with pathological myopia often lead to vision-threatening complications.

Appearance and Layers Involved

Pathological myopia presents in two stages that are age dependent, the developmental and degenerative stages. Ocular alterations during the developmental stage are the direct result of axial length changes, while the degenerative phase is secondary to vascular changes.

In pathological myopia, the primary alteration is a posterior elongation of the eyeball. This alteration is often age related and as such can be divided into stages. The earliest stages present between

TABLE 3–2. OCULAR AND SYSTEMIC DISEASES ASSOCIATED WITH PATHOLOGICAL MYOPIA

Infantile glaucoma	Ehlers-Danlos syndrome
Ocular albinism	Low birth weight
Pigmentary retinal degeneration	Marfan's syndrome
Retrolental fibroplasia	Maternal alcoholism
Down's syndrome	

birth to the age of 30 years. About 30 percent of patients with pathological myopia have onset at birth, while about 60 percent of patients present from the ages of 6 to 12 years. About 10 percent of patients with pathological myopia present early changes after the age of 12 years.

The elongation of the eyeball in the posterior segment occurs as a result of progressive thinning of the sclera, resulting in a bulge or ectasia. This thinning seems to be the result of meridional collagen-bundle thinning and deformity. The posterior staphylomas (Fig. 3–13) are a poor visual prognostic sign, with over 50 percent of eyes with staphylomas over the age of 60 years being considered legally blind. Some feel that there is a genetic factor involved that initiates abnormal RPE changes leading to scleral degeneration.

The elongation of the globe continues with age, resulting in chorioretinal changes manifesting as patches of choriocapillaris and choroidal atrophy. These patches may coalesce, creating a very dramatic picture. As the choriocapillaris and choroidal complex breaks down, rifts may develop in Bruch's membrane that appear as jagged lines that are known as lacquer cracks. These cracks are known to be mobile from one visit to the next and certainly open an avenue for the genesis of choroidal hemorrhages. Lacquer cracks are seen most often in young men. These lacquer cracks, or breaks, in Bruch's membrane also open the channel for the development of choroidal neovascular nets. These nets usually develop with overlying retinal pigment epithelial hyperplasia and are classically known as Fuch's spots. The onset of the Fuch's spot is typically in the fourth to sixth decade and may be preceded by sensory retinal elevations. The Fuch's spot is similar to the choroidal neovascular net associated with other varieties of exudative maculopathies but has more of a tendency toward hyperplasia of the retinal pigment epithelium. The Fuch's spot may hemorrhage or develop into a disciform scar. Slightly over 5 percent of eyes with degenerative myopia develop a Fuch's spot. Unfortunately, as with other choroidal neovascular nets, there is a predilection for the macular area.

In addition to the extensive choroidal atrophy of the posterior pole (Fig. 3–14), there are peripheral retinal changes that predispose to retinal detachment. Because of the continual stretching of the retina and tugging at the vitreoretinal interface, several retinal changes may develop. These changes include white without pressure, lattice degeneration, atrophic and operculated retinal holes, chorioretinal cobblestone degeneration, retinal breaks, and retinal detachment. The risks of detachment rise significantly with an increase in the extent of myopia.

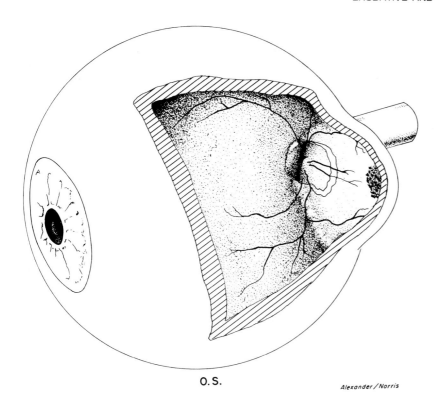

O.S.

Alexander/Norris

Figure 3–13. A schematic illustrating a posterior staphyloma in a left eye in the macular area. The bulging pulls on the edge of the nerve head, creating a temporal scleral crescent and straightening or "dragging" of the vessels exiting the disc.

Structural changes also occur at the optic nerve head but are of no direct threat to vision. With ectasia in the macular area, there is a pulling away of the choroid and retinal pigment epithelium from the edge of the optic nerve head. This results in the classical scleral crescent (Fig. 3–15). Because of this physical tugging, the vessels emanating from the disc that run temporally are also stretched. The disc may also appear tilted toward the ectatic area, with the nasal aspect of the nerve head slightly elevated, known as supertraction. If a posterior staphyloma encircles the disc, the lamina is displaced an-

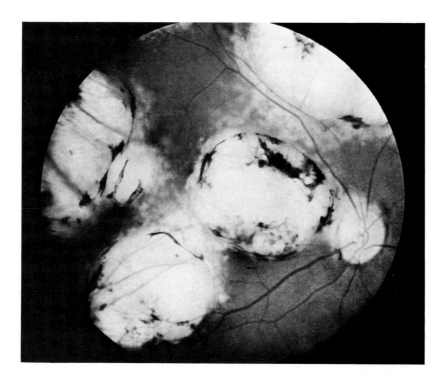

Figure 3–14. Areas of gross choroidal atrophy in pathological myopia.

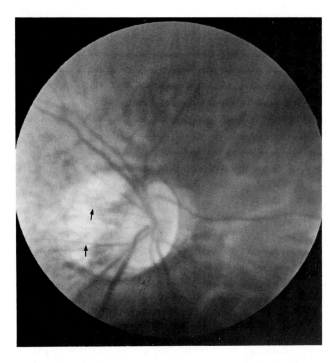

Figure 3–15. A scleral crescent in a highly myopic eye. The small arrows point to straightened disc vessels.

teriorly, and the optic nerve head is elevated above the retina.

Anterior chamber alterations are often present in patients with high myopia secondary to posterior staphylomas. These alterations are iris remnants and increased iris processes. These alterations may lead toward an increased incidence of primary open angle glaucoma in the patient with pathological myopia.

Signs and Symptoms
Pathological myopia is a continuing spectrum of change. Initially the clinician must be concerned about optimizing the refraction. As the degeneration progresses, the retinal changes increase the threat of neovascular nets and retinal detachment. The overall incidence of open-angle glaucoma is also significantly higher, and its detection is complicated by the gross refractive errors and the physically altered disc appearance. The inevitability of some vision compromise is omnipresent.

Prognosis and Management
The patient with pathological myopia must be monitored constantly, especially as he or she ages. With age the incidence of Fuch's spot, peripheral retinal degenerative changes, and glaucoma all increase. With the threat of glaucoma, fields must be performed with a contact lens prescription and a lot of attention to detail. Intervention must be pro-

vided at the first sign of destructive peripheral retinal disease or glaucoma. Intervention with laser application to Fuch's spots provides only equivocal results, but all patients with Fuch's spots should have fluorescein angiography performed. A retinology consultion is advised when a Fuch's spot develops.

DEGENERATIVE MYOPIA—PEARLS

- Developmental stage
  - Posterior elongation of the globe
  - Development of scleral crescent and vessel straightening
  - Peripheral vitreoretinal degenerations
  - Disc tilting and supertraction
- Degenerative stage
  - Patches of choriocapillaris/choroidal atrophy
  - Lacquer cracks
  - Choroidal neovascularization—Fuch's spot
- Increased incidence of primary open-angle glaucoma secondary to anterior chamber alterations
- Management
  - Provision of best possible prescription in protective eyewear
  - Routine monitoring for development of peripheral vitreoretinal disease
  - Routine monitoring for development of neovascular nets
  - Retinology consultation if a Fuch's spot develops

ANGIOID STREAKS

Introduction
Angioid streaks (Fig. 3–16) are an anatomical phenomenon secondary to pathological changes in the retinal pigment epithelium, Bruch's membrane, and the choroid/choriocapillaris. There seems to be a higher prevalence of angioid streaks in whites with an increase in appearance with age. The majority of patients have pseudoxanthoma elasticum, while some patients have Paget's disease, Ehlers-Danlos syndrome, or sickle cell disease. There are, however, some patients with no systemic association whatsoever.

Appearance and Layers Involved
Angioid streaks are manifestations of breaks in thickened and calcified Bruch's membrane. There is then a loss or migration of pigment granules in the RPE. When full thickness breaks occur in Bruch's membrane, there is a disruption of the choriocapillaris, atrophy of the retinal pigment epithelium, and loss of overlying photoreceptor cells. The cracks in Bruch's membrane result in leakage or,

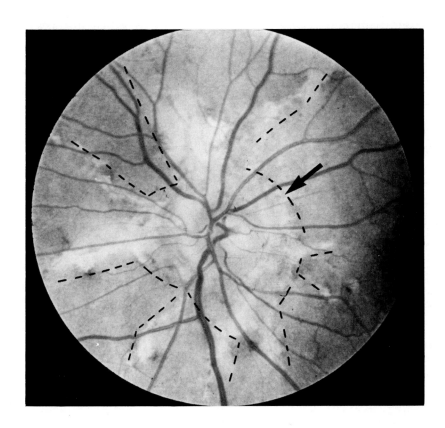

Figure 3–16. An illustration of angioid streaks. The arrow points to the "hub" around the disc, while the dotted lines follow the contour of the streaks emanating from the "hub."

coupled with hypoxia, in development of choroidal neovascular nets. The nets may then develop into disciform scars or hemorrhage, creating a classical exudative maculopathy.

The ophthalmoscopic signs of angioid streaks develop in a characteristic pattern, but all seem to have individuality in their clinical appearance. **See color plate 54.** An area of circumpapillary degeneration appears as the hub for the outward radiation of spokes of irregularly placed, jagged lines. The lines often vary in color from gray, red gray, red brown, to red, depending on the overall ocular pigmentation. In black patients the lines may be enhanced by extensive retinal pigment epithelial migration and proliferation. A mottled fundus appearance (peau d'orange) temporal to the macula may present with or actually precede the development of the streaks. This mottled appearance may extend to the temporal equator. The author has observed this mottled appearance throughout the entire retina with the exception of the macula.

In some cases poorly defined red-brown spots occur in pairs on either side of the light-colored area along the margins of the streaks. These spots are usually less than ½ disc diameter (DD) in size. Another characteristic that may be seen is peripheral focal chorioretinal lesions that are salmon in color and resemble histo spots. When these spots occur along with the peripapillary atrophy and

macular lesions, presumed ocular histoplasmosis may be suspected. Two other fundus characterisitcs, disc drusen and short, verticle lines concentric to the disc margins, may also be present with angioid streaks.

Signs and Symptoms

Often signs and symptoms are not present initially with angioid streaks. The patient may enter the office for a routine eye examination, and the streaks may be found on routine binocular indirect ophthalmoscopy. Unfortunately the patient may present at the first sign of vision loss either to a moderate degree, associated with macular degeneration, or to a more severe degree, associated with disciform maculopathy.

Prognosis and Management

Visual compromise can occur in angioid streaks secondary to progression and extension of the cracks in Bruch's membrane into the macular area. A very high percentage of patients develops some form of macular degeneration (dry), creating some vision loss, while others develop choroidal neovascular nets leading to severe vision loss. There seems to be an association of vision loss to trauma even though this may be difficult to elicit in a case history. Studies vary regarding the presence of neovascular membranes, as does the success rate for treating the membrane with photocoagulation. While choroidal neovascularization is a treatable lesion, one must remember that photocoagulation will only further break down an already weakened Bruch's membrane. This further breakdown of Bruch's membrane enhances future development of neovascular nets. If indications and methods are well chosen and there is no alternative, photocoagulation is indicated to abort the development of the net.

In addition to being watchful for the development of neovascular nets with routine examination and home monitoring of vision, it is important to rule out the possibility of associated systemic disease. Pseudoxanthoma elasticum presents in the second to fourth decade of life as changes in the skin of the neck, axillae, inguinal areas, and periumbilical zone. These changes appear as thickened, grooved, inelastic areas. The disease is *autosomal recessive*, so a pedigree may assist in the differential diagnosis. Paget's disease, Ehlers-Danlos syndrome, and sickle cell disease must also be ruled out. The systemic implications of all of these conditions must be addressed. The patient should also be prescribed polycarbonate lenses and be advised against potentially traumatic situations, such as contact sports or occupations at high risk of trauma.

ANGIOID STREAKS—PEARLS

- Associations include pseudoxanthoma elasticum, Paget's disease, Ehlers-Danlos syndrome, sickle cell disease, or associated with no identifiable systemic disease
- Area of circumpapillary degeneration serves as the hub for outward radiation of spokes or breaks in Bruch's membrane.
- Possible peau d'orange appearance temporal to macula and peripheral focal chorioretinal lesions
- May develop macula degeneration and/or choroidal neovascular nets
- Management
  - Watch for development of neovascular nets
  - Schedule retinology consult when indicated
  - Rule out systemic diseases
  - Recommend safety lenses and advise about trauma

ICSC

Introduction
ICSC (Fig. 3–17) is an enigma in that there are transient episodes of serous retinal or pigment epithelial detachments in the posterior pole of eyes of young patients, with none of the common predisposing conditions, such as drusen. The average age in years of onset of ICSC is the mid 30s, with a range in the late 20s to the late 50s. ICSC seems to affect males more than females and whites more than nonwhites.

Appearance and Layers Involved
The initial problem in ICSC seems to originate at the level of the retinal pigment epithelium. The RPE cells are typically strongly adherent to one another and to Bruch's membrane. They are only loosely adherent to the overlying sensory retina. This tight bond prevents leakage from the spongy choroidal layer from seeping up under the sensory retina. Should the RPE be compromised by poor circulation, the cells may break down, allowing the seepage to occur, which creates a sensory retinal detachment. Further breakdown of the RPE bonds may allow a separation from the underlying Bruch's membrane. This precipitates a retinal pigment epithelial detachment. **See color plate 55.**

The breakdown of the RPE has been hypothesized to occur secondary to vasomotor instability or sympathetic nervous excitation. This may create a localized breakdown in choriocapillaris blood supply to the RPE. The propensity of ICSC for the macula speaks to the high hemodynamic activity at the macula. Because of the compromise of the RPE, the practitioner will often find pigmentary migration and hyperplasia associated with ICSC as well as some microcystic changes.

The ophthalmoscopic view of the active condition is variable. Binocular indirect ophthalmoscopy gives the best overall view of the dome of elevated retina. The change is subtle, and the clinician must rely on color variation and reflections from the internal limiting membrane. There is a loss of foveal reflex. The details of the dome are best observed under high magnification with a Hruby or Volk lens. The dome can also be transilluminated to enhance the view. Should the detachment be longstanding, the dome may present with yellow precipitates. The appearance of the precipitates indicates a poorer prognosis for visual recovery as these are a sign of longevity.

Evidence of past bouts of ICSC present as RPE disturbances or cystlike areas in the macula. In most cases of ICSC, the clinician can observe a one third DD or less area of RPE detachment beneath the detached retina. This area is usually yellow and is referred to as a lemon-drop nodule. This nodule may transilluminate as a golden glow. Infrequently this nodule may be larger, sometimes up to 1 DD, and may even lie outside the area of retinal detachment.

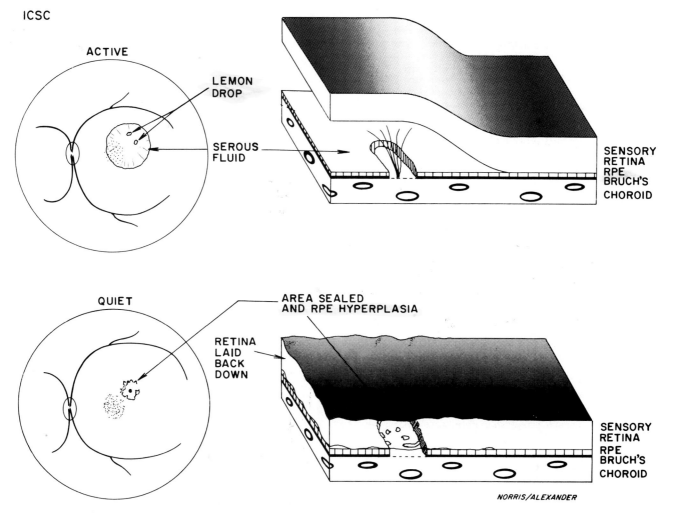

Figure 3–17. A schematic illustrating both active and quiet stages of idiopathic central serous choroidopathy.

In all cases of ICSC, fluorescein angiography (FA) offers the definitive diagnosis. In most cases of ICSC the FA starts as a focal punctate stain that grows in size and holds its fluorescence into the late stages. Ultimately, the stain diffuses into the area of the sensory retinal detachment. The FA will demonstrate no leakage in cases where the RPE has resealed itself.

Signs and Symptoms

ICSC typically presents as a sudden onset of unilateral distortion (metamorphopsia) or slight loss of central vision. The patient may also complain of a haze over vision or a slight color perception problem. Contrast sensitivity will be altered as well as macular photostress recovery time. There may be a unilateral hyperopic shift. General health is usually good, with no particular association with systemic disease. There is, however, often an association with anxiety or stress. Past bouts of ICSC may present as areas of RPE migration and hyperplasia.

Prognosis and Management

ICSC carries a relatively good prognosis with no intervention whatsoever. A very high percentage of patients recover vision to a 20/40 level within one to six months after the onset of symptoms. Up to 60 percent recover vision to the 20/20 level. When associated with the stress of pregnancy, the symptoms typically resolve by the third trimester.

There is always some residual metamorphopsia, but it is rarely noticed by the patient. The major problem associated with ICSC is recurrence. Up to 50 percent of patients have recurrences that may progress to reduced vision associated with RPE atrophy. It is, however, very rare to have permanent vision loss below 20/40. The fellow eye may develop ICSC even after a considerable time delay, but this occurrence is also very rare.

Localized photocoagulation affords the only proven mode of therapeutic intervention. It is believed that under certain circumstances photocoagulation may be effective in sealing the site of RPE damage and leakage. As there is a very strong tendency for excellent spontaneous recovery, photocoagulation must be applied only after strong consideration. Indications for photocoagulation are (1) a patient who is intolerant of symptoms and is willing to take a risk, (2) accumulation of turbid subretinal fluid, (3) severe bouts of recurrence with a direct threat to vision, (4) long-standing cases where photocoagulation is not a direct threat to macular function (ie, leakage point outside of the foveal avascular zone [FAZ], and (5) cases where there is a defect in the fellow eye from recurrent bouts of ICSC.

ICSC—PEARLS

- ICSC occurs in young patients associated with anxiety or stress
- Dome of elevated retina is associated with loss of foveal reflex
- If long-standing, there are yellow precipitates in the area
- The area of swelling shows RPE disturbance and may have a lemon-drop nodule within
- Fluorescein angiography is diagnostic
- Metamorphopsia, delayed photostress recovery, and vision loss are symptoms
- Percentage recovery of vision is high one to six months after bout
- Recurrence rate is high
- Management
  - Reassurance
  - Possible photocoagulation

CYSTOID MACULAR EDEMA

Introduction

Cystoid macular edema (CME) may be secondary to many ocular conditions. These include retinal vaso-occlusive disease, postcataract surgery (Irvine-Gass syndrome), pars planitis, severe carotid or ophthalmic artery disease, retinitis pigmentosa, progressive pigmentary degeneration, YAG laser posterior capsulotomy, relaxing corneal incision, retinal surgery, radiation retinopathy, ocular inflammatory conditions, and ocular tumors. The macular area is very sensitive to fluid accumulation, and as such even remote lesions such as angiomatosis retina can precipitate cystoid macular edema. The clinician must also rule out toxic substances such as epinephrine, as their use may be related to the accumulation of edema in the macular area.

When CME occurs secondary to cataract extraction (Irvine-Gass syndrome), there is usually a delay in onset of the edema. The peak occurrence is usually at about the sixth postoperative week. By using fluorescein studies it has been shown that up to 50 percent of postsurgical aphakic eyes develop CME, but only an extremely small percentage of these are symptomatic. There seems to be no race, age, or sexual predilection for CME.

Appearance and Layers Involved

CME usually is secondary to fluid seeping into the unusual arrangement of fibers in Henle's layer. The etiology of fluid accumulation is sometimes obscure.

The ophthalmoscopic picture is rarely dramatic. Often all that is evident is loss of foveal reflex. When CME is suspected, fluorescein angiography is the definitive diagnostic test. On fluorescein, the radiating cystoid spaces present a glow simulating the petals of a flower.

If the CME is chronic, the cystoid spaces may coalesce, allowing for the development of a lamellar or through-and-through macular hole.

Signs and Symptoms

The patient with CME may complain of variable reduction in vision. This reduction would be most obvious with contrast sensitivity. Slight metamorphopsia may be evident on Amsler grid, and a prolonged photostress recovery time will occur.

As CME is associated with many other ocular conditions, numerous other unrelated signs and symptoms may be present.

Prognosis and Management

Prognosis for untreated Irvine-Gass syndrome is very good, as about 50 percent of eyes recover normal vision in about 6 months. Twenty percent of these patients will, however, have the condition for up to 5 years.

Several studies support use of prostaglandin inhibitors for the treatment of aphakic and pseudophakic CME. Topical indomethacin (1 percent) drops given four times a day for 1 to 4 months to treat or prophylax against CME has been effective. The prostaglandin inhibitor coupled with 1 percent topical corticosteroids may also be of some value. The question still exists as to whether intervention or prophylactic treatment is indicated, as such a small percentage of angiographically proven CME ever creates any visual problem at all. When CME is secondary to another ocular or systemic condition, the associated conditions must always be managed.

If CME stands alone as the primary condition, the intervention question becomes even more clouded. Oral inhibitors of prostaglandins, oral corticosteroids, and topical steroids all have variable efficacy and unpreditable side effects. Periocular corticosteroid injections are likewise unpredictable. Pars plana vitrectomy may be considered if vitreoretinal traction is present. Grid photocoagulation has also produced some positive results.

CME—PEARLS

- Occurs secondary to many ocular or systemic conditions
- Usually loss of foveal reflex as the elevation is subtle
- Fluorescein angiography gives definitive diagnosis—petalliform
- Reduced vision, metamorphopsia, and prolonged photostress recovery may occur along with the signs and symptoms of the precipitating conditions
- Management
  - High percentage of spontaneous recovery
  - Controversy as to the benefit of prostaglandin inhibitors or corticosteroids
  - Possible grid photocoagulation intervention
  - Retinology consult is indicated

MACULAR HOLES

Introduction

The etiology of macular hole formation is somewhat confusing. Trauma with subsequent cystoid macular edema was originally considered the primary causative factor. It is now considered that any condition that precipitates cystoid macular edema may be implicated in the genesis of the macular hole. There is also some thought that macular hole formation may be related to the tugging at the macular area secondary to posterior vitreous detachment. Macular holes usually occur in patients over 60 years of age.

The important aspect of macular hole management is the differentiation of through-and-through macular holes, lamellar holes, and macular cysts, as each condition carries a different prognosis (Figs. 3–18 and 3–19).

Appearance and Layers Involved

A macular hole is a circular to oval depression in the avascular area of the macula. The color variation from the surrounding edematous retina makes identification with the binocular indirect ophthalmoscope quite obvious. Macular cysts are often the result of coalescence of macular cystoid areas into a larger cavity.

Macular holes are usually divided into two distinct entities, lamellar holes and full thickness holes. The lamellar hole is the result of the rupture of the thin, inner retinal layer of a macular cyst. There is a slight reddish coloration of the hole and often a surround of a preretinal membrane. This makes the lamellar hole a partial-thickness macular excavation with some maintenance of visual acuity.

A full-thickness macular hole is an excavation that is either entirely devoid of retinal tissue or has a nondistinguishable outer retinal layer. The classic full-thickness hole is one fourth to one third DD in size, appearing as a reddish area often with a surround of grayish retinal elevation appearing like a doughnut. There are yellowish deposits in the base of the hole that may be migratory. Macular cysts and lamellar holes do not have the dramatic color of a through-and-through hole, but visual acuity and stereoscopic observation are necessary to validate the diagnosis. Retinal glial membranes may also grow onto the surface of the retina surrounding a lamellar or through-and-through macular hole.

In the early arteriovenous phase of fluorescein angiography, a through-and-through hole will demonstrate hyperfluorescence, while a lamellar hole or cyst will hypofluoresce. In the late stages, cysts may hyperfluoresce like true holes. **See color plate 56.**

The end results of solar maculopathy may simulate a true macular hole, but the small size and variable visual acuity of 20/25 to 20/80 often assist in the differential diagnosis. Foveomacular retinitis may also simulate a macular hole. Foveomacular retinitis presents as macular edema followed by a macular cyst surrounded by a one-half to 1 disc diameter gray area. This lesion may then progress to further macular degeneration, resulting in an irregular macular hole and acuity between 20/25 and 5/200.

Signs and Symptoms

Patients with lamellar holes and macular cysts will present with slightly reduced acuity and metamorphopsia in addition to the classic ophthalmoscopic picture. The true macular hole will create significantly reduced visual acuity, a central scotoma, and the potential for the effects of a retinal detachment.

Prognosis and Management

If a patient presents with a macular cyst, there is about a 50 percent chance that this will develop into a hole. Hole development is associated with a posterior vitreous detachment (PVD). The presence of a PVD is a pretty good indicator of stability.

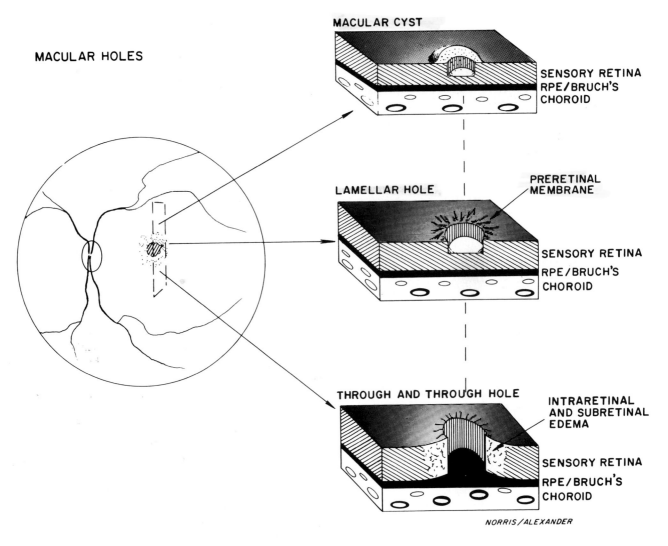

MACULAR HOLES

MACULAR CYST

SENSORY RETINA
RPE/BRUCH'S
CHOROID

LAMELLAR HOLE

PRERETINAL
MEMBRANE

SENSORY RETINA
RPE/BRUCH'S
CHOROID

THROUGH AND THROUGH HOLE

INTRARETINAL
AND SUBRETINAL
EDEMA

SENSORY RETINA
RPE/BRUCH'S
CHOROID

NORRIS/ALEXANDER

Figure 3–18. A schematic illustrating the differences between macular cysts, lamellar macular holes, and through-and-through macular holes.

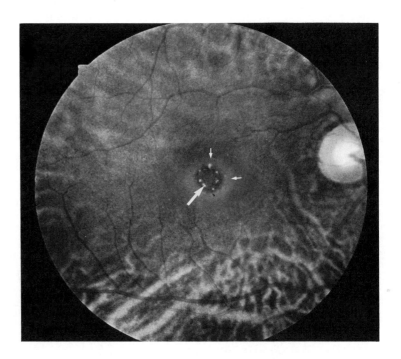

Figure 3–19. A through-and-through macular hole. The small arrows point to the surrounding retinal "edema," while the large arrow points to the yellow deposits in the base of the hole.

184

If a patient has a true macular hole in one eye, there are predictors of hole formation in the fellow eye. If PVD is present in the fellow eye, there is little to no risk of development of a true macular hole. If a PVD is not present, 28 to 44 percent of fellow eyes have been reported to develop macular holes. Patients with pigment epithelial defects in the macula of the fellow eye to a macular hole showed an 80 percent risk of developing a macular hole. Posterior vitreous detachment, RPE defects/disturbances in the macula, and retinal thinning at the macula all represent risk factors for the development of macular holes.

It is not advisable to treat patients with macular holes until retinal detachment has occurred or is an immediate threat. Medical therapy has not proven effective. Secondary retinal detachment of the retina caused by liquefied vitreous seeping under the retina through the hole occurs at a very low rate. When detachment does occur, there is a fairly good success rate with reattachment. Prophylactic photocoagulation is indicated in myopic eyes over 6 D because of the high incidence of secondary detachment.

The clinician has the responsibility of explaining the condition to the patient, mentioning the risk factors for involvement of the fellow eye, providing polycarbonate lenses for protection, advising against avoidable trauma, and re-evaluating at frequent intervals.

MACULAR HOLES—PEARLS

- Usually occurs in patients over 60 years of age
- Lamellar holes
  - Result of rupture of macular cyst, reddish color
  - Partial thickness excavation with metamorphopsia and slightly reduced acuity
  - Often a surround of a preretinal membrane
- Through-and-through hole
  - One fourth to one third DD reddish area with a surround of gray edema
  - Yellow deposits at base
  - Severely reduced acuity and a central scotoma
- Management
  - 50% chance of cyst developing into a hole
  - If macular hole in one eye and PVD in other, little chance of fellow eye developing hole
  - If macular hole in one eye and no PVD in other, 28 to 44% chance of fellow eye developing hole
  - RPE disturbances in fellow eye to macular hole are an 80% risk factor
  - Retinal thinning in fellow eye to macular hole is a risk factor
  - Possibility of retinal detachment but only prophylax in patients over 6 D of myopia
  - Safety lenses and educate to avoid trauma

INFLAMMATORY MACULOPATHIES

Presumed Ocular Histoplasmosis Syndrome

Introduction. Presumed ocular histoplasmosis syndrome (POHS) is a fungal disease endemic in many river valleys of the world. Histoplasmin sensitivity is particularly prevalent in the United States. It is believed that the ocular syndrome is the result of bloodborne histoplasma capsulatum organisms reaching choroidal circulation during a bout of systemic dissemination. It is thought that the fungus is inhaled. Systemic histoplasmosis has a wide variety of presentations, from a flulike illness to a disseminated disease in the young, aged, and immunosuppressed. It must be remembered that Acquired immunodeficiency syndrome (AIDS) has the potential to create reactivation of POHS. Signs of disseminated disease and ocular manifestations do not usually coexist.

Patients typically present with POHS between ages 20 and 50, with rare occurrences outside this range. Macular involvement associated with POHS usually occurs more frequently in patients over the age of 30 years. POHS only rarely occurs in blacks, and when it does occur macular involvement is less than 20 percent of that in whites. POHS has no sexual predilection. Involvement in both maculae occurs more frequently in men than women. It is also important to note that the macular form of the disease may not occur until up to 30 years after the disseminated form appears. It is also of note that the macular form is often precipitated by stress.

Appearance and Layers Involved. POHS is characterized by a triad of circumpapillary choroidal scarring, peripheral atrophic histo (choroidal) spots, and macular compromise secondary to choroidal neovascularization. There is neither the anterior uveitis nor the vitritis, which often accompanies other intraocular inflammatory processes.

The lesions surrounding the optic nerve head resemble the histo spots spread throughout the periphery. The diffuse choroidal inflammation results in choroidal degenerative changes and retinal pigment epithelial hyperplasia. This ring of scarring can be up to 0.5 DD in width. Up to 10 percent of POHS patients develop hemorrhage secondary to choroidal neovascularization in the circumpapillary area. Those who do hemorrhage have a poor prognosis for vision. The changes surrounding the optic nerve head are at the level of the choroid and retinal pigment epithelium, which eventually compromises the overlying retina.

The choroidal granulomatous lesions can also occur spread throughout the retina. The majority of atrophic histo spots occur posterior to the equator and may number up to 70. **See color plate 57.** Bilaterality is the rule (over 60 percent). It is assumed that the histoplasma capsulatum or its byproducts reach the choroidal circulation, creating a granulomatous inflammatory mass that may create breaks in Bruch's membrane on the way to scarring. The active peripheral choroiditis is usually so mild that it is not clinically observable. The lesion typically heals in a few weeks. If these lesions are outside the major temporal vascular supply, the eye will not suffer any associated visual loss. The breaks in Bruch's membrane in peripheral scars rarely lead to neovascularization or serous retinopathy. The peripheral scars are usually 0.2 to 0.7 DD diameters in size and may present with or without retinal pigment epithelial hyperplasia.

Macular lesions of POHS seem to progress through specific stages of development (Figs. 3–20 through 3–23). While the basic pathogenesis is similar to wet ARM, there are usually no drusen as precursors. In stage 1 of POHS maculopathy, a yellowish focus of active choroiditis occurs near the macular area. This may also be considered a choroidal infiltration, as the activity is characterized by fuzzy white borders. These infiltrates are less than 1 DD in size and may remain in a holding pattern indefinitely; but the majority will progress toward the development of exudative macular disease. The clinicopathology of this stage is characterized by a small choroidal granulomatous mass that extends through Bruch's membrane to the retinal pigment epithelium. There is no leakage during fluorescein angiography at this stage.

Stage 2 is characterized by a pigment ring or pigment nodule in the macular area with an overlying sensory retinal serous detachment. These changes occur because of the choroidal neovascular growth through the compromised Bruch's membrane and the reactive retinal pigment epithelial hyperplasia in the area of the lesion. The RPE actually attempts to envelop the growing net and retard its growth. The growing, leaking neovascular net only adds to the development of serous sensory retinal elevation. This stage will be obvious in all stages of fluorescein angiography. This stage may also stop and regress, leaving only a small scotoma.

Stage 3 of POHS consists of hemorrhages emanating from the neovascular net of stage 2. If the hemorrhage occurs under the retinal pigment epithelium, it is gray green, and if it dissects through to the subsensory retinal space, it will appear red. At this stage, lipid exudates may accumulate around the area of serous elevation. The lipid exudate accumulation is considered by some to indicate longevity of the lesion and is often referred to as stage 4.

Stage 5 is considered to be the end stage of the development of maculopathy. This stage usually indicates maculopathy of 2 years or more duration. This is the stage of scarring that is seen as a white elevated lesion, indicating a chronic disciform detachment of the sensory retina with microcystic degeneration. The lesions vary in size up to 1 DD. If hemorrhage has occurred, the scar may be fibrotic

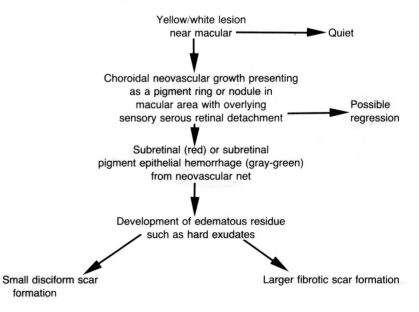

Figure 3–20. A flow chart illustrating the stages in the development of maculopathy of presumed ocular histoplasmosis syndrome.

DEVELOPMENT OF MACULAR LESIONS IN POHS

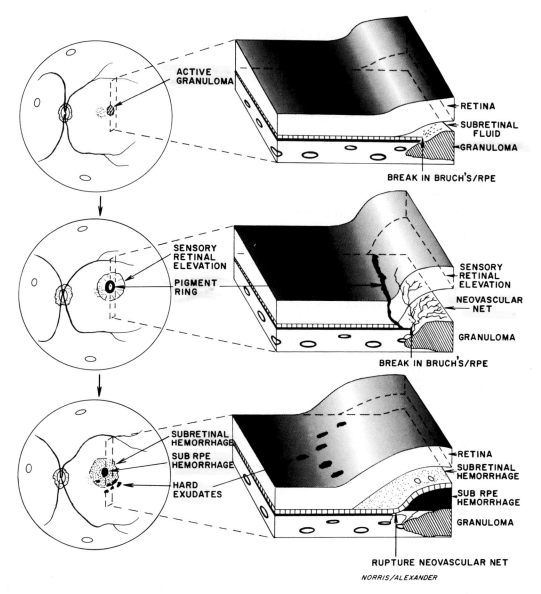

Figure 3–21. A schematic illustrating the stages in the development of macular lesions in presumed ocular histoplasmosis syndrome.

and may have less distinct characteristics. The fibrotic scarring usually occupies more territory than the disciform scar, creating a larger scotoma.

Signs and Symptoms.

The patient with POHS is usually asymptomatic until the macula or circumpapillary area is involved. At that point, vision reduction and metamorphopsia are variable, depending on the proximity of the lesion to the macula. Symptoms of flashing lights, waviness, and field loss may occur with active circumpapillary choroidopathy. Laboratory diagnostic tests are of no value in the differential diagnosis of POHS.

Prognosis and Management.

Once choroidal neovascularization begins near the macular area, the prognosis for good vision is poor. Resultant vision of less than 20/200 occurs in over 60 percent of untreated cases. Bilateral loss of vision occurs in 20 to 30 percent of patients, with a mean onset of the second eye 6 to 7 years after the first. Involvement of the second eye usually results in better acuity than the first.

The key to successful management of POHS is the early detection of stages 1 and 2 macular involvement. In general, the peripheral lesions and the circumpapillary chorioretinal lesions are of no threat to vision. All patients with POHS should be

THE MACULAR SCARS IN POHS

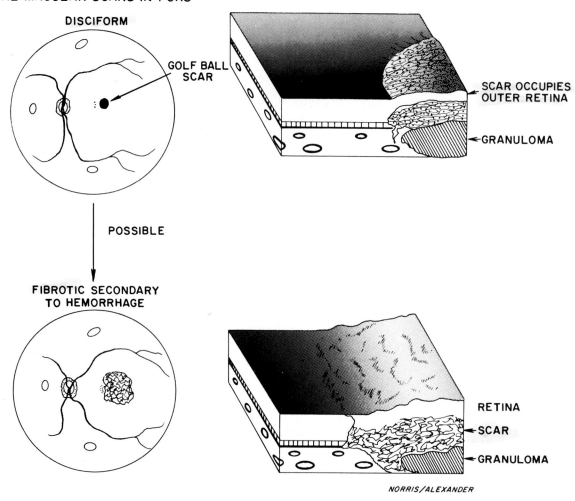

Figure 3–22. A schematic illustrating the development of two types of macular scarring in presumed ocular histoplasmosis syndrome.

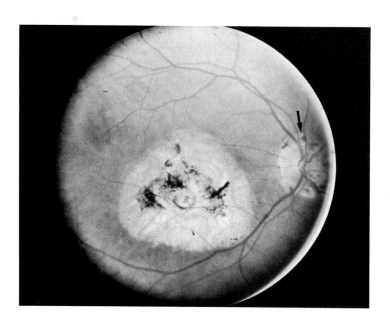

Figure 3–23. A photograph illustrating a large fibrotic macular scar and circumpapillary choroiditis **(arrow)** in presumed ocular histoplasmosis syndrome.

on routine follow-up and home Amsler grid monitoring, especially during the high risk years of ages 30 to 50. Once the macular vision is threatened, fluorescein angiography is indicated.

Two modes of therapy are accepted for the prevention of severe vision loss secondary to POHS. Corticosteroids, both oral and depot injection, are used often to quiet the inflammatory reaction of the disease process. The use of corticosteroids is also of benefit in the management of recurrences of macular POHS. Numerous studies including the Ocular Histoplasmosis Study have demonstrated the benefit of photocoagulative intervention for patients with POHS who are developing neovascular nets outside the foveal areas. Patients who meet certain criteria have a significant reduction in the potential for severe loss of vision over untreated eyes when photocoagulation is properly applied. At the first sign of macular involvement, fluorescein angiography is indicated in addition to a consultation with a retinologist.

POHS—PEARLS

- Usually presents between 20 and 50 years of age, with macular involvement over 30 years of age
- Bilateral macular involvement more common in men than in women
- Circumpapillary choroidal scarring, peripheral atrophic histo spots, and exudative maculopathy
- Patient is asymptomatic until macular involvement, which shows as vision reduction and/or metamorphopsia
- Management
  - Educate patient
  - Routine follow-up and home monitoring of vision
  - FA and retinology consult at first sign of macular involvement

---

Ocular Toxoplasmosis

Introduction. Toxoplasmosis gondii is an obligate intracellular protozoan parasite that produces either a congenital or acquired retinochoroiditis. Toxoplasmosis (Figs. 3–24 through 3–27) is one of the more likely causes of posterior uveitis in the United States. Reactivation of both ocular and cerebral toxoplasmosis is also a common occurrence associated with AIDS. In general, compromise of the patient's immune status is the basis for reactivation that creates the inflammatory response.

Fewer than 1 percent of patients with documented acquired toxoplasmosis with lymph node involvement develop retinitis, but over 80 percent of patients with congenitally acquired toxoplasmosis develop retinitis at some time. Congenital toxoplasmosis is an omnipresent threat, with 60 to 70 percent of females at risk during the childbearing years. Congenital infection occurs because of primary maternal infection during pregnancy. It is important to realize that toxoplasmosis can only be transmitted to the fetus during maternal parasitemia. The most common route of maternal infection is exposure to cat feces. The second child of an exposed mother stands no chance of transplacental infection. The rate of fetal infection increases throughout pregnancy, and the incidence of congenital infection is 0.01 percent of live births.

Appearance and Layers Involved. The toxoplasmic protozoa enters the eye via the circulatory system but then locates within the nerve fiber layer. Once the organism is within the nerve fiber layer, it may actively invade cells, which burst and allow for infection of nearby cells. If the host's resistance is high, the cells may encyst the still viable organisms. The organisms may remain viable within the cysts for over 25 years. These cysts are, however, liable to rupture when the host is immunocompromised, allowing for active spread of the inflammatory process. The cysts often encircle old toxoplasmic focal scars.

A granulomatous anterior uveitis usually accompanies a reactivation of congenital toxoplasmosis. The anterior uveitis is an extension forward of the posterior inflammation that is believed to be a manifestation of hypersensitivity. The organism has never been recovered from the anterior chamber. **See color plate 58.**

When inactive, a toxoplasmosis scar is often indistinguishable from other chorioretinal scars. When active, the lesion usually appears as a white lesion next to a pigmented scar with overlying vitreous cells. These cells will cast a haze on the underlying retinal structure. The active lesion may also appear with no apparent accompanying pigmented scar. The lesions may also be multiple and may have an accompanying optic-nerve head locus.

There may be an accompanying posterior-vitreous detachment, retinal arteritis, occlusive vasculitis, optic neuritis (papillitis), granulomatous anterior uveitis or macular edema. The arteritis may be so severe as to obscure all other retinal signs, especially in very large inflammatory foci.

It is also well established that reactivation of congenital toxoplasmosis can manifest itself neurologically. The neurological lesions are a very common complication of AIDS.

Signs and Symptoms. The patient with active toxoplasmic retinitis may present with blurred vision or floaters secondary to the vitritis, vision or

TOXOPLASMIC RETINOPATHY
INACTIVE SCAR

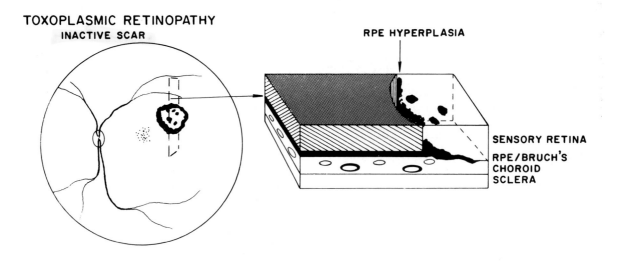

RPE HYPERPLASIA

SENSORY RETINA
RPE/BRUCH'S
CHOROID
SCLERA

REACTIVATION OF SCAR

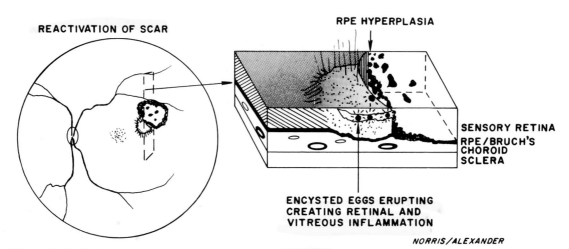

RPE HYPERPLASIA

SENSORY RETINA
RPE/BRUCH'S
CHOROID
SCLERA

ENCYSTED EGGS ERUPTING
CREATING RETINAL AND
VITREOUS INFLAMMATION

NORRIS/ALEXANDER

Figure 3–24. A schematic illustrating both an inactive toxoplasmosis scar and a reactivated toxoplasmosis scar.

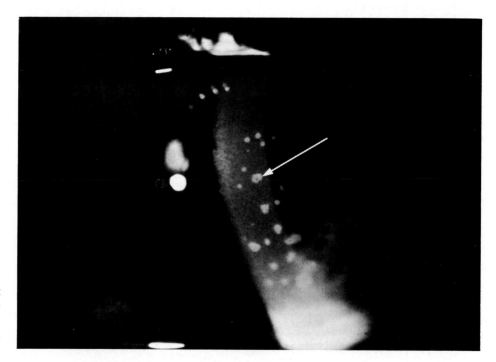

Figure 3–25. The greasy mutton-fat keratitic precipitates **(arrow)** seen in granulomatous anterior uveitis often associated with active ocular toxoplasmosis.

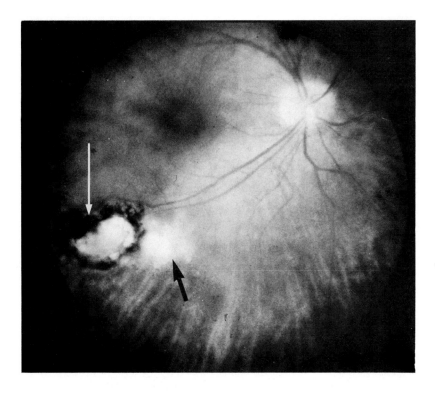

Figure 3–26. The white arrow points to the pigmented toxoplasmosis scar, while the black arrow points to the "headlight in the fog" area of reactivation.

visual field loss secondary to optic nerve inflammation or retinal inflammation near the macula, or a red eye secondary to the anterior uveitis. All granulomatous anterior uveitis should be investigated by a dilated fundus examination to rule out toxoplasmic retinitis.

Prognosis and Management. Recurrent attacks of congenital toxoplasmic retinitis can occur between ages 5 and 60 years, with the first attack often occurring in the 20s. The duration of each attack averages 4 months, with most patients having no more than three attacks. Retinal scarring occurs

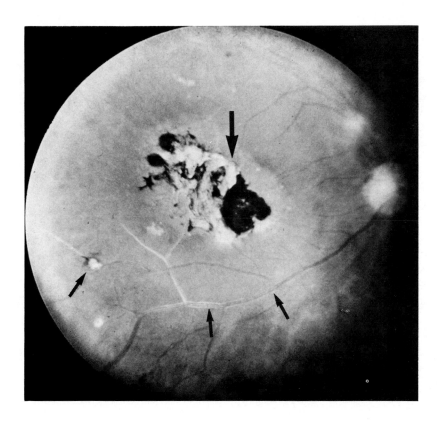

Figure 3–27. The large arrow in this photograph points to an inactive macular toxoplasmosis scar, while the small arrows point to areas of active vasculitis secondary to toxoplasmosis.

with each attack. The scarring can compromise vision if it occurs near the macula or within the optic nerve.

Retinal tears near scars open the channel for retinal detachment. Choroidal neovascularization provides a threat for disciform macular disease. The brain and eye share a common vascular system, allowing for neurological involvement, including convulsions and intracranial calcifications.

The proper diagnosis must be made, as virtually all active toxoplasmic retinitis should be treated. Several laboratory tests may be used to assist in the diagnosis, including the Sabin-Feldman methylene blue dye test (SFDT). The SFDT is, however, of limited value in congenital toxoplasmosis, as the mother's antibodies cross the placenta whether or not the infection is transmitted. The complement fixation test measures antibodies of comparatively short duration and therefore has value in children who have been infected during the first 6 years of life. Fluorescent antibody testing is of value because the IgM antibody will not pass the placental barrier, therefore indicating infection by the toxoplasmic organism.

Toxoplasmic retinitis must be treated because of the associated necrosis of retinal tissue. Indications for treatment include (1) lesions near or threatening the optic nerve or peripapillary bundle, (2) lesions severe enough to cause vitreous traction or retinal detachment, and (3) active lesions near the macula. In fact, there are only *rare* instances when aggressive therapy should not be instituted.

Systemic therapy consists of the synergistic employment of triple sulfonamides with pyrethamine and oral corticosteroids to suppress the inflammatory reaction. The therapy is not without risk, as the antitoxoplasmic agents may alter white blood cell and platelet production. Other agents, such as chlortetracycline, clindamycin, and spiramycin, may also be used. The accompanying anterior uveitis should be managed by mydriatic/cycloplegic agents combined with topical corticosteroids with high ocular penetrability.

Surgical treatment of the active lesions has value only when all medical modalities have been exhausted. Even then, photocoagulation is of limited benefit, as the burn intensity must be extremely high to penetrate the hazy vitreous. This high intensity is often very destructive. Cryopexy offers more opportunity for eradication of the lesion because of the organism's sensitivity to cold.

Ocular Parasititis

Introduction. Migration of parasitic larvae to the eye is an important cause of blindness in many parts of the world. The most common of these par-

---

OCULAR TOXOPLASMOSIS—PEARLS

- Congenital toxoplasmosis is most common resulting from primary maternal infection during pregnancy
- Organism in nerve fiber layer that may encyst awaiting immunocompromise
- Organisms may remain viable surrounding old scars for up to 25 years
- Active toxo presents as anterior granulomatous uveitis, focal white fuzzy retinitis, and overlying vitritis
- May have focus of inflammation in nerve head
- Patient complains of hazy vision, floaters, field loss, or a red eye
- Management
    - Educate patient regarding inactive scars and follow at routine intervals
    - Schedule retinology consult for active lesions
    - Manage anterior uveitis
    - Watch for retinal tears near scars
    - Order toxo titre for diagnosis

---

asites in the United States is the nematode larvae of Toxocara canis. This parasite infects dogs and other canids and is transferred to humans by fecal material (Fig. 3–28). Cysticercus cellulosae is the larval form of the pork tapeworm that may also infect the ocular area. Many other parasites, including giardiasis and onchocerciasis, have been implicated in eye infections.

Human infestation by the toxocara larvae manifests as ocular larval migrans and visceral larval migrans. **Table 3–3 summarizes the differences between ocular and visceral forms.** The infestation usually presents between the ages of 2 and 40 years and is most commonly diagnosed in the south central and south eastern regions of the United States. The infestation is usually associated with ingestion of the eggs of the parasite and is often associated with eating dirt. The ingested eggs may remain viable for years and develop into viable larvae at any point in time. These larvae then enter the lymph and blood systems to form foci of granulomas throughout the host's body.

Appearance and Layers Involved. The ocular manifestations of toxocara (Fig. 3–29 and 3–30) may present as peripheral focal lesions, posterior pole focal lesions, or diffuse vitreous involvement with associated retinal detachment. Anterior uveitis, hypopyon, and vascular occlusion secondary to neuroretinitis have also been reported. Virtually any condition associated with an inflammatory response may present.

The choroid may be involved with extension into the retina and vitreous, or the retina may be the focus of infestation. The nematode may be present both within or below the retina. The retinal

Route of Human Infestation by Toxocara

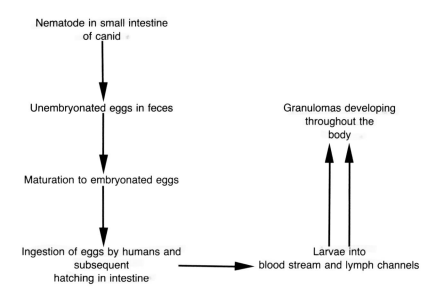

Nematode in small intestine
of canid

Unembryonated eggs in feces

Maturation to embryonated eggs

Ingestion of eggs by humans and
subsequent
hatching in intestine

Granulomas developing
throughout the
body

Larvae into
blood stream and lymph channels

Figure 3–28. A flow chart illustrating the route of human infestation by the Toxocara organism.

lesion is typically round, raised, white, and about 1 DD in size. **See color plate 59.** There is often an associated reactive retinal-pigment epithelial hyperplasia and fibrotic bands radiating from the lesion.

Signs and Symptoms.

The visceral form of toxocara is associated with a cough, chest pain, intermittent fever, loss of appetite, and, at times, right upper abdominal pain. In children, eruptions and nodules may present over the trunk and lower extremities.

Ocular toxocara may present with a mild iritis but is often discovered when a child is examined because of decreased vision or strabismus or both. It is rare to have any systemic manifestations.

The clinical diagnosis is based upon the ELISA (enzyme-linked immunosorbent assay) test, which gives a diagnostic sensitivity of 78 percent with a specificity of 92 percent.

Prognosis and Management.

Should the inflammatory process invade the posterior pole and the granuloma become established, hopes for recovery of vision are poor. If the larva is active and seen away from the capillary free zone, several modes of therapy may be attempted. Corticosteroid therapy by mouth may act to suppress the inflammatory response. Thiabendazole, photocoagulation, and cryopexy have all been attempted with variable success. Clearly the most effective measure against ocular parasititis is prevention. The public must be educated regarding the eating of dirt by children and the consumption of all undercooked meat.

TABLE 3–3. CHARACTERISTICS OF OCULAR AND VISCERAL TOXOCARA INFESTATION

Characteristics	Ocular Larval	Visceral Larval
Age at onset	7½ years	2 years
Ocular findings	Posterior retinal granuloma	None
	Peripheral retinal granuloma	
	Anterior uveitis	
White count	Normal	Elevated
Eosinophil count	Normal	Elevated
Enzyme-linked immunosorbent assay	Low < 1:512	High < 1:16
Visceral signs	None	Present

OCULAR PARASITITIS—PEARLS

- Result of children eating dirt and of eating undercooked meat
- Visceral and ocular form
- Ocular form presents as a round, raised, white lesion that is about 1 DD in size
- Ocular form may have anterior uveitis and vitritis
- A cause of decreased vision and strabismus in children
- ELISA for diagnosis
- Management
  - Prevention and education
  - Retinology consult if active
  - Best possible correction if established

OCULAR TOXOCARA

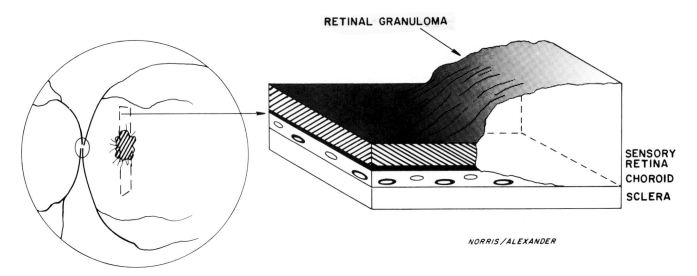

Figure 3–29. A schematic illustrating a granuloma created by the Toxocara organism.

Ocular Manifestations of Sarcoidosis

Introduction. Sarcoidosis is a systemic disease suspected to be an antigenic reaction of the reticuloendothelial system. The disease is granulomatous with a multifaceted presentation. Age of onset is usually between 20 to 60 years, with approximately 27 to 50 percent of patients having ocular involvement. Blacks are afflicted more often than whites.

Appearance and Layers Involved. Granulomatous anterior uveitis is often the most prevalent ocular manifestation, and 25 to 37 percent of patients manifest retinal involvement (Fig. 3–31). Periphlebitis in equatorial retinal veins is the most common retinal sign. The periphlebitis appears as creamy white perivascular exudations. Focal choroidal granulomas may occur elsewhere in the retina. Whitish fluffy infiltrates may also occur in the vitreous over the choroidal nodules. Optic disc edema or choroidal neovascularization may also be

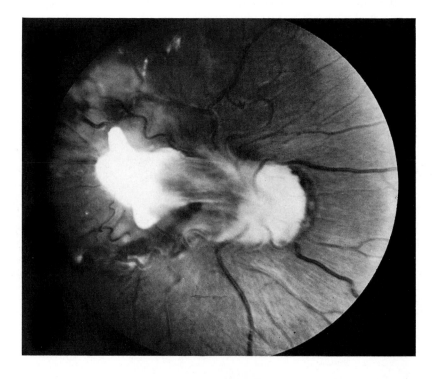

Figure 3–30. A photograph of a retinal granuloma created by Toxocara. *(Photo courtesy of R. Coshatt.)*

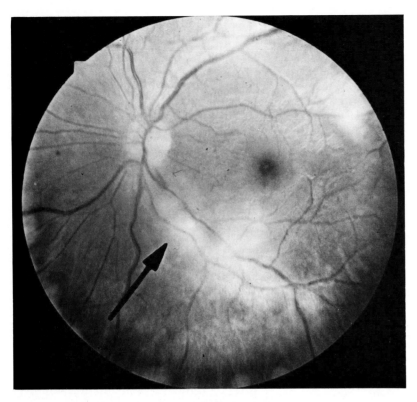

Figure 3–31. The arrow points to a choroidal granuloma of the posterior pole. It is larger and more posterior than sarcoid lesions. Diagnosis by blood tests determined this to be a toxoplasmosis lesion.

a part of the picture of sarcoid ophthalmopathy. The author has also seen a preganglionic Horner's syndrome secondary to an apical lung granuloma. Conjunctival granulomas may also occur with sarcoidosis.

Diagnosis of sarcoidosis may be made by laboratory techniques. The Kveim biopsy is the most effective test, but chest radiographs will pick up lung changes.

Elevation of serum angiotensin-converting enzyme (ACE) occurring in patients with the manifestations of sarcoid is strongly suggestive of the disease. Limited gallium scans of the head, neck, and chest may be of use in diagnosing patients suspected of having sarcoidosis.

Signs and Symptoms. Sarcoidosis is a disease of remissions and exacerbations. The remissions occur more frequently in the first 3 years, ultimately leading to chronicity. Visual signs and symptoms recur and must be managed to prevent long-term tissue damage. Blurred vision, discomfort, redness, and photophobia accompany the anterior uveitis. Long-term vision loss may occur with the choroidal granulomas and neovascularization.

Prognosis and Management. A final visual acuity of at least 20/30 can be expected if ocular inflammation is properly controlled and if choroidal and retinal neovascularization is held at bay. If vision threatening sarcoid retinopathy occurs, oral corticosteriod therapy is indicated. If unresponsive to corticosteroids, chlorambucil may be tried as well as phenylbutazone, oxyphenbutazone, and chloroquine. The accompanying anterior uveitis must also be managed appropriately. Should choroidal neovascularization occur, fluorescein angiography is indicated as well as a retinology consult.

Sarcoidosis is a multisystem disease, and as such one must never ignore the potential systemic morbidity of the disease. Sarcoidosis must be managed by the entire health care team.

Table 3–4 lists the characteristics of inflammatory lesions of the posterior pole.

OCULAR MANIFESTATIONS OF SARCOIDOSIS—PEARLS

- Granulomatous disease with age of onset at 20 to 60 years with 27 to 50% of patients having some ocular involvement
- More prevalent in blacks
- Signs include granulomatous anterior uveitis, equatorial periphlebitis, and equatorial choroidal granulomas
- Diagnosis by Kveim biopsy, chest radiographs, ACE
- Vision compromise may occur from tissue destruction and/or choroidal neovascular nets
- Management
  - A disease to be managed by many disciplines
  - Control the anterior uveitis
  - If vision threatening sarcoid retinopathy occurs, systemic pharmaceutical management is indicated
  - If choroidal neovascularization occurs, FA and a retinology consult are indicated

TABLE 3—4. COMPARISON OF INFLAMMATORY LESIONS OF THE POSTERIOR POLE (MACULA)

	Toxoplasmosis	Histoplasmosis	Toxocariasis	Sarcoid Ophthalmopathy
Typical Age Range	All ages average 25 years	20—50 years	6—30 years	20—40 years (blacks)
Layer of primary affectation	Retina	Choroid	Retina/Choroid	Retina/Choroid
Anterior uveitis	Yes	No	Yes	Yes
Vitritis	Yes	No	Yes	Yes
Exudative maculopathy	Rare	Yes	Rare	No
Characteristic appearance	White area 0.2—15 DD, hazy white when active	Pigment ring at macula ↓ Exudative macula, Atrophic histo spots, Circumpapillary scarring	1 DD granuloma (white) raised	Yellow 0.25 DD nodules near vessels

AIDS AND THE EYE

Introduction

In the United States alone as of December 1987, the Centers for Disease Control (CDC) had on file over 47,000 reports of adult or adolescent cases of AIDS. There were at that time over 700 pediatric cases. Over 57 percent of the reported cases had died. Of these totals in the adult and adolescent category, approximately 70 percent have presented in homosexual and bisexual males and about 14 percent in intravenous (IV) drug users. The heterosexual numbers are, however, on the rise.

The CDC defines a case of AIDS as an illness characterized by (1) the presence of one or more opportunistic diseases as outlined in Table 3–5 that are at least moderately indicative of immunodeficiency, (2) absence of all known underlying causes of immunodeficiency, and (3) absence of all other possible causes of reduced resistance ordinarily associated with the opportunistic diseases.

The recognized cause of AIDS is a retrovirus of the human T-cell lymphotropic class (HTLV-III). The virus has also been called the lymphadenopathy-associated virus (LAV) and is referred to as HTLV-III/LAV by the CDC or, more recently as human immunovirus (HIV). Very few of the persons now infected with HTLV-III have the AIDS syndrome. Approximately 25 percent of infected individuals have the lymphadenopathy syndrome, which is characterized by fever, fatigue, night sweats, malaise, weight loss, thrush, or diarrhea. Somewhere between 10 and 30 percent of patients with lymphadenopathy syndrome progress to AIDS within 2 to 3 years. Patients with AIDS can be expected to live about 3 years.

Transmission of the HTLV-III/LAV is by (1) sexual contact with exchange of bodily fluids, (2) infusion of blood or blood products, or (3) passage from infected mother to child.

Appearance

Individuals with AIDS will probably have at least one ocular or neuro-ocular manifestation at some point. Cotton wool spots occur in about 67 percent of patients and last 4 to 6 weeks. Flame, white-centered, or dot/blot hemorrhages are seen in up to

TABLE 3–5. CONDITIONS SUGGESTIVE OF UNDERLYING IMMUNODEFICIENCY

Conditions	Symptoms/Signs
Protozoal and helminthic infections	
Cryptosporidosis	Diarrhea for over one month
Pneumocystis carinii	Pneumonia
Strongyloidosis	Disseminated infection
Toxoplasmosis	Cerebral infection, retinitis
Fungal infections	
Candidiasis	Esophagitis
Cryptococcosis	Central nervous system or other infection
Viral infections	
Herpes zoster	Vessicular eruptions/pain
Cytomegalovirus	Infection, retinitis
Herpes simplex	Persistent (one month) mucocutaneous lesions
Bacterial infections	
Mycobacterium avium or intracellulare	Disseminated infection
Mycobacterium tuberculosis, kansasi	Disseminated infection
Cancer	
Kaposi's sarcoma	Reddish/blue skin lesions
Lymphoma/diffuse lymphoma	
Hodgkin's disease	
Miscellaneous	
Histoplasmosis	Ocular reactivation

40 percent of patients. Ischemic macular edema is seen in up to 6 percent of patients with AIDS.

Vision-threatening changes associated with AIDS include cytomegalovirus (CMV) retinopathy, toxoplasmosis, and histoplasmosis. CMV retinopathy is the most common severe ocular manifestation of AIDS, affecting up to 45 percent of patients. Most adults have been exposed to CMV, but the immunosuppressive system subdues the virus. When allowed to proliferate, CMV causes a necrotizing retinopathy, creating full-thickness retinal destruction. The early stage of CMV retinopathy consists of white, granular lesions near major vessel arcades near the disc. The destruction spreads outward, accompanied by hemorrhages engulfing the entire retina within 6 months.

While toxoplasmosis can reactivate within the eye in AIDS, it is a far more common neurological complication. Toxoplasmosis is, in fact, the most common neurological complication of AIDS. All other opportunistic infections may affect the eye. Kaposi's sarcoma may present in the ocular area, often as reddish-purple tumors near the medial canthus or inferior cul-de-sac. Kaposi's sarcomas occur in 24 percent of AIDS victims, with 18 percent of those also having the conjunctival lesions.

Neuro-ocular disorders such as cranial nerve palsies may occur in AIDS. Papilledema and visual field loss may present secondary to intracranial infection or intracranial tumors. Pupillary abnormalities may also occur.

TABLE 3–6. RECOMMENDATIONS TO PREVENT THE TRANSFER OF HUMAN IMMUNO VIRUS

General
1. Exercise special care regarding sexual contacts.
2. Wear goggles when there is potential for infected fluids to be splashed into the eyes.
3. Wear masks when examining patients suspected of having airborne opportunistic organisms.
4. Dispose of all needles and syringes in "contaminant" containers.

Ocular
1. Glove when there is potential contact with bodily secretions or blood.
2. Wash hands after each patient contact.
3. Disinfect tonometer tips and all other instruments that make contact with the eye.
   Note: HTLV-III/LAV may be inactivated by
   (1) Five- to ten-minute exposure to 3% hydrogen peroxide,
   (2) 1:10 dilution of household bleach, or
   (3) 70% ethanol or isopropyl alcohol.
4. Disinfect rigid gas permeable and PMMA contact lenses with hydrogen peroxide.
5. Disinfect soft contact lenses with heat or hydrogen peroxide disinfection systems.

Laboratory diagnosis of HTLV-III/LAV is made by using the ELISA. Positive results on ELISA should then be confirmed by either the Western blot test or immunofluorescent assay (IFA).

Prognosis and Management
Currently prognosis for AIDS and its related ocular complications is grim. Many drugs are under investigation and may create a brief state of quiescence in the systemic or ocular manifestations; but there is a high recurrence rate at cessation of treatment.

The best management modality for AIDS is prevention. **Table 3–6 summarizes current recommendations for prevention of or prophylaxis against infection by HTLV-III/LAV.**

AIDS—PEARLS

- Immunosuppression allowing for destruction by opportunistic infections
- Transmission of virus by
  - Sexual contact with exchange of bodily fluids
  - Infusion of blood or blood products
  - Passage from infected mother to child
- Ocular manifestations include cotton wool spots, retinal hemorrhages, ischemic macular edema, cytomegalovirus retinopathy, toxoplasmosis, histoplasmosis, Kaposi's sarcomas, papilledema, nerve palsies
- Diagnosis by ELISA, Western blot test, or IFA
- Management
  - Education
  - Prevention
  - Suppression of opportunistic infections

THE NONHEREDITARY RETINAL PIGMENT EPITHELIOPATHIES

Acute Posterior Multifocal Placoid Pigment Epitheliopathy

Introduction. Acute posterior multifocal placoid pigment epitheliopathy (APMPPE) is a relatively benign bilateral process that usually affects young adults (typically between the ages of 20 and 40 years). There appears to be no sexual predilection. The disease appears to affect the retinal pigment epithelium and is thought to be secondary to some underlying vascular problem of the choroid/choriocapillaris. There is a strong association with recent bouts of systemic viral disease. Table 3–7 summarizes conditions reported to be associated with APMPPE.

TABLE 3–7. SYSTEMIC AND OCULAR CONDITIONS REPORTED TO BE ASSOCIATED WITH THE DEVELOPMENT OF APMPPE

Systemic	Ocular
Toxoplasmosis	Papillitis
Meningoencephalitis	Posterior uveitis/anterior uveitis
Tuberculosis	Retinal vasculitis
Cerebral vasculitis	Serous retinal detachment
Headache	Harada's disease
Erythema nodosum	Marginal corneal thinning
Thyroiditis	Choroidal neovascularization
Adenovirus type 5	Episcleritis
Spinal fluid pleocytosis	Keratitis

Appearance and Layers Involved. The sudden appearance of dirty yellow-white (creamy) multiple placoid lesions in the posterior pole followed by the same in the fellow eye is the characteristic of APMPPE. The lesions occur deep in the retina, and there may be associated retinal/optic nerve disease.

Fluorescein angiography exhibits a characteristic pattern that strongly implicates the retinal pigment epithelium as the layer of primary affectation. In the early phases of FA there is a blockage of background choroidal fluorescence by the altered RPE. The late stage of FA demonstrates an accumulation of dye in the diseased RPE. Old lesions appear, as do all RPE defects on FA. There is some possibility that the RPE disturbance could be secondary to focal disease of the underlying choriocapillaris. The fundus lesions resolve rapidly over 7 to 10 days, leaving evidence of mottled RPE. Should the *rare* recurrence occur, there may be the appearance of new lesions or enlargement of previously existing lesions.

Signs and Symptoms. See color plate 60. APMPPE presents as a rapid loss of vision eventually affecting both eyes. Scotomas will present corresponding to the locations of the lesions. As mentioned previously, there may be a relationship to a recent nondescript illness.

Laboratory testing is usually nonproductive in the diagnosis of underlying conditions associated with APMPPE. Anterior uveitis or cells in the vitreous are present in approximately 50 percent of affected patients.

Prognosis and Management. APMPPE is a process that demonstrates rapid resolution of the fundus lesions over 1 to 2 weeks. Remnants of vision compromise or field defects may persist for up to 6 months. There is a low incidence of recurrence, and the large majority of patients recover to an acuity level between 20/20 to 20/30. There is no reason to intervene therapeutically.

There is the possibility of long-term development of choroidal neovascularization secondary to the altered metabolic state of the retinal pigment epithelium. There are also some suggestions that APMPPE is a part of a continuum resulting in extensive chorioretinal disease. This theory is, however, not well-supported at this point in time.

Should an accompanying anterior uveitis be present and symptomatic, it must be treated appropriately.

APMPPE—PEARLS

- Bilateral condition in young adults
- Yellow-white multiple placoid lesions in posterior pole
- FA shows early hypofluorescence and late hyperfluorescence
- Visual acuity reduction and scotomas are quick to develop
- Fundus lesions resolve over 7 to 10 days, but vision reduction or scotomas may persist 6 months
- Possibility of anterior uveitis
- Management
  - Proper diagnosis
  - Manage anterior uveitis
  - Patient education
  - Watch for long-term development of choroidal neovascular nets

---

Geographical Helicoid Peripapillary Choroidopathy

Introduction. Geographical helicoid peripapillary choroidopathy (GHPC) is also known as serpiginous choroidopathy and geographical choroiditis. It is a bilateral disease of the choriocapillaris and RPE. There is the characteristic of recurrence to differentiate GHPC from APMPPE. The involvement of the second eye may be after a time delay and may be asymmetrical. GHPC shows no apparent sexual preference but has been reported more often in whites than blacks. The age range for onset is 30 to 70 years of age, with the average 45 to 50 years of age. Associated ocular findings are rare but may include serous sensory retinal detachment, anterior uveitis, vitritis, and choroidal neovascular nets. There are no apparent related systemic diseases. Severe visual loss can occur if the macular area is affected. The exact cause of the disease has not been determined.

Appearance and Layers Involved. GHPC is a chronic, progressive disease that usually involves the circumpapillary RPE, choriocapillaris, and choroid (Fig. 3–32). In the acute phase, pseudopods extend out from the optic nerve head in a propellerlike fashion (centrifugal). The pseudopods represent subretinal scarring. The scarring may be noncontinuous with "skip zones." During activity, gray or cream lesions will develop at the advancing edge of the scar at the level of the RPE. The active lesion usually persists only several weeks. Should the pseudopods crawl into the macular area, vision will be compromised.

There is a variant of the "classical" GHPC in which the lesions start away from the disc and extend inward toward the disc (centripetal). The disease is characterized by remissions and exacerbations. During the stage of inactivity, the ophthalmoscopic picture is that of extensive irregular scars and occasional choroidal neovascularization. The choroidal neovascularization may create more extensive disciform scarring. The loss of overlying RPE often results in easy visualization of the large choroidal vessels around the optic nerve head.

The fluorescein pattern is characteristic in GHPC. Early in the angiogram, the central part of the inactive lesion hypofluoresces and is surrounded by hyperfluorescence. During the later phase the fluorescein seeps into the scar, creating spotty fluorescence. The active lesion is hypofluorescent and demonstrates variable fluorescence late in the angiogram. The fluorescein pattern strongly implicates the choriocapillaris as the initial site of the disease. The fellow eye, while usually involved, may present nothing more than mild circumpapillary changes that are certainly capable of progression.

Signs and Symptoms. In the active phase the patient may report the sudden onset of reduced vision or a paracentral scotoma if the pseudopods have encroached upon the macular area. There is usually no accompanying pain, photophobia, or lacrimation. Recurrence is the rule. Patients may report symptoms early if they have been placed on a home monitoring system.

Prognosis and Management. GHPC is characterized by multiple recurrences with development of new scars and extensions of old scars. Active development has been documented as occurring over a 10-year period. During the active lesion, vision drops. In some cases there does seem to be some improvement in acuity with quiescene of the lesions. The time to recovery seems to vary between 2 and 22 months. Some of the patients may, however, have an irreversible drop in visual acuity. Final visual acuity seems to be unpredictable, but GHPC does not inevitably result in severe visual loss.

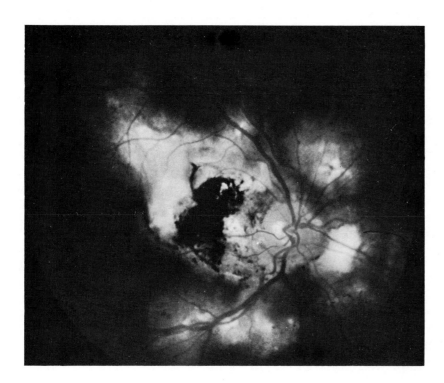

Figure 3–32. A photograph illustrating the destruction of geographical helicoid peripapillary choroidopathy. Diagnosis by F. LaRussa.

The issue of management seems to be controversial, as some practitioners advocate aggressive corticosteroid intervention when the lesions become active, while others point out that no clinical trials are available to support efficacy. The patient nonetheless should be placed on a home vision monitoring system and should report reactivation. Should choroidal neovascularization occur in the scarred areas, fluorescein angiography should be performed to determine if laser photocoagulation would be of benefit.

GHPC—PEARLS

- Bilateral, recurrent choriocapillaris/RPE disease with asymmetrical presentation
- Average age of onset 45 to 50 years
- Acute phase presents as propellarlike pseudopods extending out from optic nerve head
- Creamy lesions develop at the edges of the pseudopods and persist for several weeks (RPE disease)
- When the pseudopods creep into the macula, vision is lost, scotomas occur at sites of pseudopods
- FA shows early hypofluorescence of central scar and hypofluorescence early in active creamy lesions
- Management
  - Disease characterized by recurrences and there is controversy regarding efficacy of corticosteroid intervention
  - Patient education and routine follow-up with home monitoring of vision
  - Choroidal neovascular nets can develop. Should this occur order fluorescein angiography

---

Recurrent Multifocal Choroiditis

Introduction. Recurrent multifocal choroiditis (RMC) is a newly described clinical entity affecting young (14 to 34 years of age, one reported over 34 years of age), mildly myopic, female patients. The condition may be unilateral or bilateral, and recurrences are common. One eye may follow the other in development of the lesions. There appears to be no particular relationship to systemic diseases, and laboratory diagnosis appears to be of no value. Because of the positive response to corticosteroid therapy, the lesions are thought to be inflammatory.

Appearance and Layers Involved. Ophthalmoscopic findings include small, multiple, yellow-white lesions that may have a surround of pigment proliferation. During activity these areas become gray and fuzzy and may be accompanied by vitritis, anterior uveitis, and optic disc edema. These lesions of the retinal pigment epithelium and cho-

riocapillaris are usually confined to the clinical posterior pole but may encroach upon the macular area. The lesions hyperfluoresce early and remain fuzzy throughout the duration of an angiogram. Recurrences often occur next to older lesions.

Because of the compromise to the RPE/Bruch's membrane zone, there is a significant threat for the development of choroidal neovascularization or progressive subretinal fibrotic scarring (reports of 30 to 40 percent). A variable percentage of patients may develop cystoid macular edema.

Signs and Symptoms. The condition may be found on routine eye examination if the lesions have not impacted on the macular area. When macular function is compromised, visual acuity is rapidly reduced, and metamorphopsia occurs. Isolated scotomas may be demonstrated on visual field testing.

Prognosis and Management. As RMC is a newly described condition, there is considerable variation in the reports on prognosis. Both choroidal neovascularization and subretinal fibrosis carry a poor prognosis, and intervention must occur should either of these complications arise. Acute fundus lesions do respond positively to systemic corticosteroids, but again the response is variable. It appears that laser treatment of the choroidal neovascular nets does not afford excellent results.

All patients suspected of having RMC must have all other causes of choroiditis ruled out. In addition, the patients should be on some form of home monitoring system. Should activity occur, it is imperative that systemic corticosteroid therapy be instituted immediately at least on a trial basis.

RMC—PEARLS

- Affects young (14–34 years of age), myopic females
- Small, multiple, yellow-white lesions (in posterior pole) that become gray and fuzzy during activity
- During activity there may be vitritis, anterior uveitis, optic disc edema, loss of vision, and scotomas
- FA shows early hyperfluorescence of active lesions
- Recurrences often are next to older lesions
- With continued scarring there is a threat for choroidal neovascularizaton or progressive subretinal fibrotic scarring
- Management
  - Education and home monitoring of vision
  - Systemic therapy when reactivation occurs
  - Watch for choroidal neovascularization—poor prognosis
  - Routine examinations

Multiple Evanescent White Dot Syndrome

Introduction. Multiple evanescent white dot syndrome (MEWDS) is a newly reported posterior uveitis that involves the retinal pigment epithelium, eventually affecting the overlying photoreceptors. It occurs primarily in young (ages 17 to 38 years) females. This unilateral transient disease appears to have no particular association with systemic abnormalities, but some patients report a prior "flulike" illness. There appears to be no racial predilection.

Appearance and Layers Involved. Ophthalmoscopically, MEWDS appears as a unilateral presentation of several small, discrete, white dots concentrated in the clinical posterior pole but sparing the fovea. The dots appear to be at the RPE level, with their activity causing transient interference in the photoreceptor function. There is a granularity to the macula in the affected eye that appears as tiny white to light orange specks. Cells occur in the vitreous, and fluorescein staining presents in the macula in most cases. There is hyperfluorescence of the disc with FA in some cases and occasional venous sheathing.

Fluorescein angiography performed during the active stage shows early hyperfluorescence of the lesions with late-stage patchy staining. Electroretinogram testing reveals both a decreased a-wave and ERP amplitude in the active phase, implying impaired photoreceptor function.

With quiescence of MEWDS, the white dots and macular granularity tend to fade. Subtle RPE window defects always will be the sequelae of the process.

Signs and Symptoms. The patient with MEWDS usually presents because of acute unilateral reduction in visual acuity. Acuity during activity varies between 20/50 (6/12) to 20/200 (6/60).

Prognosis and Management. Prognosis for MEWDS is excellent. Vision typically recovers to the 20/20 to 20/30 level within 1 to 16 weeks. There are no reports of recurrences and no reports of secondary complications such as choroidal neovascularization. The responsibility of the clinician is to rule out all other causes of acute unilateral vision loss.

MEWDS—PEARLS

- Occurs primarily in young females (17 to 38 years of age)
- Unilateral transient disease appearing as multiple white dots in clinical posterior pole but sparing the fovea
- Granularity to affected macula with staining in FA
- Patients present because of acute unilateral vision decrease (20/50–20/20)
- Management
  - Proper diagnosis and patient education
  - Vision recovery to 20/20–20/30 in 1–16 weeks
  - No recurrence

■ Clinical Note: Acute Retinal-Pigment Epitheliitis

Acute retinal-pigment epitheliitis may also cause an acute reduction in acuity in young and middle-aged patients. This condition may be bilateral. The lesions in acute retinal epitheliitis are hyperpigmented, presenting as one to four discrete clusters with an irregular halo of white. These clusters are about 1/4 DD. Spontaneous resolution of vision from the 20/100 level occurs in 6 to 12 weeks without therapeutic intervention. RPE abnormalities remain after the active phase.

■ Clinical Note: Birdshot Retinochoroidopathy

Birdshot retinochoroidopathy occurs in patients aged 40 to 60 years. There are multiple, discrete, depigmented or creamy spots in the mid periphery that are arranged near large choroidal vessels. During early fluorescein angiography, these lesions at the level of the RPE hypofluoresce, accumulating some dye in the later phases. Patients have chronic vitritis, retinal vasculitis, optic disc edema, and, ultimately, cystoid macular edema. Birdshot is similar to pars planitis without the snowbanks at the ora. The disease is chronic and protracted. This is thought to be an autoimmune disease and as such may benefit from corticosteroids.

Pigmented Paravenous Retinochoroidal Atrophy

Introduction. Pigmented paravenous retinochoroidal atrophy (PPRA) was at one time considered a rare occurrence. Many case reports have surfaced lately, and the author has personally seen several cases. The age range for presentation of PPRA has been reported as 4 to 70 years, although one report suggests congenital onset. The majority of reported cases are males, which suggests a hereditary nature. The author has seen both males and females with PPRA. The disease has also been reported to be passed from mother to son. The disease presentation is extremely variable, which suggests that if it is hereditary in nature, there is variable penetrance. There appears to be no racial predilection.

Cases of PPRA have been reported to be associated with measles, which suggests that an infectious process cannot be ruled out. There have been several suggestions alluding to PPRA as being an incomplete, self-limited form of retinitis pigmentosa.

In spite of the dramatic ophthalmoscopic presentation, PPRA is considered to be a relatively benign process that rarely affects macular vision in spite of the fact that it may be progressive. PPRA is usually bilateral and symmetrical, but unilateral cases have been reported.

Appearance and Layers Involved. The origin of this condition seems to be in the retinal pigment epithelium. There appears to be atrophy of the RPE surrounding the optic nerve head and the veins. These corridors of RPE atrophy hyperfluoresce on fluorescein angiography but do not leak. There is marked bone-spiculelike cuffing of pigment surrounding the retinal veins. However, as the disease is highly variable, many variations of the classic picture can present.

The ophthalmoscopic signs rarely progress to involve the macula in PPRA (Fig. 3–33). It does seem that changes do start to invade the clinical posterior pole with time and may even resemble gyrate atrophy. Should progression occur to the stage of resembling the scalloping of gyrate atrophy, serum and urine ornithine levels will help in the differential diagnosis. Serum and urine ornithine levels are elevated in gyrate atrophy.

Signs and Symptoms. PPRA is usually asymptomatic. PPRA is usually found during a routine ophthalmoscopic examination. Visual field defects correspond to the areas of RPE atrophy and may demonstrate overall constriction or a ring scotoma. Dark adaptation and electroretinography may be normal or abnormal. Electro-oculograms are usually abnormal but have also been reported as normal. There does not appear to be any strong relationship to positive findings on routine laboratory diagnostic tests.

Prognosis and Management. Visual acuity is usually unaffected in PPRA, even in cases judged to be severe by ophthalmoscopy. There is, however, a progressive constriction of visual fields in some cases associated with progressive fundus changes.

Some reported cases of PPRA have a severe, progressive loss of vision. As such it would be prudent in cases of suspected PPRA to (1) establish a pedigree, (2) perform visual fields, (3) obtain retinal photographs, (4) perform electrodiagnostic testing to rule out other similar conditions, and (5) follow the patient on routine intervals.

Table 3–8 lists the characteristics of the retinal pigment epitheliopathies.

PPRA—PEARLS

- Broad range of age presentation
- Usually bilateral, symmetrical atrophy and migration of the RPE surrounding the optic nerve head and corridors along the veins
- Bone-spicule cuffing of veins
- May progress toward macula but rarely affects vision
- Usually asymptomatic but affected areas will demonstrate field compromise
- Electrodiagnosis is normal to abnormal
- Management
  - Establish a pedigree
  - Educate patient
  - Perform visual fields
  - Monitor on routine intervals

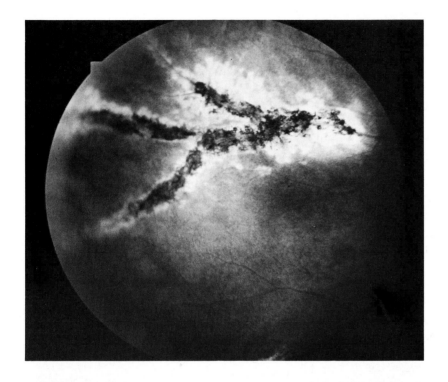

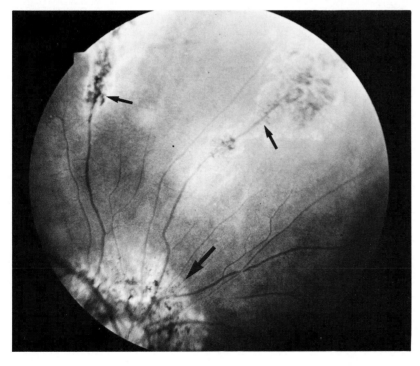

Figure 3–33. Top. Significant paravenous pigment associated with PPRA. **Bottom.** The arrows point to circumpapillary and paravenous changes associated with PPRA.

TABLE 3–8. RETINAL PIGMENT EPITHELIOPATHIES

	Acute Posterior Multifocal Placoid Pigment Epitheliopathy	Geographical Helicoid Peripapillary Choroidopathy	Recurrent Multifocal Choroiditis	Multiple Evanescent White-Dot Syndrome	Acute Retinal Pigment Epitheliitis	Birdshot Retinochoroid-opathy	Pigmented Paravenous Retinochoroidal Atrophy
Average age of onset (years)	20–40	45–50	13–34	17–38	Young to middle age	40–60	4–70
Sex	—	—	Females	Females	—	—	Usually males
Active lesion acuity	Rapid reduction	Sudden scotoma or vision loss if pseudopods in macula	Sudden scotoma or vision loss if near macula	Sudden unilateral vision loss to 20/50–20/200	Sudden loss to 20/100	No loss until cystoid macular edema	Asymptomatic
Final visual acuity	20/20–20/30 over 6 months	Variable from good to severe vision loss	Variable from good to severe vision loss	20/20–20/30 within 16 weeks	Good VA within 12 weeks	Variable	Rare progression to severe loss of vision
Clinical appearance	Creamy multiple placoid lesions in posterior pole; anterior uveitis and vitritis in 50%	Pseudopod subretinal scarring extending out from the disc in a propellerlike pattern, gray lesions develop at scars during activity, choroidal neo may develop	Small multiple yellow-white lesions that are gray when active; occur in posterior pole; may develop choroidal neo or subretinal fibrosis	Several small white dots in posterior pole with a granular macula. With resolution, granularity and dots fade.	Hyperpigmented clusters with a white halo (1/4 DD) in macular area. With resolution, defects in RPE remain.	Multiple creamy spots midperiphery; chronic vitritis, optic disc edema, vasculitis cystoid macular edema	Symmetrical circumpapillary RPE atrophy. Corridors of RPE atrophy along veins; bone-spicule cuffing of veins
Recurrence	Rare	Common	Common	No	Rare	Chronic	Chronic
Laterality	Bilateral	Bilateral	Unilateral or bilateral	Unilateral	Unilateral or bilateral	Bilateral	Bilateral
Management	No intervention except in anterior uveitis	Corticosteroids of questionable value; laser neovascular nets	Corticosteroids of value in active lesions	No intervention	No intervention	Possible corticosteroids -Autoimmune?-	No intervention

REFERENCES

Aaberg TM: Macular holes: A review. *Surv Ophthalmol* 1970;15:139–162.

Ajamian PC, Coughran J: Acute posterior multifocal placoid pigment epitheliopathy. *S J Optom* 1983;9:28–30.

Alexander LJ: Choroidal rupture. *Rev Optom* 1978;115: 33–34.

Alexander LJ: The prevalence of macular drusen in a population of patients with known insulin-dependent diabetes mellitus. *J Am Optom Assoc* 1985;56:806–809.

Alexander LJ: Diseases of the retina, in Bartlett JD, Jaanus SD (eds): *Clinical Ocular Pharmacology.* Boston, Butterworths, 1984.

Alexander LJ, Jones W, Potter JW: *Retina, Retina, Retina.* Philadelphia, Primary Eye Care, 1985.

Anderson CJ, Zauel DW, Schlaegel TF, Meyer SM: Bilateral juxta papillary subretinal neovascularization and pseudopapilledema in a three-year-old child. *J Pediatr Ophthalmol Strab* 1978;15:296–299.

Annesley WH, Shields JA, Tomer T, Christopherson K: The clinical course of serpiginous choroidopathy. *Am J Ophthalmol* 1979;87:133–142.

Aubsburger JJ, Benson WE: Subretinal neovascularization in chronic uveitis. *Albrecht von Graef es Arch Klin Ophthalmol* 1980;215:32–51.

Avila MP, Weiter JJ, Jalkh AE, et al: Natural history of choroidal neovascularization in degenerative myopia. *Ophthalmology* 1984;91:1573–1581.

Beck RW, Sergott RC, Barr CC, Annesley WH: Optic disc edema in presumed ocular histoplasmosis syndrome. *Ophthalmology* 1984;91:183–185.

Berger JR, Maskowitz L, Fisch IM, Kelley RE: Neurologic disease as the presenting manifestation of acquired immunodeficiency syndrome. *South Med J* 1987;80:683–686.

Blumenkranz MS, Russell SR, Robey MG, et al: Risk factors in age-related maculopathy complicated by choroidal neovascularization. *Ophthalmology* 1986;93:552–558.

Bressler NM, Bressler SB, Fine SL: Age-related macular degeneration. *Surv Ophthalmol* 1988;32:374–413.

Bronstein MA, Trempe CL, Freeman HM: Fellow eyes of eyes with macular holes. *Am. J. Ophthalmol* 1981; 92:757–761.

Brooks DN, Potter JW, Bartlett JD, Nowakowski R. Pigmented paravenous retino choroidal atrophy. *J Am Optom Assoc* 1980;51:1097–1101.

Brown DH: Ocular toxocara canis. *J Pediatr Ophthalmol* 1970;7:182–191.

Burgess DB: Ocular histoplasmosis syndrome. *Ophthalmology* 1986;93:967–968.

Cantrill HL, Folk JC: Multifocal choroiditis associated with progressive subretinal fibrosis. *Am J Ophthalmol* 1986;101:170–180.

Carter AD, Frank JW: Congenital toxoplasmosis epidemiologic features and control. *Can Med Assoc J* 1986; 135:618–623.

Centers for Disease Control: Recommendations for prevention of HIV transmission in health care settings. *MMWR* 1987;36(suppl 25):3–18.

Chandra SR, Bresnick GH, Dovis MD, et al: Choroidal neovascular ingrowth after photocoagulation for proliferative diabetic retinopathy. *Arch Ophthalmol* 1980;98: 1593–1600.

Condon PI, Jampol M, Ford S, Sergeant GR: Choroidal neovascularization induced by photocoagulation in sickle cell disease. *Br J Ophthalmol* 1981;65:192–197.

Coscas G, Guadric A: Natural course of nonaphakic cystoid macular edema. *Surv Ophthalmol* 1984;28(suppl): 471–484.

Curtain BJ, Karlin DB: Axial length measurements and fundus changes of the myopic eye. *Am J Ophthalmol* 1971;71:41.

Den Beste BP, Hummer J: AIDS: A review and guide for infection control. *J Am Optom Assoc* 1986;57:675–682.

Dreyer RF, Gass DJ: Multifocal choroiditis and panuveitis. A syndrome that mimics ocular histoplasmosis. *Arch Ophthalmol* 1984;102:1776–1784.

Ebert EM, Fine AM, Markowitz J, et al: Functional vision in patients with neovascular maculopathy and poor visual acuity. *Arch Ophthalmol* 1986;104: 1009–1012.

Elman MJ, Fine SL, Murphy RP, et al The natural history of serous retinal pigment epithelium detachment in patients with age related macular degeneration. *Ophthalmology* 1986;93:224–230.

Federman JL, Shields JA, Tomer TL: Angioid streaks. *Arch Ophthalmol* 1975;93:951.

Ferris FL, Fine SL, Hyman L: Age-related macular degeneration and blindness due to neovascular maculopathy. *Arch Ophthalmol* 1984;102:1640–1642.

Fine SL: Early detection of extrafoveal neovascular membranes by daily central field evaluation. *Ophthalmology* 1985;92:603–609.

Flach AJ, Dolan BJ, Irvine AR: Effectiveness of ketorolac tromethamine 0.5% ophthalmic solution for chronic aphakic and pseudophakic cystoid macular edema. *Am J Ophthalmol* 1987;103:479–486.

Folk JC: Aging macular degeneration clinical features of treatable disease. *Ophthalmology* 1985;92:594–602.

Frederick AR: Multifocal and recurrent (serous) choroidopathy (MARC) syndrome: A new variety of idiopathic central serous choroidopathy. *Doc Ophthalmol* 1984;56:203–235.

Fung WE: Vitrectomy for chronic cystoid macular edema. Results of a national, collaborative, prospective, randomized investigation. *Ophthalmology* 1985;92:1102–1111.

Gass JDM: *Stereoscopic Atlas of Macular Disease.* St. Louis, Mosby, 1970.

Gass JDM: Pathogenesis of disciform detachment of the neuroepithelium. I-IV. *Am J Ophthalmol* 1967;63:573–711.

Gass JDM: Photocoagulation treatment of idiopathic central serous choroidopathy. *Trans Am Acad Ophthalmol Otolaryngol* 1977;83:456–463.

Gass JDM, Clarkson JG: Angioid streaks and disciform macular detachment in Paget's disease. *Am J Ophthalmol* 1973;75:576–586.

Geeraets WJ, Guerry D: Angioid streaks and sickle cell disease. *Am J Ophthalmol* 1960;49:450.

Goen TM, Terry JE: Acute posterior multifocal placoid pigment epitheliopathy. *J Am Optom Assoc* 1987;58: 112–117.

Green WR, McDonnell PJ, Yeo JH: Pathologic features of senile macular degeneration. *Ophthalmology* 1985;92: 615–627.

Guyer DR, Fine SL, Maguire MG, et al: Subfoveal choroidal neovascular membranes in age-related macular degeneration. Visual prognosis in eyes with relatively good initial visual acuity. *Arch Ophthalmol* 1986;104: 702–705.

Hardy RA, Schatz H: Macular geographic helicoid choroidopathy. *Arch Ophthalmol* 1987;105:1237–1242.

Henderly DE, Freeman WR, Smith RE, et al: Cytomegalovirus retinitis as the initial manifestation of the acquired immunodeficiency syndrome. *Ann Ophthalmol* 1987;103:316–320.

Hotchkiss ML, Fine SL: Pathologic myopia and choroidal neovascularization. *Am J Ophthalmol* 1981;91:177–183.

Inslor MS: AIDS and Other Sexually Transmitted Diseases and the Eye. Orlando, Fla, Grune & Stratton, 1987.

Jabs DA, Johns CJ: Ocular involvement in chronic sarcoidosis. *Am J Ophthalmol* 1986;102:297–301.

Jampol LM: Pharmacologic therapy of aphakic and pseudophakic cystoid macular edema. 1985 update. *Ophthalmology* 1985;92:807–810.

Jampol LM, Sanders DR, Kraff MC: Prophylaxis and therapy of aphakic cystoid macular edema. *Surv Ophthalmol* 1984;28(Suppl):535–539.

Kanski JJ, Morse PH: *Disorders of the Vitreous, Retina and Choroid*. Boston, Butterworths, 1983.

Kaplan HJ, Aaberg TM: Birdshot retinochoroidopathy. *Am J Ophthalmol 1980;90:773–782.*

Kegarise JL: Diagnosis and management of macular holes. *J Am Optom Assoc* 1988;59:411–421.

Kraff MC, Sanders DR, Jampol LM, et al: Prophylaxis of pseudophakic cystoid macular edema with indomethacin. *Ophthalmology* 1982;89:886–889.

Levy JH, Pollock HM, Curtain BJ: The Fuch's spot: An ophthalmoscopic and fluorescein angiographic study. *Ann Ophthalmol* 1977;1433–1443.

Levy RM, Rosenbloom S. Perrett LV, Neuroradiologic findings in AIDS: A review of 200 cases. *AJR* 1986; 147:977–983.

Lewis H, Straatsma BR, Foos RY: Chorioretinal juncture. Multiple extramacular drusen. *Ophthalmology* 1986;93: 1098–1112.

Macular Photocoagulation Study Group: Argon laser photocoagulation for neovascular maculopathy. Three-year results from randomized clinical trials. *Arch Ophthalmol* 1986;104:694–701.

Macular Photocoagulation Study Group: Argon laser photocoagulation for senile macular degeneration. Results of randomized clinical trial. *Arch Ophthalmol* 1982;100:912–918.

Macular Photocoagulation Study Group: Argon laser photocoagulation for ocular histoplasmosis. *Arch Ophthalmol* 1983;101:1347–1357.

Macular Photocoagulation Study Group: Recurrent choroidal neovascularization after argon laser photocoag-

ulation for neovascular maculopathy. *Arch Ophthalmol* 1986;104:503–512.

McDonald HR, Schatz H: Grid photocoagulation for diffuse macular edema. *Retina* 1985;5:65–72.

Melrose MA, Margargal LE, Donoso LA, et al: Vision parameters in krypton laser photocoagulation of subfoveal neovascular membranes. *Ophthalmic Surg* 1985;16: 495–502.

Meredith JT: Toxoplasmosis of the central nervous system. *Am Fam Physician* 1987;35:113–116.

Michelson JB, Michelson PE, Chisari FV: Subretinal neovascular membrane and disciform scar in Behçet's disease. *Am J Ophthalmol* 1980;90:182–185.

Michelson JB, Chisari FV: Behçet's disease, review. *Surv Ophthalmol* 1982;26:190–203.

Miller H, Miller B, Ryan SJ: The role of pigment epithelium in the involution of subretinal neovascularization. *Invest Ophthalmol Vis Sci* 1986;27:1644–1652.

Miller SA, Stevens TS, Myers F, Nieder M: Pigmented paravenous retinochoroidal atrophy. *Ann Ophthalmol* 1978;10:867–871.

Mills J: Pneumocystis carnii and toxoplasma gondii infections in patients with AIDS. *Rev Infect Dis* 1986;8:1001–1011.

Mizuno K, Takahashi J: Sarcoid cyclitis. *Ophthalmology* 1986;93:511–517.

Morgan CM, Schatz H: Recurrent multifocal choroiditis. *Ophthalmology* 1986;93:1138–1147.

Morris PD, Katerndahl DA: Human toxocariasis. Review with report of a probable cause. *Postgrad Med* 1987;81:263–267.

Murphy RP: Age-related macular degeneration. *Ophthalmology* 1986;93:969–971.

Noble KG, Carr RE: Pigmented paravenous chorioretinal atrophy. *Am J Ophthalmol* 1983;96:338–344.

O'Connor GR: Protozoan diseases of the uvea. *Int Ophthalmol Clin* 1977;17:163–176.

Olk RJ, Burgess DM, McCormick PA: Subfoveal and juxtafoveal subretinal neovascularization in the presumed ocular histoplasmosis syndrome. *Ophthalmology* 1984;91: 1592–1602.

Olk RJ, Burgess DB: Treatment of recurrent juxtafoveal subretinal neovascular membranes with red laser photocoagulation. *Ophthalmology* 1985;92:1035–1046.

Peduzzi M, Guerrieri F, Torlai F, Prampolini ML: Bilateral pigmented paravenous retino-choroidal degeneration following measles. *Int Ophthalmol* 1984;7:11–14.

Perkins ES: Ocular toxoplasmosis. *Br J Ophthalmol* 1973;57:1–17.

Poliner LS, Olk RJ, Burgess D, Gordon ME: Natural history of retinal pigment epithelial detachments in age-related macular degeneration. *Ophthalmology* 1986; 93:543–551.

Pruett RC, Weiter JJ, Goldstein RB: Myopic cracks, angioid streaks, and traumatic tears in Bruch's membrane. *Am J Ophthalmol* 1987;103:537–543.

Rothberg DS, Cibis GW, Trese M: Paravenous pigmentary retinochoroidal atrophy. *Ann Ophthalmol* 1984;16:643–646.

Ryan SJ, Dawson AK, LIttle HL: *Retinal Diseases*. Orlando, Fla, Grune & Stratton, 1985.

Ryan SJ, Maumenee AE: Birdshot retinochoroidopathy. *Am J Ophthalmol* 1980;89:31–45.

Schlaegel TF, Kenny D: Changes around the optic nerve head in presumed ocular histoplasmosis. *Am J Ophthalmol* 1966;62:454.

Schlaegel TF: *Ocular Histoplasmosis.* New York, Grune & Stratton, 1977.

Schlaegel TF: Perspectives in uveitis. *Ann Ophthalmol* 1981;13:799–806.

Sieving PA, Fishman GA, Jampol LM, Pugh D: Multiple evanescent white dot syndrome. II. Electrophysiology of photoreceptors during retinal pigment epithelial disease. *Arch Ophthalmol* 1984;102:675–679.

Sigelman J. *Retinal Diseases. Pathogenesis, Laser Therapy, and Surgery.* Boston, Little, Brown, 1984.

Singerman LJ, Wong B, Ai E, Smith S. Spontaneous visual improvement in the first affected eye of patients with bilateral disciform scars. *Retina* 1985;5:135–143.

Smiddy WE, Fine SL: Prognosis of patients with bilateral macular drusen. *Ophthalmology* 1984;91:271–277.

Snyder DA, Tessler HH: Vogt-Koyanagi-Harada syndrome. *Am J Ophthalmol* 1980;90:69–75.

Spalton DJ, Sanders MD: Fundus changes in histologically-confirmed sarcoidosis. *Br J Ophthalmol* 1981;65:348–358.

Spencer WH: *Ophthalmic Pathology. An Atlas and Textbook.* Philadelphia, Saunders, 1985.

Theodossiadis GP: Choroidal neovascularization after cryoapplication. *Albrecht von Graefes Arch Klin Ophthalmol* 1981;215:203–208.

Traboulsi EI, Maumenee IH: Hereditary pigmented paravenous chorioretinal atrophy. *Arch Ophthalmol* 1986;104:1636–1640.

Tso MO: Pathogenetic factors of aging macular degeneration. *Ophthalmology* 1985;92:628–635.

Watzke RC, Burton TC, Woolson RF: Direct and indirect laser photocoagulation of central serous choroidopathy. *Am J Ophthalmol* 1979;88:914–918.

Weiter JJ, Delori FC, Wing GL, Fitch KA: Relationship of senile macular degeneration to ocular pigmentation. *Am J Ophthalmol* 1985;15:185–187.

Wright BE, Bird AC, Hamilton AM: Placoid pigment epitheliopathy and Harada's disease. *Br J Ophthalmol* 1978;62:609–621.

Yanuzzi LA: A perspective on the treatment of aphakic cystoid macular edema. *Surv Ophthalmol* 1984;28(Suppl):540–553.

Yanuzzi LA, Gitter KA, Schatz H: *The Macula. A Comprehensive Text and Atlas.* Baltimore, Williams and Wilkins, 1979.

Young NJA, Bird AC, Sehmi K: Pigment epithelial disease with abnormal choroidal perfusion. *Am J Ophthalmol* 1980;90:607–608.

Anomalies of the Vitreous and Peripheral Retina

THE HUMAN VITREOUS

Introduction

The adult human vitreous is often overlooked in the analysis of diseases of the retina. It is, however, very important to understand the vitreous, diseases of the vitreous, and the vitreous connection to the retina. Vitreous/retina connections are extremely important in the genesis of the various diseases of the peripheral retina.

Anatomy and Attachments

The vitreous occupies about 67 percent to 75 percent of the ocular volume. The vitreous is a type of connective tissue that is semisolid to liquid consistency and is composed of approximately 99 percent water. The vitreous is attached in a few places within the eye (Fig. 4–1). Among these attachments is the anterior vitreous attachment at the posterior lens surface. This anterior vitreous attachment is called Weiger's adhesion. Weiger's adhesion is very strong in a young person, creating potential complications should intracapsular extraction be performed for a congenital cataract. Weiger's adhesion weakens with age, enabling safe intracapsular cataract extraction. The line demarcated on the posterior lens capsule representing Weiger's adhesion is called Egger's line. The anterior vitreous also attaches at the vitreous base, which is a very strong connection, 2 to 3 mm wide, straddling the ora serrata. It holds the vitreous cortex, sensory retina, and pars plana together. This adhesion can be disturbed, usually by trauma, resulting in a giant retinal tear or perhaps a retinal dialysis. The posterior portion of the vitreous is attached at the optic disc margin. This is most evident subsequent to a posterior vitreous detachment because the attachment then becomes an annular opacity floating in front of the optic nerve head. Sometimes the force of the posterior vitreous detachment at the optic nerve head can result in preretinal hemorrhages occurring near the disc. The posterior vitreous is also attached in the macular area in an oval form. This is usually a weak attachment that weakens even more with age. Detachment at the macula can create transient macular edema with metamorphopsia. This can be recurrent in a case of incomplete posterior vitreous detachment with repeated traction at the macular area. The posterior vitreous also may have weak connections at retinal vessels. This vascular connection is most evident in the case of posterior vitreous detachment with a subsequent preretinal bleed.

One other aspect of the vitreous that must be considered is Cloquet's canal. Cloquet's canal is a tubular structure running from the crystalline lens to the optic nerve head containing the primary vitreous. Cloquet's canal is bounded by condensations of the vitreous, referred to as plicated membranes. A hyaloid membrane is a thin, glasslike structure that surrounds the cortex of the vitreous like a crust on bread. This hyaloid membrane is thought to be a modified collagen fiber structure from the outer layer of the cortex of the vitreous.

ANATOMY AND ATTACHMENTS OF THE VITREOUS—PEARLS

- Attachments include
  - Weiger's Adhesion
  - 2- to 3- mm zone at the vitreous base, very strong
  - Optic disc margins, strong
  - Macular area, loose
  - Retinal vessels, loose
- 99 percent water occupying 67% to 75% of ocular volume
- Cloquet's canal bounded by plicated membranes
- Hyaloid membrane surrounds vitreous cortex

Vitreous Consistency and Transparency

The vitreous remains clear throughout most of the patient's life because the retinal vasculature is prevented from leaking into the vitreous cavity by the internal limiting membrane of the sensory retina and the vitreous cortex. Both of these structures act as selective barriers to prevent passage of blood components into the vitreous. Because the vitreous gel is approximately 99 percent water, it allows for maximum light transmission. The majority of the material within the vitreous that is considered to be solid is smaller than the wavelengths of visible light. As such, light scatter is minimized.

The consistency of the vitreous is determined by the concentration of collagenlike material called vitrosin. The viscosity of the vitreous is about four times that of water because of the concentration of hyaluronic acid macromolecules. The combination of hyaluronic acid and vitrosin forms the elasticity of the vitreous. Liquefaction or increased viscosity occurs when the hyaluronic acid macromolecules depolymerize. This liquefaction increases the chances of rapid volume shifts, movement of the vitreous through breaks in the hyaloid membrane, and movement of the vitreous through retinal tears and holes. The liquefied vitreous does

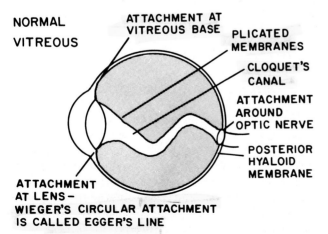

Figure 4–1. A schematic demonstrating the anatomy of the "normal" vitreous.

create a change in the retinal pigment epithelium once penetration of the retinal tissue occurs. The liquefied vitreous acts to break the mucopolysaccharide bonds of the retinal pigment epithelium, allowing for escape of the pigment granules into the vitreous. This escape of the pigment granules into the vitreous is characteristically a sign of impending or active retinal detachment and is known as the tobacco dust sign.

VITREOUS CONSISTENCY—PEARLS

- Transparency is maintained by internal limiting membrane and hyaloid membrane
- Consistency is determined by vitrosin (V) concentration
- Viscosity is determined by hyaluronic acid (HA) macromolecule concentration: V + HA = elasticity
- Liquefaction occurs when HA macromolecules depolymerize
  - Breaks down RPE
  - Allows for rapid volume shifts
  - Allows for movement of vitreous through breaks in hyaloid
  - Allows for movement of vitreous through breaks in retina

Examination of the Vitreous

Clinical examination of the vitreous is difficult because it is a clear substance and as such makes standard examination techniques very difficult. The vitreous can, however, be examined under magnification with the use of a fundus contact lens or some other device coupled with the variable power of the slit lamp. The slit lamp examination technique allows for microscopic examination of the vitreous. However, this is often an inadequate examination technique because the clinician must rely on subtle shadows and movement to properly diagnose vitreous alterations. It sometimes becomes necessary to incorporate the direct and binocular indirect ophthalmoscopy into the examination technique. The binocular indirect often will be unsuitable for examination of the vitreous contents. However, it can be used to pick up shadows of shifting vitreous that may be cast on the retina. The most effective examination technique of the vitreous, at least from a screening standpoint, is use of the direct ophthalmoscope. The direct ophthalmoscope held a few inches from the eye with proper magnification can be a very effective tool in screening for disorders of the vitreous. The clinician is using the back lit pupil while observing for breaks and shadows in the normal red reflex. Any examination technique of the vitreous is, however, enhanced by

maximal dilation of the pupil in addition to proper dark adaptation of both the clinician and the patient.

■ Clinical Note: Complete Examination of the Vitreous

A complete examination of the vitreous is both time consuming and requires a tremendous amount of skill. It uses all of the aspects available to the practitioner by way of the Goldmann three-mirror contact lens. A. The posterior portion of the Goldmann three-mirror contact lens can be used to scan the vitreous from immediately behind a crystalline lens to the retina interface. A wide beam in the slit lamp should be used, coupled with the lowest magnification possible. The beam should be variable, from vertical to oblique to a horizontal beam, to enhance total examination of the vitreous content. The slit is then narrowed, and the posterior portion of the Goldmann lens is used to examine the anterior vitreous more critically. B. While maintaining a narrow slit and low magnification, the central portion of the vitreous may now be examined. The slit should be focused very slowly and carefully as it is moved through the vitreous, which at this point includes Cloquet's canal. Again, for complete examination, vertical, oblique, and horizontal beams should be used to examine the entire vitreous. C. Still using the narrow slit beam, the posterior vitreous may now be evaluated. To properly examine the posterior vitreous, maintain a narrow slit beam and relatively low magnification. The red-free filter may also be used to attempt to enhance the view. It is important to remember that vitreous examination is a dynamic examination procedure. As such it is necessary to move the slit beam, the practitioner's view, the patient's fixation, as well as the Goldmann three-mirror lens. Movement enhances a situation known as the ascension phenomenon. The ascension phenomenon refers to the movement of the plicated Cloquet's canal. It is important to remember that anything viewed within the vitreous is going to be seen because of reflection of light from the beam. In theory the vitreous is optically empty, and as such one must remember that all things seen are obstructions to this free passage of light. D. To examine the vitreous using the mirrors, the practitioner must remember that the widest mirror is the equatorial mirror and should be used first. To come forward into the retina (the anterior retina), the clinician must use the more squared mirror. The U-shaped gonioscopy mirror may be tilted to examine pars plana and the vitreous base. It is extremely important to remember when using the mirrors that minimal magnification is necessary to enhance the view. In addition to that, it is necessary to manipulate the beam and mirror considerably to get to the area of interest. An indenter is available on some three-mirror lenses to enhance the view.

The Aging Vitreous

The aging vitreous becomes more easily viewed because of an increased density of fibers usually occurring after the age of 40 years. There is also an increase in the mobility of Cloquet's canal (the structure surrounding the primary vitreous). As mentioned before, this is known as the ascension phenomenon. The mobility of the structure within the vitreous becomes much more apparent with age because of liquefaction of the vitreous. This increased liquefaction with age manifests as lacunae, or optically empty spaces. It is important to remember that liquefaction of the vitreous does occur at a slightly earlier age in myopic patients than in other patients. It is also very important to remember that extensive liquefaction at a young age is usually an indication of a *pathological condition*. In addition to an increase in liquefaction, there is also a condition known as syneresis, or shrinkage of the vitreous, caused by separation of the liquids and solids. Age-related vitreous liquefaction and syneresis together are known as fibrillary degeneration. It is important to recognize the fact that fibrillary degeneration is a crucial prerequisite to the genesis of posterior vitreous detachment. Retinal manifestations of aging vitreous—liquefaction and syneresis—are many. They include white without pressure, retinal edema, and retinal tears. Figure 4–2 illustrates a schematic of the aging vitreous.

AGING VITREOUS—PEARLS

- Increased density of fibers after 40 years of age
- Increased liquefaction manifesting as lacunae and increased mobility of Cloquet's canal
- Syneresis, or shrinkage, caused by separation of the liquids and solids
- Fibrillary degeneration = liquefaction + syneresis

POSTERIOR VITREOUS DETACHMENT

Posterior vitreous detachment (PVD) is undoubtedly one of the more common occurrences that a clinician will experience in practice. It is, however, an extremely difficult process to view clinically. From an epidemiological standpoint, PVD rarely occurs until the age of 45 years. It does occur very

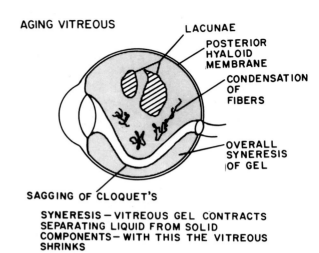

Figure 4–2. A schematic demonstrating vitreous changes typical of the aging vitreous.

commonly in up to 90 percent of aphakic eyes. Assuredly PVD increases in frequency with age, with a prevalence approximately equal to the person's age over 50 years. PVD can occur in younger patients and is usually related to trauma or chorioretinitis. PVD occurs as a result of several factors associated with aging. Table 4–1 illustrates a flow pattern for the genesis of posterior vitreous detachment.

PVD implies that the vitreous behind the vitreous base and hyaloid membrane is separated from the sensory retina. There can be several different categories of PVD. Under most circumstances, vitreous detachment is classified as a complete PVD and an incomplete PVD. This can be further broken down into subcategories with collapse of the vitreous gel and without collapse of the vitreous gel. Figures 4–2 through 4–6 illustrate various types of PVD.

The most frequently occurring PVD is a PVD with collapse of the vitreous gel. In this variety the

TABLE 4–1. HISTOPATHOLOGY OF PVD

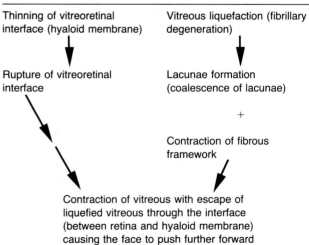

Thinning of vitreoretinal interface (hyaloid membrane)

Vitreous liquefaction (fibrillary degeneration)

↓

↓

Rupture of vitreoretinal interface

Lacunae formation (coalescence of lacunae)

+

Contraction of fibrous framework

Contraction of vitreous with escape of liquefied vitreous through the interface (between retina and hyaloid membrane) causing the face to push further forward

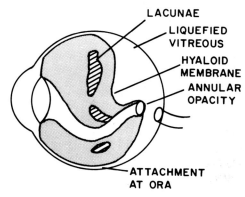

Figure 4–3. A schematic demonstrating vitreous changes typical of a complete posterior vitreous detachment with collapse.

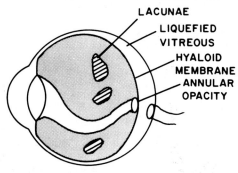

Figure 4–5. A schematic demonstrating vitreous changes typical of a complete posterior vitreous detachment without collapse.

vitreous is completely separated from the sensory retina up to the vitreous base. The vitreous base collapses upon itself but remains attached at the very strong anterior oral attachment. Clinically this creates the appearance of the posterior hyaloid membrane and vitreous cortex hanging down from the vitreous base. This also creates the common annular opacity floating in front of the optic nerve head. The incomplete posterior vitreous detachment does not represent a complete separation of the vitreous cortex from the sensory retina. This variety may occur with or without collapse of the vitreous gel. This variety may result in continued tugging in the macular area, resulting in macular edema.

Symptoms of PVD are fairly classical. Floaters are common, especially those of sudden onset with well outlined shadows cast on the retina from debris. If insect shaped, these floaters may indicate an operculated retinal tear. If they are cobweb in appearance, they may indicate an associated vitreous hemorrhage. Photopsia is reported to occur in 25 to 50 percent of cases. Photopsia usually occurs

as lightning streaks in the far periphery of the field of vision. These lightning streaks are due to vitreoretinal traction that causes physical stimulation of the photoreceptors. Photopsia may continue for weeks to years. The cessation of photopsia indicates that there is no longer traction and tugging on that vitreoretinal adhesion. Metamorphopsia, or distorted vision, may also result from macular edema secondary to the tugging of the vitreoretinal adherence at the macula. In addition, you must remember that the vitreoretinal adherence in oval form at the macula may tug with enough strength to precipitate transient macular edema and may help to create a macular hole. The classical shower of floaters that may occur is either a vitreous hemorrhage or possibly a retinal tear associated with the vitreous detachment.

The signs of PVD include vitreous opacities, the most common and classical being the annular ring in front of the optic nerve head. This annular ring represents the previous adherence of the vitreous face around the optic nerve. It must be remembered, however, that vitreous opacities may occur in any shape. Hemorrhages may occur around the disc associated with mild tears of the loosely adherent vitreous face to retinal vessels. These hemorrhages are transient. Vitreous hemorrhages may also occur associated with PVD and classically occur in the retrovitreous space. As mentioned previously, PVD may cause transient retinal edema (especially in the macula area), white without pressure, retinal tears, macular holes, and the long-term effects of traction (folds of the retina). The actual detection of the corrugated hyaloid membrane collapsed forward into the cortex is also a reasonably good sign of a posterior vitreous detachment.

Acute symptomatic PVD is associated with the onset of retinal breaks in about 10 percent of cases.

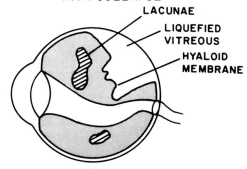

Figure 4–4. A schematic demonstrating vitreous changes typical of an incomplete posterior vitreous detachment with collapse.

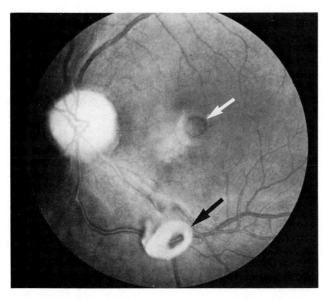

Figure 4–6. A posterior vitreous detachment as evidenced by the annular opacity **(dark arrow)** associated with a through-and-through macular hole **(white arrow).**

of retinal detachment. It is important to realize that patients with acute retinal tears usually will present a retinal detachment within 6 weeks after the onset of symptomatology. Table 4–2 will illustrate the signs, symptoms, and specific management of PVD.

PVD CHARACTERISTICS—PEARLS

- Increases in frequency with age—90 percent of aphakic patients
- Presents with sudden onset floaters—not a shower
- Often associated with photopsia that my continue for years
- May have metamorphopsia due to macular edema
- Appearance of annular ring floating over optic nerve
- May have short-lived hemorrhages around the optic nerve
- With time may see corrugated hyaloid membrane in the cortex
- May be retinal signs such as retinal breaks

PVD MANAGEMENT—PEARLS

- Maximal dilation investigating peripheral retina for tears—patients with acute retinal tears usually detach within 6 weeks after the onset of symptoms
- Advise of signs/symptoms of retinal detachment—unlikely 6 months after onset of PVD
- Follow-up according to these guidelines assuming no observable retinal tear:
  - No observable PVD but photopsia and vitreous degeneration—follow-up 6 months
  - PVD observed and ring or line floater—follow-up monthly for 3 months
  - PVD observed and photopsia—follow-up monthly for 3 months
  - PVD observed and pigment in vitreous—follow-up weekly for 6 weeks

See color plate 61.

It is important to note that approximately 50 percent of patients with retinal detachments do not have any history of flashes or floaters. About one third to one half of symptomatic retinal breaks progress on to retinal detachments. About 2.5 percent of symptomatic PVDs have traction at the posterior pole and may result in transient macular edema. It is also important to note that retinal detachment is highly unlikedly 6 months after a PVD has occurred. If a patient presents with symptoms of PVD, do the following! Perform a case history and visual acuity. Dilate the patient maximally, and try to find the signs of PVD. As discussed before, the practitioner must use a combination of the direct ophthalmoscope, binocular indirect ophthalmoscope, and Goldmann-type fundus lens. It is important to investigate the peripheral retina carefully for tears using scleral indentation. Assuming that there are no retinal tears, the practitioner must educate the patient about the signs and symptoms

---

TABLE 4–2. SIGNS, SYMPTOMS, AND MANAGEMENT OF PVD

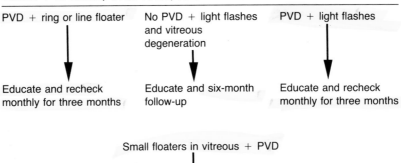

PVD + ring or line floater	No PVD + light flashes and vitreous degeneration	PVD + light flashes
↓	↓	↓
Educate and recheck monthly for three months	Educate and six-month follow-up	Educate and recheck monthly for three months

Small floaters in vitreous + PVD

↓

Educate + observe weekly for six weeks

ANTERIOR VITREOUS DETACHMENT

Anterior vitreous detachment is a relatively rare condition. Anterior vitreous detachment is rare because of the very strong attachment of the vitreous to the oral area of the retina. As such, most anterior vitreous detachments are typically associated with trauma or lens dislocation associated with specific conditions such as Marfan syndrome. The symptoms of anterior vitreous detachment include floaters and veils coming in front of the line of sight. The signs that the practitioner may observe are cells out into the vitreous cortex and an increase in the visibility of fibers. Management of anterior vitreous detachment would include assuring that there are no retinal tears. Retinal tears are highly likely because trauma that would cause an anterior vitreous detachment would more than likely also cause a retinal tear. If there are signs and symptoms of retinal traction, recheck the patient in three months and have the patient report at the onset of any new or changing symptoms. If a patient is asymptomatic and there are no retinal tears, the patient may be rechecked in one year. It is of course necessary in all of these cases to make the patient aware of the signs and symptoms of retinal detachment.

ANTERIOR VITREOUS DETACHMENT—PEARLS

- Associated with trauma and/or lens dislocation
- Symptoms include floaters and veils
- Signs include an increase in visibility of vitreous fibers and the appearance of cells
- Management.
  - Rule out retinal tears, especially near ora
  - If signs/symptoms of continued retinal traction present, follow-up in 3 months and advise of signs/symptoms of retinal detachment
  - If asymptomatic and no signs of traction, follow-up yearly and advise of signs/symptoms of retinal detachment

---

BASAL VITREAL DETACHMENT

Basal vitreal detachment (Fig. 4–7) is extremely rare but again is associated with trauma and retinal dialysis occurring at the ora serrata. It is important to manage the retinal dialysis by photocoagulative sealing or cryopexy.

BASAL VITREOUS DETACHMENT

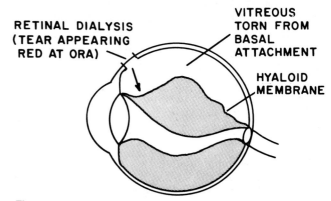

Figure 4–7. A schematic demonstrating vitreous changes typical of a basal vitreous detachment.

ASTEROID BODIES

Asteroid bodies are a relatively common finding in the vitreous. These asteroid bodies are classically described as Benson's bodies. They usually occur in patients over the age of 60 years, with approximately 90 percent unilaterality. While arguable, most studies point to the fact that there is no particular association with systemic-based diseases. From a histopathological standpoint, it is known that asteroid bodies are composed of calcium soaps that are 0.01 to 0.1 mm in diameter. The patients are often symptomless; however, the author has personally observed patients who complain of floaters in some of the more dramatic cases. From a clinical standpoint, the practitioner can observe small yellow-white spheres within the vitreous body. These spheres are adherent to the vitreous framework and always return to their original position after initiation of the ascension phenomenon. The clinician will also notice, when comparing one eye to the other, an increase in the vitreous density. From a management standpoint, it is only important that the patient be aware of the fact that he or she has asteroid bodies and that he or she realizes that asteroid bodies are a benign self-limited condition that will not lead to blindness.

ASTEROID BODIES—PEARLS

- Usually over the age of 60 years and most often unilateral
- Composed of calcium soaps
- Patient may complain of floaters
- Small yellow-white spheres adherent to vitreous framework and as such return to original position in ascension phenomenon
- Increased vitreous density
- Self-limiting and benign

Synchisis Scintillans

Synchisis scintillans is classically described as a bilateral vitreous disorder in the young. Synchisis scintillans is thought to be an accumulation of flat crystals of cholesterol (cholesterolosis bulbi). It is thought that these flat crystals sink to the bottom of the vitreous. What is probably truly being described only occurs in blind, severely damaged eyes. It is highly likely that synchisis scintillans is a very rare condition.

Paravascular Vitreous Attachments

Paravascular vitreous attachments may be acquired or congenital. They are also known as retinal tufts and will be discussed in more detail under the heading of retinal tufts. It is important to recognize, however, that they represent a strong adhesion of the posterior vitreous cortex to the equatorial zone in the form of granular tissue. These adhesions are considered to be proliferated glial cells. They are typically asymptomatic; however, they may have an associated phosphene, indicating an impending tear.

PARAVASCULAR VITREOUS ATTACHMENTS—PEARLS

- Strong adhesion of vitreous cortex to equatorial zone of retina
- Presents as white granular tissue that may demonstrate vitreous strands with potential for retinal tear
- Often symptomless unless impending tear
- A phosphene noted by a patient may be a sign of an impending tear associated with a paravascular vitreous attachment
- Management. • Advise on signs/symptoms of retinal detachment
  - Advise on sign of phosphene
  - Document and follow-up in 6 months

AMYLOID DEGENERATION OF THE VITREOUS—PRIMARY HEREDOFAMILIAL AMYLOIDOSIS

Amyloidosis is a very rare systemic disease with multiple manifestations. It can mimic several other conditions. Often amyloidosis is classified into the primary and secondary type. In the primary type, amyloid is deposited within collagen fibers usually involving the heart, thyroid, pancreas, and peripheral nerves and muscles. The primary type is usually not associated with generalized systemic disease debilitation. In the secondary type the amyloid substance is deposited in the liver,

spleen, kidneys, and adrenal glands and is associated with chronic debilitating diseases. Primary heredofamilial amyloidosis associated with the eye is the type more often seen clinically. The condition is transmitted as a dominant trait involving an extra chromosome. The condition typically presents after the second decade of life and runs a course of approximately 20 years. From the ocular standpoint, it must be realized that ocular involvement is present in 8 to 10 percent of cases including diplopia, progressive loss of vision, photophobia, blepharospasm, ophthalmoplegia, exophthalmos, vitreous opacities, retinal hemorrhages, and exudates. The vitreous may be the first area of involvement within the eye. It also may be a predecessor to organ involvement of the remainder of the body.

The amyloid typically deposits in the vessels of the choroid, optic nerve, and retina. The amyloid in the vitreous results from a break through the internal limiting membrane from retinal vessel foci. This results in fibrillar deposits within the vitreous content. The ocular signs are then vitreous opacities, typically being bilateral and slowly progressive, accompanied by retinal hemorrhages and perivascular exudates. Along with the ocular symptoms and signs, there may be the systemic manifestations of fatigue, loss of weight, progressive peripheral neuropathy, gastrointestinal (GI) disorders, as well as endocrine and cardiovascular compromise. As there is no cure for primary heredofamilial amyloidosis, management consists of supportive treatment for the systemic manifestations of the disease. Should severe vision loss occur, vitrectomy may be necessary to clean the debris from the vitreous. It is important to realize, however, that vitrectomy may cause retinal and vitreous bleeds because of the adhesion and close association of the vitreous to the foci of amyloid involvement of the retinal vessels.

AMYLOID DEGENERATION OF THE VITREOUS—PEARLS

- Rare systemic disease with dominant inheritance pattern
- Usually presents after second decade and runs 20 years
- Ocular involvement in 8 percent secondary to amyloid deposition in tissue
  - Diplopia
  - Photophobia and blepharospasm
  - Progressive loss of vision
  - Ophthalmoplegia
  - Vitreous opacities, retinal hemorrhages, and perivascular exudates
- Supportive management, as there is no cure, and genetic counseling
- Retinology consultation may be necessary at times

WAGNER'S HEREDITARY VITREORETINAL DEGENERATION

Wagner's hereditary vitreoretinal degeneration is autosomal dominant with 100 percent penetrance. This assures that 50 percent of the offspring of an affected parent will have the disease. The condition is bilateral and progressive. At birth the infant may have an entirely normal fundus. The children with Wagner's typically develop some degree of myopia under 5 diopters. As the child ages, the tessellation of the central and peripheral fundus becomes more prominent. Along with tessellation, the choroidal vessels along the distribution pattern of the retinal vessels become atrophic.

Progressive vitreous changes are observed in most patients and typically occur earlier in life. Initially there is liquefaction and fibrous condensation of the vitreous. This will eventually create a large lacuna in the posterior vitreous that appears optically empty. Preretinal gray-white membranes from the equator to the periphery then develop on the surface of the retina. Contracture of these preretinal membranes causes kinking of the vessels and edema of the retina. Associated with this there may be peripheral clumps of retinal pigment epithelium and choroidal atrophy. During adolescence and early adulthood there is shrinkage of the vitreous body resulting in the development of retinal tears with or without posterior vitreous detachment. Seventy-five percent of these patients do develop retinal tears, and 50 percent develop retinal detachment. Along with the retinal changes there is an increased incidence of cataract to more than 60 percent as the patient matures. After the age of 40 years almost all patients have cataracts.

There are no particular symptoms until the retinal or lenticular complications ensue. There may be an altered electroretinogram associated with Wagner's. There may be associated visual field contractions as well.

Management of this condition, once identified, consists of dilated fundus examinations every six months. As retinal breaks or detachments develop, it is important to intervene with photocoagulation, cryopexy, or scleral buckling. Cataract surgery is often indicated at an early age. Genetic counseling is also an important consideration.

WAGNER'S HEREDITARY VITREORETINAL DEGENERATION—PEARLS

- Bilateral progressive autosomal dominant condition
- Tessellation of central and peripheral fundus along with atrophy of the choroidal vessels associated with myopia in the child
- With progression there is fibrillary degeneration of the vitreous with development of a preretinal membrane and vitreous strands
- Contraction of membrane and strands creates retinal changes, including retinal pigment epithelium (RPE) clumping around vessels
- With further vitreous shrinkage retinal tears (75 percent) and retinal detachment occur (50 percent)
- 60 percent incidence of early-onset cataract
- Management
  - Advise of signs/symptoms of retinal detachment
  - Follow-up every 6 months
  - Retinology consultation for development of tears
  - Genetic counseling

CONGENITAL HEREDITARY RETINOSCHISIS

Congenital hereditary retinoschisis is sometimes known as juvenile retinoschisis. The disease is transmitted as a recessive sex-linked trait affecting male offspring. In rare cases, however, females may contract the disease as an autosomal recessive disease. This disease may present between the ages of 7 months to 28 years. The condition is more often than not bilateral.

Congenital hereditary retinoschisis occurs as a result of the splitting of the retina at the nerve fiber layer. Associated with this splitting of the retina is vitreous liquefaction. The patient complains of poor vision, strabismus, nystagmus (if the condition occurs at a young enough age), and floaters. The condition is stationary, with periods of slow progression that alternate with periods of spontaneous remission. Signs of progression are an increase in the extent or volume of the retinoschisis, an increase in the size or number of inner layer or outer layer breaks, decreased visual acuity, and vitreous hemorrhage. Progression of the disease is fairly rapid in the initial stages slowing at later stages. There is often a deep scotoma in the area of the schisis.

Usually congenital hereditary retinoschisis occurs in the inferotemporal quadrant but usually not all the way out to the ora. The schisis is often accompanied by a veil membrane coursing out into the vitreous carrying retinal vasculature. To differentiate this from acquired retinoschisis, the practitioner must remember that acquired retinoschisis runs all the way to the ora serrata and usually occurs in older patients. As mentioned in signs of progression, there are inner layer and outer layer breaks, or holes, that can develop in the schisis. The clinician may also notice pigmented demarcation lines along the posterior border of the retinoschisis, indicating progression and remission. There may be associated optic nerve changes in the form of pseudopapilledema, dragging of the disc vasculature, and, in some instances, descending optic atrophy. Macular changes usually involve a cystic kind of alteration, giving a depigmented star on the background of mottled pigment. Actually the macula has a beaten metallic appearance but not nearly as dramatic as Stargardt's disease. The liquefaction of the vitreous may allow for vitreous cortex bands to be attached to the retinoschisis.

There is no especially good treatment for congenital hereditary retinoschisis. Treatment of the breaks in the retinoschisis and/or the associated retinal detachment are indicated once those lesions appear. It is of course absolutely necessary that a patient with congenital hereditary retinoschisis have yearly examinations to ascertain times of progression. Should the condition progress, it is necessary to recognize complications as early as possible. Genetic counseling is indicated. The patient often becomes a candidate for low-vision rehabilitation. **See color plate 62.**

nal degeneration and congenital hereditary retinoschisis. It affects almost all retinal layers and structures within the eye. In Goldmann-Favre's there is a progressive loss of vision associated with retinoschisis and pigmented chorioretinal degeneration. The condition is more often than not bilateral, with no particular predilection for sex. It is transmitted in an autosomal recessive fashion.

Associated with a progressive loss of vision are areas of scotomas. The central and peripheral retinoschisis look entirely different. The central retinoschisis appears as it does in congenital hereditary retinoschisis as a beaten metallic alteration. The peripheral schisis will be elevated, and there can be inner layer and outer layer breaks. There may also be retinal pigment epithelial clumping—bone corpuscularlike—along the vessels. There is an extinguished electroretinogram as well as night blindness. An early onset cataract may be present associated with considerable liquefaction of the vitreous. The patient also often complains of poor day vision (hemeralopia).

There is no known effective management for Goldmann-Favre's vitreotapetoretinal degeneration. The best the clinician can hope to do is perform routine eye examinations on this patient, advise on the hereditary aspect of the disease, and attempt to treat complications as they occur.

CONGENITAL HEREDITARY RETINOSCHISIS—PEARLS

- Bilateral, slow progression with periods of remission
- Sex-linked recessive transmission
- May present between 7 months to 28 years of age
- Schisis of retina at nerve fiber layer with early-onset vitreous liquefaction
- Presents in inferotemporal quadrant with a veil membrane that does not run to ora
- Macular cystic changes may present as depigmented star on mottled background
- Management . • Advise of signs/symptoms of retinal detachment
   • Documentation and yearly follow-up
   • Retinology consult for tears
   • Genetic counseling
   • Low vision rehabilitation

GOLDMANN-FAVRE'S VITREOTAPETORETINAL DEGENERATION—PEARLS

- Bilateral progressive loss of vision
- Autosomal recessive inheritance
- Central and peripheral retinoschisis with RPE clumping along vessels
- Vitreous liquefaction
- Possible early-onset cataract
- Management . • Advise of signs/symptoms of retinal detachment
   • Documentation and yearly follow-up
   • Retinology consultation for complications
   • Genetic counseling

GOLDMANN-FAVRE'S VITREOTAPETORETINAL DEGENERATION

Goldmann-Favre's vitreotapetoretinal degeneration is a rare condition that seems to be a combination of the signs and symptoms of Wagner's vitreoreti-

FAMILIAL EXUDATIVE VITREORETINOPATHY

Familial exudative vitreoretinopathy is inherited in an autosomal dominant pattern. It occurs bilaterally in relatively young patients. There are no associated systemic manifestations, and the disease process involves primarily the vitreous and the retina. Visual loss is slow and progressive.

Patients with exudative vitreoretinopathy may run the full gamut of fundus signs. There can be excessive white without pressure or white with pressure, unusual peripheral vessels, and vitreous shrinkage with band formation. As the condition becomes more severe, dilated tortuous peripheral vessels present with neovascularization. Associated with the neovascularization may be recurrent hemorrhages. As neovascularization has accompanying fibrotic scaffolding, there may be formation of traction retinal detachments and/or retinal tears. There is a minimal liquefaction of the vitreous, and vitreous haze occurs as the result of cells that have been liberated. In the end stages the patient can develop retinal detachments and optic atrophy.

Familial exudative vitreoretinopathy demonstrates relatively poor results with attempts at prophylactic treatment. The accepted mode of management at this time is treatment of the retinal detachment and/or holes when they do occur and treatment of the vitreous hemorrhage when it occurs. It is, of course, necessary to provide genetic counseling to these patients as well as routine ocular examinations.

FAMILIAL EXUDATIVE VITREORETINOPATHY—PEARLS

- Bilateral presentation in young patients with slowly progressive loss of vision
- Autosomal dominant inheritance
- Excessive WWOP, vitreous shrinkage, and band formation
- Dilated tortuous peripheral vessels and peripheral neovascularization
- Tugging may present as vitreous hemorrhage, retinal tears, and traction retinal detachment resulting in loss of vision and optic atrophy
- Management is treatment of complications and genetic counseling

---

SYSTEMIC CONDITIONS ASSOCIATED WITH VITREOUS DEGENERATION

There are several systemic conditions that have been associated with vitreous degeneration. Among those conditions are Marfan's syndrome, homocystinuria, Ehlers-Danlos syndrome, pseudoxanthoma elasticum, and retinitis pigmentosa. Marfan's syndrome presents with liquefaction of the vitreous, posterior vitreous detachment, and crystalline lens dislocation. Homocystinuria presents with vitreous liquefaction, posterior vitreous detachment, and crystalline lens dislocation. Ehlers-Danlos syndrome is characterized by a PVD. The pseudoxanthoma elasticum complex presents with vitreous liquefaction, PVD, and brown cells liberated into the vitreous. Retinitis pigmentosa presents with vitreous liquefaction, PVD, and brown cells in the vitreous. Characteristics of homocystinuria and Marfan's syndrome are presented in Table 4–3. All of the associate conditions carry potentially severe systemic disease implications and as such must be carefully diagnosed and managed.

HEMORRHAGE INTO THE VITREOUS

Retrovitreous Hemorrhage
Vitreous hemorrhages occur in two categories, retrovitreous and intravitreous hemorrhages. Retrovitreous hemorrhages typically occur in eyes with PVD. Retrovitreous hemorrhages are associated with trauma, diabetic retinopathy, retinal breaks without a detachment, and rhegmatogenous retinal detachment. Retrovitreous hemorrhages can also occur in retinal vein occlusive disease. The patient who presents with a retrovitreous hemorrhage will typically complain of floaters and/or loss of vision,

---

TABLE 4–3. THE DIFFERENTIAL DIAGNOSTIC FEATURES OF HOMOCYSTINURIA AND MARFAN'S SYNDROME

Feature	Homocystinuria	Marfan's Syndrome
Inheritance	Autosomal recessive	Autosomal dominant
Skeletal abnormalities	Osteoporosis, fractures, rarely arachnodactyly	Arachnodactyly and loose joints
Vascular disease	Dilatation with thrombosis in intermediate-sized arteries and veins	Dilatation or dissection of aorta
Ectopia lentis	Often observed in children; lens displaced inferiorly and often dislocated into anterior chamber or vitreous cavity	Often detected in children; lens displaced superiorly and seldom dislocated into anterior chamber or vitreous cavity

depending upon the particular location of the hemorrhage.

Retrovitreous hemorrhages present as bright red, unclotted blood that shifts readily with eye movements. They are often keel shaped or boat shaped when they settle. It is always possible to view the vitreous base when a retrovitreous hemorrhage occurs. The clinician may also notice red blood cells perfused into the vitreous gel. Retrovitreous hemorrhages occur as a result of vitreous strands that pull on retinal vessels when a posterior vitreous detachment occurs. It is believed that there is a normal, loose adherence of the vitreous base to retinal blood vessels in addition to the standard zones of attachment at the ora, the optic nerve head, and the macula.

Retrovitreous hemorrhages eventually disappear with hemolysis and phagocytosis. It is important, however, to ascertain the cause of a retrovitreous hemorrhage should there be a threat of rehemorrhage. It is at times necessary to hospitalize the patient and to consider the possibility of vitrectomy in cases of retrovitreous hemorrhages. It is important, therefore, to consult a qualified retinologist in cases of retrovitreous hemorrhage.

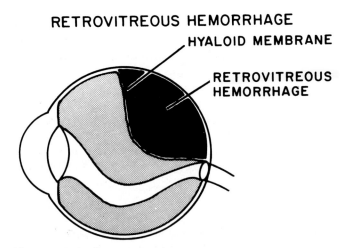

Figure 4–8. A schematic illustrating a retrovitreous hemorrhage.

to a grey coloration more rapidly than the clotted blood within the cortex. The patient with an intravitreous hemorrhage may complain of floaters or sudden loss of vision of variable degree.

Signs of intravitreous hemorrhage vary considerably according to the extent of the hemorrhage. A long-standing intravitreous hemorrhage will present with intravitreal membranes projecting out into the vitreous cortex. These intravitreal greylike membranes occur in the inferior portion of the vitreous body. Intravitreous hemorrhages take a long time to resorb and with resorption change color from the top to the bottom of the vitreous cavity. Gravity will pull most of the coagulated blood down into the inferior vitreous, creating a longer resorption time in that particular area. It is important to attempt to ascertain the cause for an intravitreal hemorrhage. This is often difficult because the extent of the blood within the cavity will prevent effective evaluation of the *retina*. Patients with intravitreal hemorrhages often need hospitalization, with the consideration of vitrectomy once enough blood has cleared from the cavity to evaluate the retina. It is important to consult a qualified

---

> **RETROVITREOUS HEMORRHAGE—PEARLS**
>
> - Occurs in eyes with PVD
> - Associated with trauma, diabetic retinopathy, retinal breaks without retinal detachment, rhegmatogenous retinal detachment, and retinal vein occlusion
> - Presents as bright red blood that is keel shaped with settling and shifts readily with eye movements
> - It is always possible to view the vitreous base
> - Management. • Ascertain cause
>   - Retinology consultation should be strongly considered

Intravitreous Hemorrhage

Intravitreous hemorrhage (Figs. 4–8 and 4–9) may or may not have a posterior vitreous detachment associated with it. Intravitreous hemorrhage is secondary to trauma and diabetic retinopathy (34.1 percent), retinal break without detachment (22.4 percent), rhegmatogenous retinal detachment (14.9 percent), and retinal vein occlusion (13.0 percent). Intravitreous hemorrhage occurs secondary to a ruptured blood vessel that may have associated vitreous traction. The blood within the vitreous gel clots very quickly, forming fixed projections. Blood may collect within lacunae, which are more liquefied than the cortex and as a result of that appear as a denser red. The blood in the lacunae changes

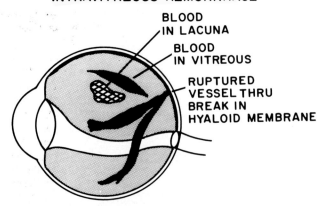

Figure 4–9. A schematic illustrating the possibilities associated with an intravitreous hemorrhage.

retinologist concerning patients with intravitreal hemorrhages. It is also important to note that it is possible to have a combination of retrovitreous and intravitreous hemorrhages and that the combinations are often associated with trauma.

INTRAVITREOUS HEMORRHAGE—PEARLS

- Associated with diabetic retinopathy (34 percent), retinal break without retinal detachment (22 percent), rhegmatogenous retinal detachment (15 percent), and retinal vein occlusion (13 percent)
- Blood clots quickly forming fixed projections within cortex but stay very red in lacunae
- Slow resorption from superior to inferior with formation of dense membranes inferiorly
- Management
  - Ascertain cause
  - Retinology consultation should be strongly considered

PERSISTENT HYPERPLASTIC PRIMARY VITREOUS

Persistent hyperplastic primary vitreous (PHPV; Figs. 4–10 and 4–11) occurs in full-term infants that have had no exposure to oxygen therapy. Histopathologically, PHPV represents a failure of regression of the structures of the primary vitreous. there are two basic forms of PHPV, anterior and posterior. The anterior form of PHPV presents with leukocoria, unilateral affliction, microcornea, strabismus at times, a retrolental membrane that may progress to a cataract, congenital glaucoma, microophthalmia, and a normal retina. The ciliary processes may be drawn to the periphery of the crystalline lens and are easily seen with dilation. The posterior form presents with unilateral microcornea, often a pale hypoplastic disc, a normal crystalline lens, vitreous membranes containing hyaloid artery remnants, vitreoretinal adhesions, and peripapillary retinal-pigment epithelial changes. In the posterior form it is important to remember that the vitreous membranes that remain have the potential to cause retinal folds and subsequent decrease in visual acuity.

Management of the anterior form is early surgical intervention to prevent ultimate blindness and possible loss of the eye. In the posterior form it is important to watch the patient yearly for the development of glaucoma and/or retinal breaks.

Perhaps the most important feature of PHPV is the differentiation of this condition from other ocular disease anomalies. It is important to differentiate PHPV in the anterior form from retinoblastoma. In the posterior form, PHPV may simulate retinopathy of prematurity. The primary differentiating feature from retinopathy of prematurity is the fact that PHPV occurs in full-term infants who have had no oxygen therapy. The leukocoria of the anterior form becomes a bit more of a diagnostic dilemma, perhaps necessitating the implementation of higher-level diagnostic procedures. When in doubt, consult a retinologist concerning the differential diagnosis of PHPV, retinoblastoma, and retinolental fibroplasia.

Norrie's disease is a condition that may be confused with PHPV. Norrie's disease is an x-linked disorder associated with a hearing disorder, ocular appearance similar to PHPV, and cerebral dysplasia (retardation). The ocular disorder is characterized by leukocoria, retinal folds, shallow anterior chambers, synechiae, retinal detachment, micro-ophthalmos, corneal degeneration, cataract, and pthisis balbi. Differentiation of Norrie's disease from PHPV is important because of the genetic implications.

PERSISTENT HYPERPLASTIC PRIMARY VITREOUS

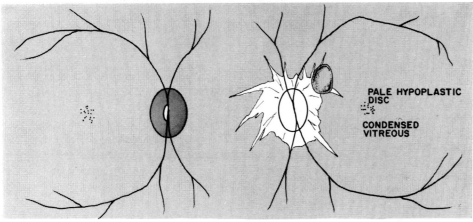

PALE HYPOPLASTIC DISC

CONDENSED VITREOUS

Norris/Alexander

Figure 4–10. A schematic illustrating optic-nerve head changes associated with persistent hyperplastic primary vitreous.

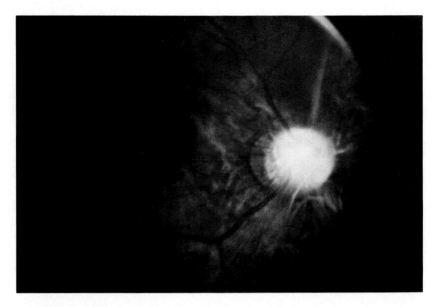

OD

A. PIGMENT DYSTROPHY
B. VITREAL CONDENSATION
C. VITREO - RETINAL MEMBRANE
D. TORTUOUS VESSELS
E. HYPOPLASTIC DISC
F. MACULA DRAGGED TOWARD
   DISC

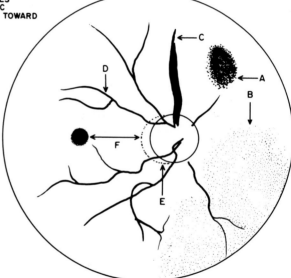

Figure 4–11. Top. A black and white photograph of PHPV with the schematic **(bottom)** illustrating the changes. *(Photo and figure from T. Madgar.)*

PERSISTENT HYPERPLASTIC PRIMARY VITREOUS—PEARLS

- Failure in the regression of the primary vitreous
- Full-term nonoxygenated history
- Anterior form—leukocoria, unilateral, strabismus, retrolental membrane, cataract, microcornea, shallow anterior chamber, congenital glaucoma, normal retina
- Posterior form—microcornea, unilateral, vitreous membranes and vitreoretinal adhesions, retinal folds, peripapillary RPE changes, pale hypoplastic disc
- Management anterior—early surgical intervention and patient education
- Management posterior—monitor yearly for the development of retinal breaks or glaucoma and patient education

ANATOMICAL CHARACTERISTICS OF THE PERIPHERAL RETINA

Figure 4–12 is a schematic representation of retinal layers in the posterior pole. Variations in these layers occur in the peripheral retina. The retinal periphery is defined as the zone from the equator to the ora serrata and is approximately 3 disc diameters (DD) or 1 condensing lens (20 D) in width. This retinal periphery has several anatomic landmarks that can guide the practitioner in the examination and location of various lesions. The vortex vein ampullae mark the equator of the eye. There is usually one vortex vein per quadrant, but there may be up to ten in each eye. These vortex vein

MAGNIFIED SCHEMATIC RETINAL CROSS SECTION

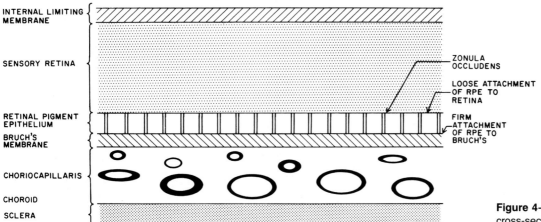

Figure 4–12. A schematic retinal cross-section of a normal retina.

ampullae vary in appearance from reddish to orange and take on the shape of an octopus. These vortex vein ampullae often have a significant amount of pigment surrounding them. There may be several tributaries emptying into a single ampulla. The ampullae may dilate with pressure created in changing direction of gaze or by making a postural change. When they dilate they assume a darker color and become elevated. These variations are known as vortex vein varices.

The long posterior ciliary nerves and arteries often serve as a good anatomic landmark in the peripheral retina. The long posterior ciliary nerves and arteries run at the 3 o'clock and 9 o'clock positions from the ora to the equator of the posterior pole. The long posterior ciliary nerves are typically yellowish to white in color, often with pigmented borders. The artery usually runs above the ciliary nerve in the nasal retina and below the ciliary nerve in the temporal retina.

The short posterior ciliary nerves may number 10 to 20 in the peripheral retina and have a tendency to congregate near the vertical meridians. As with the long posterior ciliary nerves and arteries, the short posterior ciliary nerves are yellowish to white, again often with pigmented borders. The short posterior ciliary arteries may be scattered anywhere on the horizontal meridian and may have associated pigment margins.

Peripheral retinal vessels typically run a much different course than those in the posterior pole. Peripheral retinal vessels often run parallel to the ora serrata. The area close to the ora serrata, however, is usually devoid of any apparent retinal vasculature.

The ora serrata is the anterior limit of the neural retina. The ora serrata is scalloped more nasally than temporally. The practitioner can distinguish the temporal from the nasal ora serrata because the temporal ora serrata is usually narrower

than the nasal ora serrata. The rounded areas extending from the pars plana, which is brown in color, are called oral bays. The whitish retinal extensions into these bays are called oral teeth. The oral bays and oral teeth together are called dentate processes, of which there are 20 to 30 per eye. Dentate processes are usually absent in the temporal aspect of the peripheral retina. Deep or large oral bays may occur as anatomical variants in the ora serrata region. Bridging oral teeth with no particular contact with the pars plana can also occur as an anatomical variance.

The pars plana is an anatomical landmark that is chocolate in color, running from the ora serrata to the ciliary processes. The ciliary processes number 60 to 70 and are cream colored in indirect view but pigmented with the slit lamp view. As in the sensory retina, one can have separation of layers of the epithelium of the pars plana, which are pars plana cysts.

The vitreous base is also considered an anatomical landmark of the peripheral retina. The vitreous base is a strong connection of the vitreous to the retinal tissue, running in a 2- to 4-mm band that straddles the ora serrata. The vitreous base band is typically wider nasally than it is temporally. The posterior limit of the vitreous base is usually invisible but is the anatomical limit of a posterior vitreous detachment. The anterior limit of the vitreous base may be seen as a whitish haze on the pars plana. The entire vitreous base band may be marked by an increase in pigmentation beneath the base itself, especially if there is excessive vitreoretinal traction. This increased pigmentation is nothing more than a retinal pigment epithelial hyperplasia that is a reaction to insult to the retina. It is interesting to note that about 15 percent of retinal breaks can be seen along the posterior extensions of the vitreous base.

CLINICAL EXAMINATION OF THE PERIPHERAL RETINA

Several instruments are available for examination of the retina anterior to the equator. Monocular indirect ophthalmoscopy can get the job done but suffers from (1) a lack of stereo examination ability, (2) a relatively poor light source, (3) no method of adjusting magnification, (4) lower resolution capabilities than binocular indirect ophthalmoscopy, and (5) inability to effectively perform scleral indentation.

Examination of the peripheral retina with a three-mirror lens has the advantage of variable magnification, variable illumination, availability of filters, and stereopsis. One can perform scleral indentation with specially adapted three-mirror lenses. The primary disadvantage of this technique is the reduction in observable field of view accompanied by a reduced resolution ability. The view is similar to looking at a grainy photograph at a close distance. This technique is useful as an adjunct to binocular indirect ophthalmoscopy.

The binocular indirect ophthalmoscope is an absolute necessity for effective evaluation of vitreoretinal diseases, especially those anterior to the equator. The binocular indirect ophthalmoscope offers (1) variable field of view and variable magnification, (2) access to the farthest peripheral regions of the retina, (3) a bright light source and improved resolution, (4) excellent stereopsis, and (5) the ability to add scleral indentation for more complete fundus evaluation. There are disadvantages to binocular indirect ophthalmoscopy. The disadvantages involve adaptation to the inverted reversed image as well as the difficulty of adaptation to the instrument.

Mastering scleral indentation elevates the clinician to the highest level of diagnostic skill in peripheral retinal evaluation. In reality, it is close to impossible to discern subtleties of the retina near the ora without the benefit of scleral indentation. Not only does scleral indentation push retinal structural alterations into view but it also increases the contrast between intact retina and retinal breaks (Fig. 4–13). The indented retinal/choroidal structure is darker than the surrounding retina, which increases the contrast. It is also important to realize that there is decreased retinal translucency with indentation because the examiner is viewing the retina at a more oblique angle. Scleral indentation is a kinetic procedure as well, which enhances the discovery of subtle changes. It is far easier to see changes when the retinal structures are moving. The discovery of retinal tears and holes is facilitated with indentation as the edges roll upward and lighten while the hole darkens. The rolling of holes is illustrated in Figure 4–13.

It is important to orient oneself to retinal structure prior to the performance of scleral indentation. Figure 4–14 gives the basic ocular dimensions from the corneal limbus to facilitate orientation with common retinal landmarks. It is important to realize that to indent the equator, it is only necessary to place the indenter 13 mm or about one half inch

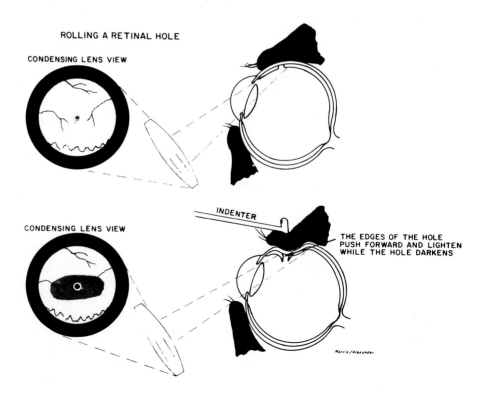

ROLLING A RETINAL HOLE

CONDENSING LENS VIEW

CONDENSING LENS VIEW

INDENTER

THE EDGES OF THE HOLE PUSH FORWARD AND LIGHTEN WHILE THE HOLE DARKENS

Norris/Alexander

Figure 4–13. A schematic illustrating the effects of applying an indenter to an eye and "rolling a retinal hole."

DISTANCE FROM LIMBUS TO EQUATOR

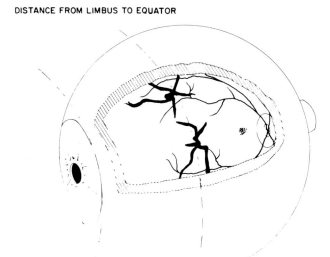

|← 11-15 mm →|

Norris/Alexander

Figure 4–14. A schematic illustrating the relatively short distance from the limbus to the equator.

posterior to the limbus. The distance back from the limbus to most structures that need to be viewed is almost always less than 13 mm.

Scleral indentation can be performed safely in most patients. Patients with active glaucoma or intraocular lenses should be indented with great care. Patients with recent intraocular surgery or those suspected of having penetrating trauma should not be indented. Choice of the type of indentor is at the discretion of the practitioner.

Technique for Scleral Indentation

1. Topical anesthesia may be applied to the eye prior to indentation but remember that this may cause mild corneal edema and sloughing. This will obviously compromise the view. Most of the time indentation is performed through the lids, which eliminates the need for anesthesia.
2. Maximal dilation is an absolute necessity.
3. Educate the patient as to the mild discomfort (pressure) experienced during the procedure.
4. Recline the patient and tilt the head forward, backward, and side to side to maximize the view. An example of this would be tilting the head back (chin up) to facilitate the view of the superior retina.
5. To view the 12 o'clock position (the easiest zone to view), ask the patient to gently close his or her eyes and to look down. Place the tip of the indenter on the upper lid at the margin of the tarsal plate (do not attempt to indent through the tarsal plate).
6. While maintaining the position of the indentor, have the patient slowly look up - the practitioner must move the indentor tip back as the eye rolls upward.
7. Remember that the indenter tip should always be tangential to the globe—not perpendicular, as this would be painful. Also remember to keep line of sight, condensing lens, and shaft of the indenter aligned. Figure 4–15 illustrates proper alignment. If any factor is out of alignment the retinal orientation is quickly lost.
8. When all factors are aligned, exert gentle pressure and view the mound created by the indentation. The necessary pressure can only be at-

PROPER ALIGNMENT OF INDENTER, CONDENSING LENS AND LINE OF SIGHT

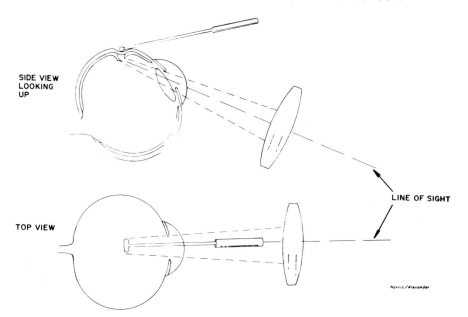

SIDE VIEW LOOKING UP

LINE OF SIGHT

TOP VIEW

Norris/Alexander

Figure 4–15. A schematic illustrating the proper alignment of the scleral indenter, condensing lens and line of sight.

tained through practice.

9. Remember that indentation is intended to be a kinetic procedure. Move the indenter gently, remembering to keep the entire observation system aligned. Also recall that the indenter must be moved opposite to what appears to be necessary when viewing through the condensing lens. Said another way, move the indenter toward the cornea to view the retina inferior in the condensing lens. Once the accessible area has been examined, move to the next quadrant.

10. To depress the 3 o'clock and 9 o'clock quadrants, it may be necessary to drag the lids up or down into position. If there is not enough laxity of the lids, it may be necessary to anesthetize and depress directly on the bulbar conjunctiva.

There is no magic to performing scleral indentation. Just remember that it is like rubbing one's stomach and patting one's head at the same time. Keep the tip tangential to the globe, exert gentle pressure, move the tip, and keep line of sight, condensing lens, and shaft of the indentor aligned.

PERIPHERAL RETINAL CHANGES THAT USUALLY DO NOT POSE AN IMMEDIATE THREAT TO VISION— EXCEPTION IS CHOROIDAL MELANOMA

Peripheral Senile Pigmentary Degeneration

Peripheral senile pigmentary degeneration (Fig. 4–16), also known as peripheral tapetochoroidal degeneration, appears as granular pigment between the ora serrata and the equator in approximately 20 percent of the population over the age of 40 years. This pigment often cuffs or surrounds the venules as macrophages carry the pigment toward the retinal vessels. This pigment may take on a reticular or bone spicule appearance, simulating the appearance of retinitis pigmentosa. This degeneration is often accompanied by benign peripheral retinal drusen. The differential diagnosis between this and retinitis pigmentosa is made by considering patient characteristics as well as performing routine visual field analysis. Peripheral senile degeneration usually is bilateral. The layers involved in peripheral senile pigmentary degeneration are degenerating retinal pigment epithelium scattering pigment throughout the sensory retina. There is ultimately loss of photoreceptors and sclerosis of the chorio-

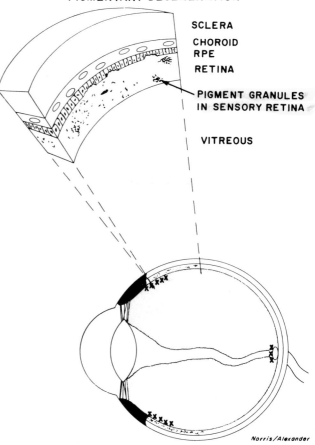

Figure 4–16. A schematic illustrating the clinicopathological changes associated with peripheral senile pigmentary degeneration.

capillaris, implicating the possibility of vascular compromise associated with aging. The prognosis of this condition is usually benign. There is typically no compromise of visual fields or dark adaptation, and the electro-retinogram (ERG) and electro-oculogram (EOG) are normal. This does help to differentiate this condition from retinitis pigmentosa or pigmented paravenous retinochoroidal atrophy. Peripheral senile pigmentary degeneration is an age-related change that requires no particular treatment except for routine visual examinations every 2 years.

The accompanying illustration will point to the specific histopathological changes associated with peripheral senile pigmentary degeneration. The clinician can see that there is essentially a breakdown in the retinal pigment epithelium with deposition of the pigment granules in the sensory retina. Loss of the retinal pigment epithelium does imply that there will eventually be loss or compromise of overlying photoreceptors.

Primary Chorioretinal Atrophy

See color plate 63. Primary chorioretinal atro-

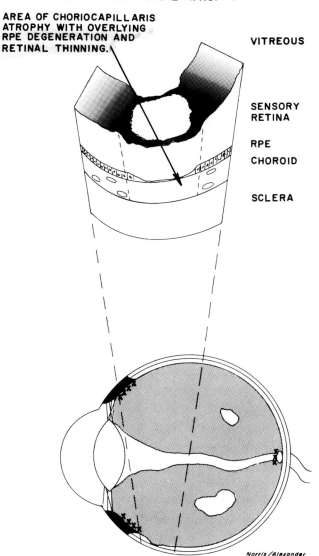

PRIMARY CHORIORETINAL ATROPHY

AREA OF CHORIOCAPILLARIS
ATROPHY WITH OVERLYING
RPE DEGENERATION AND
RETINAL THINNING.

VITREOUS

SENSORY
RETINA

RPE

CHOROID

SCLERA

Norris/Alexander

x—DENOTES STRONG VITREORETINAL
ADHESION

Figure 4–17. A schematic illustrating the clinicopathological changes associated with primary chorioretinal atrophy.

phy (Figs. 4–17 and 4–18) is also known as cobblestone degeneration and pavingstone degeneration. Primary chorioretinal atrophy occurs in over 20 percent of patients over 40 years of age. Primary chorioretinal atrophy usually appears as small (0.1 to 1.5 mm) pale yellow or depigmented non-elevated areas in the peripheral retina. Nearly 80 percent of the lesions are in the inferotemporal quadrant. These changes are typically separated from the ora serrata. The lesions may be larger when they coalesce, and they will certainly have associated pigmentary changes. The choroidal vessels may be seen within the lesion because of loss of overlying retinal pigment epithelium. This is a fairly common age-related change with prevalence increasing with age. There is a 33 percent incidence of bilaterality in primary chorioretinal atrophy. The layers involved are the choriocapillaris, with subsequent atrophy of the overlying retinal pigment epithelium and outer retina. This is thought to occur as a result of occlusion of compartments of the choriocapillaris. There is a resultant depression in the area because of retinal tissue loss. As far as prognosis is concerned, the involvement may increase with age, but it is of no long-term significance, as the inner retinal layers stay intact. That is to say that there is no particular potential toward the development of retinal holes in primary chorioretinal atrophy. From a management standpoint the primary concern is differential diagnosis including postinflammatory scars, retinal holes, and lattice degeneration. It is only necessary to examine the patient every two years.

The accompanying figure demonstrates primary chorioretinal atrophy. The clinician can see that there is a basic underlying infarct in the choriocapillaries. This infarct compromises blood flow to the retinal pigment epithelium and thus the sensory retina. This causes degeneration and atrophy of those structures, allowing for depigmentation and the genesis of the whitish circular-to-oval lesion.

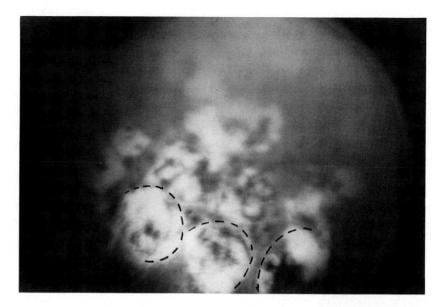

Figure 4–18. Areas of primary chorioretinal atrophy outlined by the dotted lines.

Postinflammatory Chorioretinal Scar

The postinflammatory chorioretinal scar (Figs. 4–19

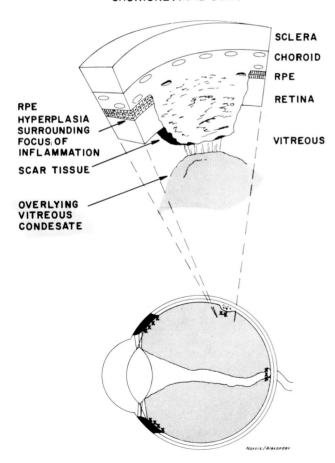

CHORIORETINAL SCAR

SCLERA
CHOROID
RPE
RETINA

VITREOUS

RPE HYPERPLASIA SURROUNDING FOCUS OF INFLAMMATION

SCAR TISSUE

OVERLYING VITREOUS CONDESATE

Norris/Alexander

x — DENOTES STRONG VITREORETINAL ADHESION

Figure 4–19. A schematic illustrating the clinicopathological changes associated with a chorioretinal scar.

and 4–20) can appear in many different ways. The scar is usually a white to yellow area of fibrosis within the retina, with reactive retinal pigment epithelial proliferation. This retinal pigment epithelial proliferation scatters dark pigmentation throughout the lesion and is nothing more than a reaction of the retinal pigment epithelium to insult. In the majority of chorioretinal scars there is overlying vitreous condensation with some strandlike attachments to the scar. **See color plate 61.**

The layers involved in chorioretinal scars can vary as well. Depending upon the severity of the lesion, one may have involvement of the choriocapillaris, retinal pigment epithelium, and the sensory retina.

The prognosis is fairly good for a chorioretinal scar. The chorioretinal scar usually is a benign finding, but there may be a retinal break associated with a posterior vitreous detachment because of the vitreoretinal condensation at the scar. One must also note that in certain chorioretinal or retinal scars there can be a reactivation of the lesion. The best example of reactivation is ocular toxoplasmosis.

In the management of chorioretinal scars, it is important that the practitioner watch for possible retinal breaks in the area of the scar. This is especially a concern when a PVD occurs. In the case of toxoplasmosis, the patient must be notified about the possibility of reactivation and the signs and symptoms of reactivation because of the importance of early incorporation of treatment in this condition. Patients with chorioretinal scars should be rechecked at yearly intervals. A schematic of a chorioretinal scar demonstrates fibrosis of the scar tissue deep into the retina and actually often penetrating out into the vitreous. There is also the presence of an overlying vitreous condensate and

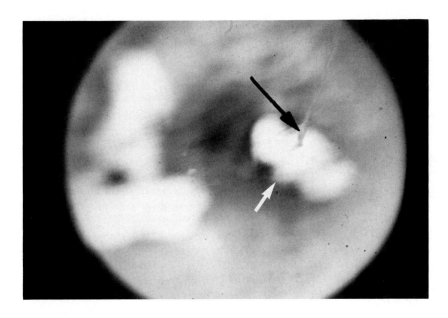

Figure 4–20. A black and white photograph of a chorioretinal scar **(white arrow)** with an overlying vitreous condensation **(black arrow).**

the vitreoretinal adhesions that are present in many of these inflammatory conditions. The vitreous condesate occurs because of an overlying inflammatory condition of the vitreous called vitritis.

POSTINFLAMMATORY CHORIORETINAL SCAR—PEARLS

- Usually white to yellow intraretinal fibrosis with accompanying RPE hyperplasia
- May be overlying vitreous condensation strands
- May involve choroid through the retina to the vitreous
- Possible traction-induced tears. If they occur, tears are usually secondary to a PVD
- Scars may reactivate in toxoplasmosis
- Management
  - Monitor yearly
  - If toxoplasmosis scar is suspected, employ home monitoring
  - Carefully investigate for retinal tears, especially in cases of PVD

Peripheral Cystoid Degeneration—Typical

Typical peripheral cystoid degeneration (Fig. 4–21) appears as an area of thickened retina extending about one half DD from the ora serrata. It can, however, extend all the way to the equator. This area appears hazy gray with enclosed hazy red dots. There may be associated vitreous strands and dots above the area. Peripheral cystoid degeneration usually appears temporally and superiorly within the retina.

Peripheral cystoid degeneration involves cystoidlike changes in the outer plexiform layer of the retina that can eventually extend to involve the entire sensory retina. These cysts may coalesce and

form larger cystic spaces causing a true splitting or schisis of the sensory retina.

The holes that potentially develop within typical peripheral cystoid degeneration are usually limited to inner-layer holes. As such they are of no threat to the development of retinal detachment. In your evaluation of the patient with peripheral cystoid degeneration, remember that cystoid is considered by some to be a precursor to the development of retinoschisis. The accompanying schematic will demonstrate the changes at a histopathological level associated with peripheral cystoid degeneration. It is to be noted that the cystoid spaces that develop within the sensory retina may coalesce and are thought by some to be precursors to retinoschisis.

Typical peripheral cystoid degeneration occurs bilaterally in virtually all patients over 8 years of age. There may be the associated finding of formation of inner-layer retinal holes. The presence of typical peripheral cystoid degeneration appears to increase with age. It is important to remember, however, that this is a very common condition and is usually of no threat to the patient whatsoever.

TYPICAL PERIPHERAL CYSTOID DEGENERATION—PEARLS

- Usually a hazy-grey area near the ora but may extend to equator
- Most evident temporally and is bilateral in everyone over 8 years of age
- May have small red dots within and strands in vitreous over the cystoid
- Intraretinal cysts may form that may coalesce to form retinoschisis
- Self-limiting and benign with occasional inner layer holes

PERIPHERAL CYSTOID DEGENERATION

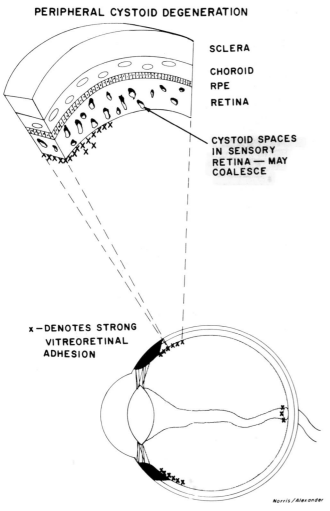

SCLERA

CHOROID

RPE

RETINA

CYSTOID SPACES IN SENSORY RETINA — MAY COALESCE

x —DENOTES STRONG VITREORETINAL ADHESION

Norris/Alexander

Figure 4–21. A schematic illustrating the clinicopathological changes associated with peripheral cystoid degeneration.

Peripheral Cystoid Degeneration—Reticular

Reticular peripheral cystoid degeneration presents as an area posterior to but continuous with typical cystoid degeneration. It occurs most commonly in the inferotemporal portion of the retina. The change presents closer to the equatorial region of the retina than typical cystoid degeneration. These areas are hazy and may be irregular, with a reticular pattern that appears like sclerotic retinal vessels. This appearance can simulate the development of the fishbone or sclerotic retinal vessel appearance of lattice degeneration. These changes are often angulated to give the practitioner some means of differential diagnosis from typical cystoid degeneration.

The layers involved are slightly different than those of typical cystoid degeneration. The cystoid spaces in reticular peripheral cystoid degeneration occur in the nerve fiber layer, and this may eventually extend into the inner plexiform layer.

Usually reticular peripheral cystoid degeneration is of no threat to vision, occurring commonly in 13 to 18 percent of adults with bilateral presen-

tation in 41 percent of affected adults. Reticular peripheral cystoid degeneration can be managed by routine eye examinations, again, looking for the potential development of holes in the retina, which may be the precursor to the development of retinal detachment. **See color plate 64.**

RETICULAR PERIPHERAL CYSTOID DEGENERATION—PEARLS

- Hazy irregular areas continuous with but posterior to typical peripheral cystoid degeneration
- Areas are reticular, appearing as fishbone sclerotic vessels
- Occurs as cystoid spaces in the nerve fiber layer
- Occurs in 13 to 18 percent of adults with 41 percent bilaterality
- Usually benign and self-limiting but must watch for hole development

---

Retinal Pigment Epithelial Window Defect

The RPE window defect (Fig. 4–22) is a relatively common occurrence in the normal population. RPE window defects appear as white to yellow, round, well-circumscribed areas often occurring in the equatorial region. They may, however, occur at any point within the retina. It is important to note that the RPE is not absent in this particular defect; however, there is an absence of melanin within the RPE cell. The RPE window defect is in and of itself no concern. Clinically they may enlarge over the years. This enlargement is of no direct threat to vision. The management includes differential diagnosis and patient education. The primary concern is the differential diagnosis from a retinal hole. This

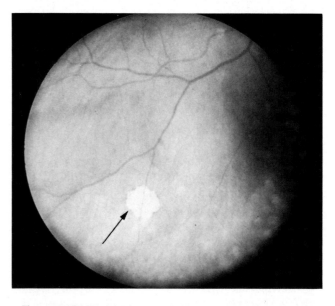

Figure 4–22. The arrow points to a retinal pigment epithelial window defect.

is very easy when considering that a RPE window defect is yellowish to white in color and is well circumscribed, whereas a retinal hole is always reddish in color and often has a surrounding cuff of white retinal edema. Routine eye examinations should be conducted on patients with RPE window defects.

RPE WINDOW DEFECT—PEARLS

- White to yellow, round, well-circumscribed areas in the retina
- Absence of melanin in the RPE
- Benign but may appear to increase in size over the years
- Management includes routine eye examinations

Congenital Hypertrophy of the Retinal Pigment Epithelium

Congenital hypertrophy of the retinal pigment epithelium (CHRPE) is also known as a halo nevus (Fig. 4–23). Also one other variant of this is the presentation of multiple isolated areas of congenital hypertrophy of the retinal pigment epithelium, called bear tracks (Fig. 4–24). Congenital hypertrophy of the retinal pigment epithelium often presents as a dark grey to black area of variable size. CHRPE can occur anywhere in the retina. The lesions typically are flat, with an area of depigmentation surrounding the lesion. This area of depigmentation is known as the halo. Often there are associated areas of chorioretinal atrophy within the lesion, known as lacunae.

The layers involved in CHRPE are primarily the RPE cells and the choriocapillaris. In this condition the RPE cells are enlarged with essentially the same amount of melanin pigment. There is an associated choriocapillaris atrophy in this condition that creates the clinical picture of the lacunae.

Congenital hypertrophy of the RPE is a benign condition. There is, however, a scotoma corresponding to the area of hypertrophy, especially when tested at threshold. As this lesion ages, the scotoma becomes more absolute because of the associated underlying chorioretinal atrophy and overlying sensory retinal changes. The clinician should observe, record, and differentiate this condition from a malignant melanoma. This should be done by routine visual examinations about every year. **See color plate 65.**

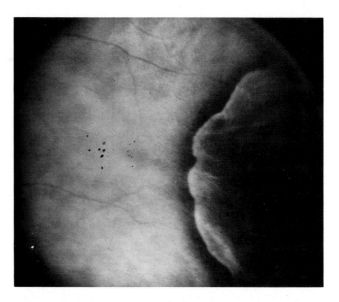

Figure 4–23. Congenital hypertrophy of the retinal pigment epithelium also known as the "halo" nevas. Note the scalloped edges.

CONGENITAL HYPERTROPHY OF THE RPE—PEARLS

- Halo nevus and bear tracks
- Flat grey to black area with a surround of depigmentation and internal areas of chorioretinal atrophy known as lacunae
- Enlarged RPE cells and choriocapillaris atrophy
- May have scotomas that become more dense with age
- Self-limiting and benign
- Routine yearly eye examinations

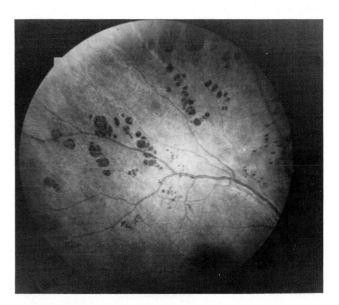

Figure 4–24. A clinicopathological variation of congenital hypertrophy of the retinal pigment epithelium, often referred to as bear tracks.

Retinal Pigment Epithelial Hyperplasia

RPE hyperplasia occurs most often as a result of insult to the retina. The clinician will see retinal pigment epithelial hyperplasia in many different condition, including chorioretinal scars, circumpapillary choroiditis, choroidal neovascularization, as well as isolated areas of RPE hyperplasia. RPE hyperplasia appears jet black with irregularly shaped areas that are variable in size. The appearance is the result of invasion of the sensory retina by replicating RPE cells. The RPE hyperplasia may cause an area of an isolated scotoma but is usually nonprogressive. It is important for the clinician to ascertain the cause for the RPE hyperplasia. If the cause is not currently active, the clinician may just follow the patient on a routine basis. If there is an active inflammatory lesion causing the RPE hyperplasia, it is important to provide the proper therapeutic intervention.

RPE HYPERPLASIA—PEARLS

- Very dense, black area
- Usually a reaction of the retinal tissue to insult the RPE cells invading the sensory retina
- Results in a scotoma
- Self-limiting but must ascertain the cause of the retinal insult
- Routine eye examinations

Benign Choroidal Melanoma

The benign choroidal melanoma is also known as a choroidal nevus and occurs in up to 30 percent of patients. The choroidal nevus or benign choroidal melanoma usually is a flat slate-grey lesion with indistinct margins. These lesions may have overlying drusen (up to 80 percent) that are a result of poor vascular supply from the choriocapillaris to the retinal pigment epithelium. The reduced blood supply occurs as the result of the barrier created by the

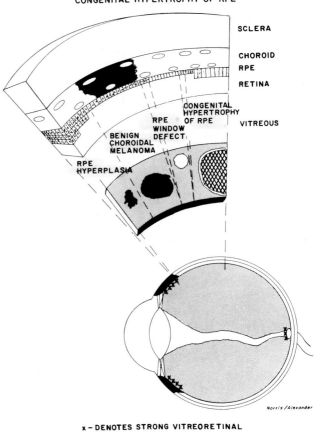

RPE HYPERPLASIA
BENIGN CHOROIDAL MELANOMA
RPE WINDOW DEFECT
CONGENITAL HYPERTROPHY OF RPE

x – DENOTES STRONG VITREORETINAL ADHESION

Figure 4–25. A schematic illustrating the clinicopathological differences between RPE hyperplasia, benign choroidal melanoma, RPE window defect, and congenital hypertrophy of the retinal pigment epithelium.

lesion. There also may be an associated serous sensory retinal detachment overlying the drusen. The benign choroidal melanoma is the result of accumulation of melanocytes within the choroid. Some believe that this nevus may convert to malignancy. Assuming that is a relatively small lesion, under 5 DD, one can be relatively well assured that it is benign and nonprogressive. Ninety-five percent of

TABLE 4–4. DIFFERENTIAL DIAGNOSIS OF MALIGNANT CHOROIDAL MELANOMA

Size	Associated Findings	Classification
0.5–2 DD	None	Benign
2–5 DD	Elevated lesion, overlying drusen, subretinal fluid	Suspicious—consider ultrasound, fluorescein angiography; photodocument, recall six months
5 DD or larger	Elevated lesion, overlying drusen, overlying orange pigmentation, photopsia, large feeder vessels	Malignant until proven otherwise

benign choroidal melanomas are under 2 DD in size. The accompanying Table 4–4 will help make the differential diagnosis and a decision as to the proper management of this condition. **See color plate 66.** It is, however, prudent to at least document the size of the lesion and to follow the patient on a routine basis to assure that there is no progression toward malignancy.

Figure 4–25 is a schematic representation of retinal epithelial hyperplasia, benign choroidal melanoma, RPE defects, and congenital hypertrophy of the RPE. The practitioner can see that a RPE hyperplasia presents because there is true proliferation of the RPE, which appears as a blackish lesion within the retina. The benign choroidal melanoma presents because of the melanocytes within the choroid and appears greyish because it is filtered by the RPE and sensory retina. The RPE window defect appears white because of the absence of melanin within the RPE. The congenital hypertrophy of the RPE presents as a greyish lesion because of swelling of the RPE cells.

BENIGN CHOROIDAL MELANOMA—PEARLS

- Flat, slate grey with indistinct margins
- May have overlying drusen and/or sensory retinal detachment
- Accumulation of melanocytes in choroid
- Management
    1. Up to 2 DD—document and follow
    2. 2DD to 5 DD—suspicious. Consider special tests and careful follow-up
    3. Over 5 DD—assume malignancy until proven otherwise

Malignant Choroidal Melanoma

The malignant choroidal melanoma (Figs. 4–26 and 4–27) appears as a mottled elevated lesion varying from whitish to a greyish-green color. The lesion is usually over 10 DD when it is discovered. This mottling may be orange due to lipofucin deposition on the surface of the lesion. There may be an accompanying RPE hyperplasia on the surface of the tumor. This RPE hyperplasia is known as "melanoma bodies" and is pathognomonic of a malignancy. After the lesion breaks through Bruch's membrane, it may be lobular in nature, taking on the formation of a collar button. There is often an associated serous retinal elevation over the top of the malignancy. This is due to the leaking of fluid through the RPE/Bruch's membrane barrier.

The malignant choroidal melanoma originates in the choroid as malignant melanocytes but may extend well into the vetreous. The extent of involvement is totally dependent upon the elapsed time of the development of the lesion.

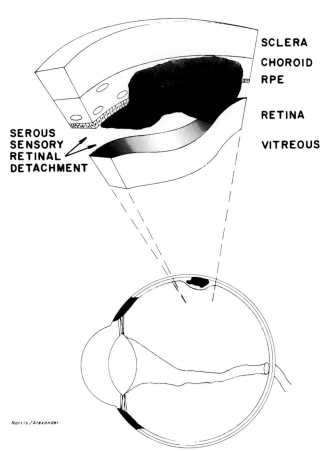

MALIGNANT CHOROIDAL MELANOMA

SCLERA
CHOROID
RPE
RETINA
VITREOUS
SEROUS SENSORY RETINAL DETACHMENT

Norris/Alexander

Figure 4–26. A schematic illustrating the clinicopathological changes associated with the development of a malignant choroidal melanoma.

The prognosis is relatively poor in malignant choroidal melanomas. There is a potential spread to the liver, lungs, and brain. There also is the potential loss of vision. Included in the management of a malignant choroidal melanoma would be diagnosis of the lesion and the performance of laboratory studies to determine whether or not there have been metastases of the lesion. These studies include carcinoembryonic antigen (CEA), liver studies, brain scans, and chest radiographs. The decision must then be made as to whether or not to irradiate the lesion or to perform careful enucleation. It is known that enucleation may cause metastasis of the lesion.

The accompanying schematic of the malignant choroidal melanoma demonstrates that the lesion is space occupying and can cause an overlying serous sensory retinal detachment. It is important that any lesion that is large, elevated, and dark in the peripheral retina have specialized studies applied to it such as ultrasound, fluorescein angiography, and photography to ascertain whether or not the lesion is malignant. **See color plate 67.**

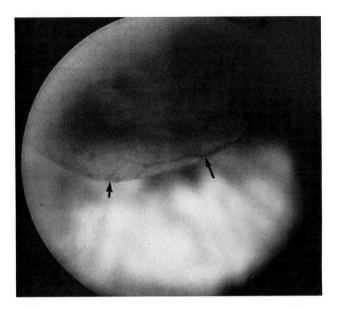

Figure 4–27. A malignant choroidal melanoma. The grossly elevated edge is demarcated by the black arrows.

MALIGNANT CHOROIDAL MELANOMA—PEARLS

- Usually over 10 DD when discovered
- Mottled, elevated lesion varying from whitish to grey-green color
- Overlying orange lipofucin, melanoma bodies, serous sensory retinal detachment may occur
- Accumulation of malignant melanocytes in the choroid
- Management
  - Rule out metastases
  - Arrange retinology consult

Oral Pearls

Oral pearls (Fig. 4–28) are also known as pearls of the ora serrata. These usually appear as single white spheres between the base and the tip of the dentate processes. They occur between the retinal pigment epithelium and Bruch's membrane, thus making them the histopathological correlates to drusen in the retina of the posterior pole. Oral pearls occur in approximately 20 percent of the population. These are benign and typically show no progression whatsoever. In fact, these would be close to impossible to find in a routine eye examination unless scleral indentation were applied. **See color plate 64.**

PEARLS OF THE ORA SERRATA—PEARLS

- White spheres between base and tip of the dentate processes
- Occur between RPE and Bruch's membrane and are the histopathological equivalent of retinal drusen
- Self-limiting and benign
- Routine eye examinations

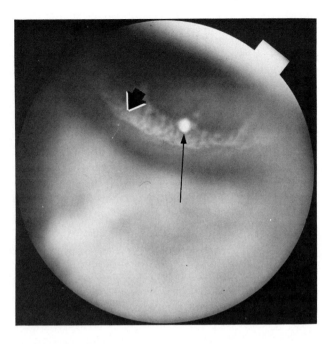

Figure 4–28. An oral pearl **(long arrow)** on an indenter in an area of cystoid degeneration **(short wide arrow).** *(Photo courtesy W. Townsend.)*

Enclosed Oral Bay

The enclosed oral bay is a brownish depression

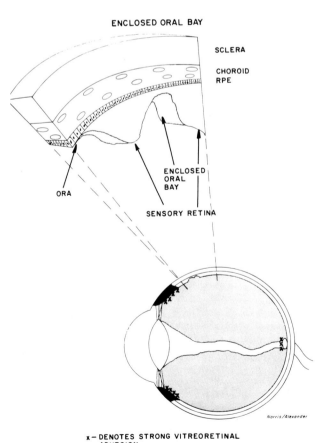

Figure 4–29. A schematic illustrating the clinicopathological changes associated with an enclosed oral bay.

surrounded by sensory retina near the ora serrata. This is found in approximately 6 percent of the population. Enclosed oral bays produce a situation in which there is nonpigmented ciliary epithelium of the pars plana surrounded by sensory retina. The schematic in Figure 4–29 demonstrates an enclosed oral bay with the surround of sensory retinal tissue. There is between a 15 to 20 percent chance of associated retinal breaks at the posterior edge of the enclosed oral bay. These breaks rarely progress to retinal detachment and are best found with indentation. Yearly examinations are indicated for the patient with an enclosed oral bay if there is an associated break. In addition, educate the patient regarding signs and symptoms of retinal detachment. Otherwise, routine eye examinations are the rule for patients with uncomplicated enclosed oral bays.

ENCLOSED ORAL BAY—PEARLS

• Brown depression surrounded by sensory retina near ora—a discontinuity in the normal outline of the ora serrata
• Perform scleral indentation to assess for breaks
• Examine yearly if retinal break at posterior edge of oral bay
• Educate patient regarding signs and symptoms of retinal detachment
• If no retinal break—routine examination
• If associated retinal detachment—retinology consult

White Without Pressure

White without pressure (Figs. 4–30 and 4–31) is also known as WWOP. White without pressure is a fairly common occurrence (reported in up to 30 percent of the general population) that appears as an area of the retina that is translucent grey bounded posteriorly by a reddish-brown line. The translucent grey area often just fades toward the ora serrata. WWOP may extend posteriorly to the equator, may have scalloped borders, and has been noted to be migratory in nature. There may be WWOP that surrounds an area of normal appearing retina. WWOP occurs in 5 percent of eyes under the age of 20 years and in 66 percent of eyes over the age of 70 years. There does appear to be a direct association with aging. WWOP occurs at a higher incidence in myopic patients and is reported as 10 times as high in black patients. There may be areas of white without pressure seen near lattice degeneration, at the borders of posterior staphylomas, associated with local retinal detachments, and seen in focal areas of the retina in PVD. White without pressure may be circumferential and usually occurs bilaterally.

White without pressure appears to be an unu-

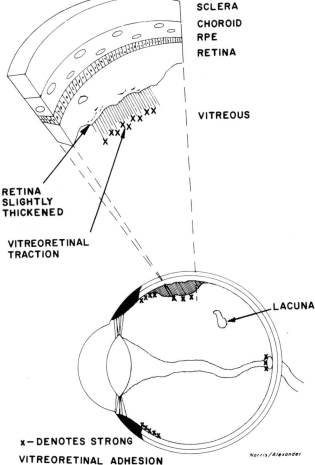

Figure 4–30. A schematic illustrating the clinicopathological changes associated with white without pressure.

sual vitreoretinal relationship that causes disorganization of the nerve fiber layer of the sensory retina even down to the RPE. Some clinicians think there may even be an associated development of retinal edema. The actual cause–effect relationship in white without pressure is controversial.

Usually white without pressure is associated with vitreous degeneration and PVD. There is, however, a relatively low incidence of retinal tears, considering this particular relationship. Horseshoe retinal tears or linear retinal tears can develop along the posterior border of white with pressure or white without pressure, and these tears are associated with the traction of PVD. **See color plate 68.**

In your management of the patient with WWOP it is important to consider factors that are contributory to the development of retinal tears. These factors are listed in Table 4–5.

Patients with white without pressure should be followed at yearly intervals. They should be reexamined every 6 months if the posterior borders of the white without pressure are scalloped and

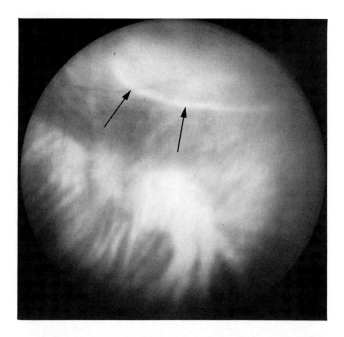

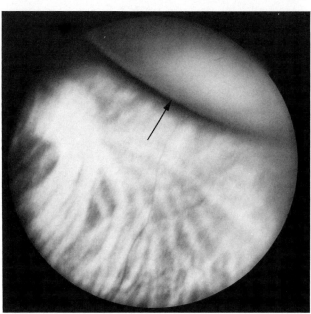

Figure 4–31. Top. Retinal white without pressure **(dark arrows)** near a vortex vein without indentation. **Bottom.** The same area as in top figure under indentation. *(Photo courtesy W. Townsend.)*

TABLE 4–5. FACTORS ASSOCIATED WITH RETINAL TEARS IN CASES OF WHITE WITHOUT PRESSURE

1. White without pressure along posterior margins of lattice degeneration
2. White without pressure with scalloped borders
3. The presence of an elevated tractional membrane adherent to the posterior margin of white without pressure
4. Progressive pathological shrinkage of vitreous

sure is an optical phenomenon of the retina similar to white without pressure. The retina appears translucent grey upon scleral indentation and is thought to be histologically similar to white with pressure. White with pressure has the same kind of prognosis and management as white without pressure, yet white without pressure is considered by some to be the more severe form.

Another clinical note should be made in regard to a phenomenon known as dark without pressure (Fig. 4–32). Dark without pressure appears as islands of homogeneous, flat, brown areas in the fundus of black patients. These areas may be migratory in nature and typically occur near the posterior pole of the eye. This is the opposite of what one would expect with white without pressure, which has more of a tendency to occur between the equator and the ora. There appears to be no particular vitreous connection in dark without pressure, but there does appear to be a relationship to sickle cell disease. Patients with dark without pressure should be considered as potential sickle cell patients, and this diagnosis should be ruled out.

It should be noted in the patient exhibiting white without pressure that the retina is thickened and that there is some associated cystic development. The most important aspect of this is the vitreoretinal traction that occurs with white without pressure. This vitreoretinal traction is strongly implicated in the genesis of retinal tears and subsequent retinal detachments.

there is extensive vitreous degeneration. The clinician must also take more precautions in patients with high myopia and in those developing PVD. It is necessary to make the patients aware of signs and symptoms of retinal detachment as well as to watch for breaks that may develop at the posterior border of the lesion. The patient should be indented to rule out retinal breaks.

A clinical note should be made at this point regarding white with pressure. White with pres-

WHITE WITHOUT PRESSURE CHARACTERISTICS—PEARLS

- Area of translucent grey retina usually between the ora and equator bounded by a reddish line
- May be migratory
- Higher incidence in black patients and myopic patients with overall incidence increasing with age
- Vitreoretinal traction causing disorganization of sensory retina
- May have associated traction retinal tears

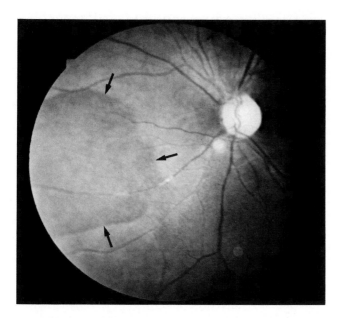

Figure 4–32. An area of dark without pressure in the posterior pole **(outlined by arrows).**

WHITE WITHOUT PRESSURE MANAGEMENT—PEARLS

- Indent to rule out breaks
- Six-month follow-up if any of the following associated factors leading to retinal tear development
  - WWOP near lattice degeneration
  - WWOP with scalloped borders
  - WWOP with elevated traction membrane
  - WWOP with progressive vitreous degeneration
- If no associated risk factors—12-month follow-up
- Watch carefully for tears when there is an associated posterior vitreous detachment
- Inform of the signs/symptoms of retinal detachment
- Retinology consult if threatening retinal tears

Pars Plana Cysts

Pars plana cysts (Fig. 4–33) are the histopathologic equivalent of a retinal detachment within the sensory retina. Pars plana cysts appear as one fourth- to 3-DD cysts that are oval to oblong. Pars plana cysts usually have a smooth, rigid, semitransparent surface. The cysts may have a small amount of pigment on the inner surface. The cavities are thought to contain hyaluronic acid similar to a retinoschisis. They may extend from the ora serrata to the ciliary processes. According to various studies, these are present in 3 to 18 percent of all patients. Because of the location, it is obvious that pars plana cysts are seen best with scleral indentation.

Pars plana cysts are an acquired separation of the nonpigmented epithelium from the pigmented

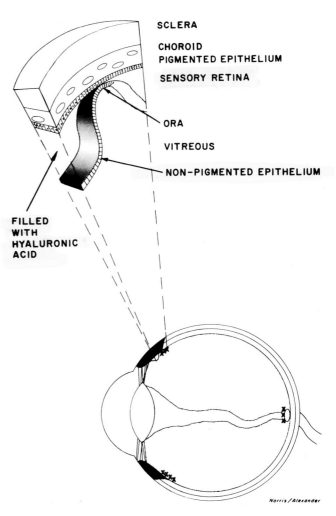

PARS PLANA CYST

SCLERA
CHOROID
PIGMENTED EPITHELIUM
SENSORY RETINA
ORA
VITREOUS
NON-PIGMENTED EPITHELIUM
FILLED WITH HYALURONIC ACID

Norris/Alexander

x – DENOTES STRONG VITREORETINAL ADHESIONS

Figure 4–33. A schematic illustrating the clinicopathology of a pars plana cyst.

epithelium of the pars plana. It is important to remember that the sensory retina becomes nonpigmented epithelium at the pars plana so that this condition is the histopathologic equivalent of a retinal detachment.

Pars plana cysts are often associated with traumatic retinal detachment, posterior uveitis, and perhaps multiple myeloma. In and of themselves, pars plana cysts are relatively benign. No treatment is indicated in isolated pars plana cysts, assuming that all other retinal problems such as tears have been ruled out. Routine eye examinations are indicated in patients with pars plana cysts.

As can be seen in Figure 4–33, which demonstrates the actual splitting of the nonpigmented epithelium from the pigmented epithelium, this simulates a retinal detachment but has none of the implications of a retinal detachment.

PARS PLANA CYSTS—PEARLS

- One fourth- to 3-DD cysts that are oval, occurring from the ora to the ciliary processes
- Transparent, taut, smooth surfaces
- Thought to be filled with hyaluronic acid
- Separation of nonpigmented and pigmented epithelium of the pars plana-histopathological equivalent of retinal detachment
- Often associated with a traumatic retinal detachment, posterior uveitis, and, perhaps, multiple myeloma
- Self-limiting and benign, assuming no other complications
- Routine eye examinations and patient education

PERIPHERAL RETINAL CHANGES THAT MAY POSE A THREAT TO VISION

Vitreoretinal Tufts

Vitreoretinal tufts (Figs. 4–34 through 4–36) are also known as retinal tufts or granular tissue. Vitreoretinal tufts appear as greyish-white pieces of tissue at the vitreoretinal interface usually located between the equator and the ora. Tufts occur more often nasally and have the tendency to accumulate within the vitreous base. There is by definition a connection to the vitreous body, and as such tufts have tendencies toward changes as the vitreous body liquefies and shrinks. Liquefaction and shrinkage of the vitreous body is primarily associated with aging but also may be associated with other vitreous diseases. Noncystic vitreoretinal tufts occur in about 72 percent of the population with about a 50 percent chance of bilaterality. Cystic tufts, on the other hand, are larger and only occur in about 5 to 7 percent of the population with a rare incidence of bilaterality. Zonular traction tufts run anterior into the vitreous with a triangular base and occur in about 15 percent of the population with a low incidence of bilaterality. **See color plate 69.**

Vitreoretinal tufts are considered to be accumulations of proliferated glial cells on the surface of the retina, causing retinal degeneration and subsequent vitreous attachment. These are often benign but may be associated with retinal tears when vitreous changes do occur.

The management of vitreoretinal tufts consists of monitoring tufts when they are associated with other potentiators of retinal detachment (Table 4–6). Indentation may be needed to assess for retinal breaks. The clinician must realize the importance of

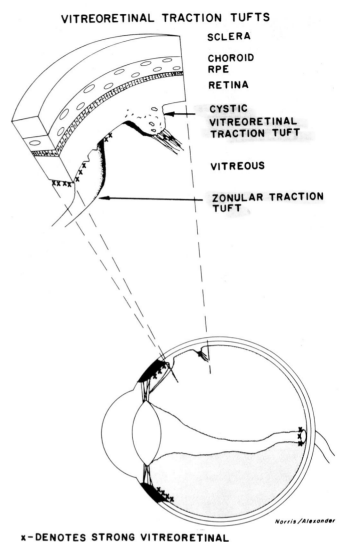

VITREORETINAL TRACTION TUFTS

SCLERA
CHOROID
RPE
RETINA
CYSTIC VITREORETINAL TRACTION TUFT
VITREOUS
ZONULAR TRACTION TUFT

Norris/Alexander

x–DENOTES STRONG VITREORETINAL ADHESION

Figure 4–34. A schematic illustrating the clinicopathology of vitreoretinal traction tufts.

the vitreoretinal adhesion in the genesis of a retinal detachment, as a tug on a vitreoretinal tuft during a PVD may precipitate a retinal tear. The clinician must make the patient aware of signs and symptoms of retinal detachment and also make the patient aware that a localized phosphene associated with a stressed vitreoretinal tuft may be a sign of an impending retinal tear. Special care must be taken during an evolving PVD. Retinal breaks may need photocoagulation or cryotherapy. A retinology consult is advised at the first sign of a tear. Prophylaxis is indicated in some cases of vitreoretinal tufts.

Figure 4–34 illustrates that the zonular traction tufts actually run forward toward the ciliary body process and are often attached to the zonules of the crystalline lens. There is also a cystic vitreoretinal traction tuft present in this particular schematic. It

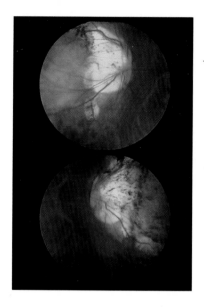

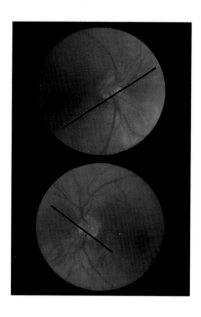

Plate 1. Bilateral posterior staphylomas involving the optic nerve heads with severe reduction in visual acuity. (See pp. 26 and 177.)

Plate 2. Bilateral tilted discs. The black lines indicate the tilting of the vertical axes of the discs. (See p. 25.)

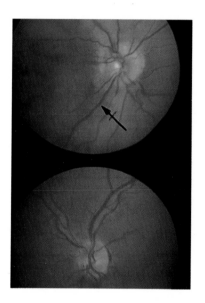

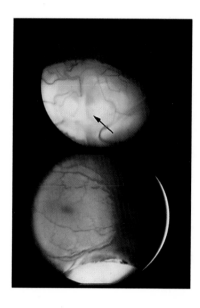

Plate 3. Top. A disc tilting into a zone of posterior staphyloma **(arrow).** When compared to the "normal" fellow disc **(bottom),** it is easy to establish that the affected disc is larger, which implies a congenital variation. (See p. 25.)

Plate 4. Top. A coloboma involving both the retinal choroidal area and the optic nerve **(arrow). Bottom.** The fellow eye has just a retinal choroidal coloboma. Both eyes are at risk for the development of a retinal detachment. (See p. 29.)

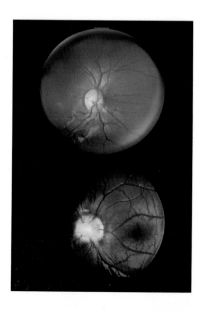

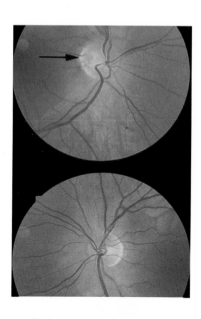

Plate 5. Top. A "normal" optic nerve head in an eye with 20/20 vision. **Bottom.** The fellow eye is amblyopic with a morning glory disc anomaly. Note the size difference between the two discs, implying a congenital variation. (See p. 32.)

Plate 6. Top. The arrow points to a congenital optic pit in the temporal aspect of the right eye. This eye is at risk for serous maculopathy. When compared to the fellow disc **(bottom),** it becomes apparent that the affected disc is larger, implying a congenital variation. (See p. 36.)

Plate 7. Top. A "normal" optic nerve head in a 20/20 eye. Note the reflections from the nerve fiber layer, especially around the macula. Contrast the nerve head and the nerve fiber layer to the figure on the **bottom.** The bottom figure is a congenital optic nerve hypoplasia with 20/200 vision. Note the absence of nerve fiber layer reflection. Again note the difference in size of the nerve heads. (See p. 37.)

Plate 8. Top. The nerve head is large but flat, with 20/20 acuity. The fellow nerve head on the **bottom** is "normal" with 20/20 vision. Again there is a nerve head-size difference, implying a congenital variation. This is an example of megalopapilla. (See p. 40.)

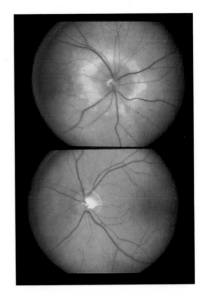

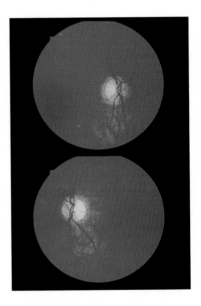

Plate 9. The glowing globules **(arrows)** represent buried drusen of the nerve head, which have a tendency to become more visible with age. (See p. 41.)

Plate 10. Temporal sector optic atrophy apparent in cases of autosomal dominant optic atrophy. (See p. 43.)

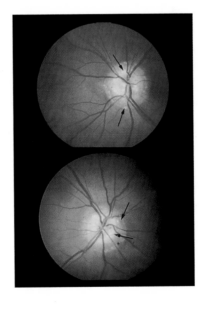

Plate 11. Top. The nerve head is edematous when compared to the fellow nerve head **(bottom).** Vision was reduced in the right eye of this young person, implicating inflammatory optic neuropathy. This is often referred to as papillitis. (See p. 48.)

Plate 12. Top. The temporal neuroretinal rim in the right eye is atrophic when compared to the temporal neuroretinal rim of the left eye **(bottom).** This occurred in a patient with other signs of demyelinizing disease and was suspected to be secondary to demyelinizing optic neuropathy in the right eye. (See p. 49.)

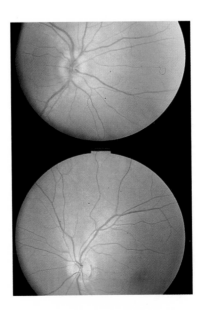

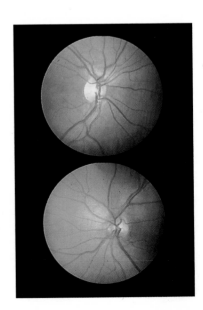

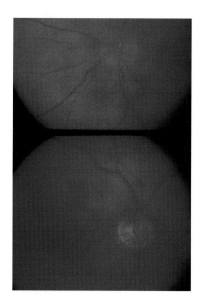

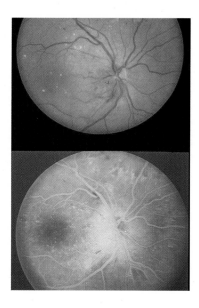

Plate 13. When comparing the top nerve head to the bottom, the top was elevated and edematous. The edema obscures underlying detail. The left **(top)** eye also had reduced acuity. This occurred in an elderly patient and was diagnosed as ischemic optic neuropathy. (See p. 52.)

Plate 14. AION in a patient with diabetes. The temporal aspect of the disc was edematous, with flame-shaped hemorrhages. The bottom photo demonstrates the leakage of AION during fluorescein angiography. (See p. 52.)

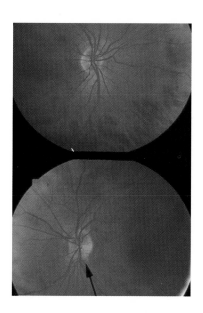

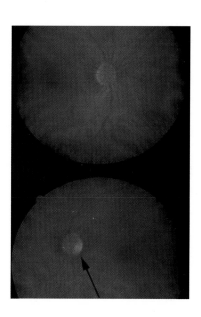

Plate 15. The subtlety of AION. The **top** photo was the "normal" eye, while the **bottom** photo was of an eye with a superior altitudinal field defect. The arrow points to the zone of the disc that was elevated and edematous. (See p. 52.)

Plate 16. The same patient as Plate 15 only 6 months later. The edematous zone of the left **(lower)** optic nerve head has since become atrophic **(arrow)** with a permanent yet reduced-in-size altitudinal field defect. Simultaneous comparison of the nerve head is crucial in the diagnosis. (See p. 52.)

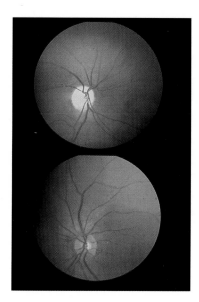

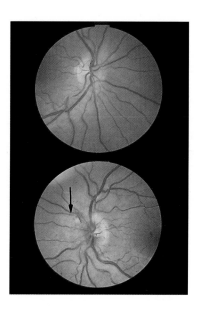

Plate 17. Top. Total optic atrophy of the right nerve head secondary to temporal arteritic ischemic optic neuropathy. The **bottom** disc is still normal in this photo but soon after became involved in spite of corticosteroid intervention. (See p. 54.)

Plate 18. Top. A normal optic nerve head in a patient with diabetes. The fellow optic nerve head **(bottom)** was edematous **(arrow)** secondary to diabetic optic neuropathy. (See p. 55.)

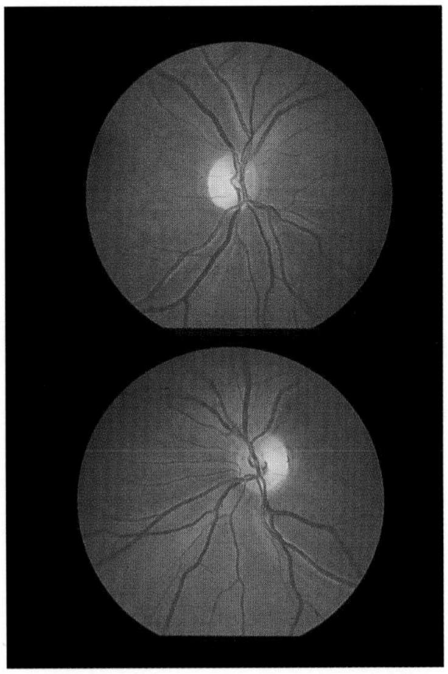

Plate 19. Toxic optic neuropathy secondary to alcohol abuse. (See p. 57.)

Plate 20. Chronic compensated papilledema secondary to benign intracranial hypertension. Note gross swelling and venous tortuosity. There is a conspicuous absence of flame-shaped hemorrhages and cotton wool spots. (See p. 60.)

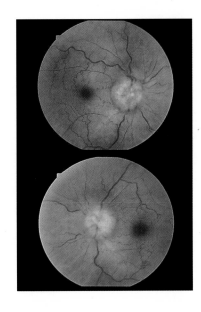

Plate 21. Bilateral, acute, noncompensated papilledema characterized by gross swelling of the optic nerves, flame-shaped hemorrhages, and cotton wool spots. The patient was shunted the next day. (See p. 60.)

Plate 22. An astrocytic homartoma of the right **(top)** nerve head **(arrow).** Note that there is no affectation of the fellow **(bottom)** nerve head. (See p. 64.)

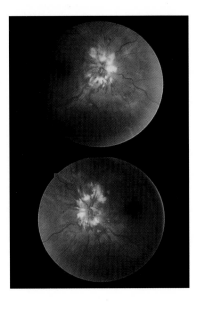
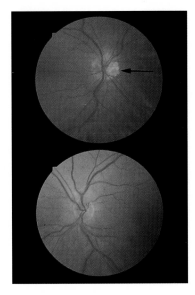

Plate 23. The arrow points to a preretinal hemorrhage in an eye with a hemicentral retinal vein occlusion. (See pp. 94 and 126.)

Plate 24. The arrow points to a flame-shaped hemorrhage near a zone of hard exudates. Other signs of diabetic retinopathy also represented in this eye. (See pp. 96 and 139.)

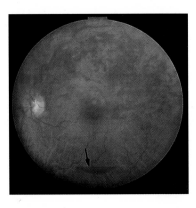
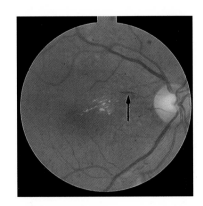

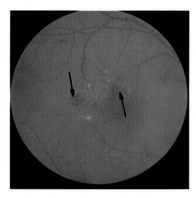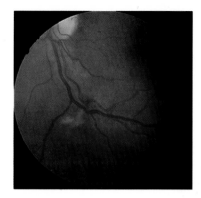

Plate 25. The arrows point to the dot/blot hemorrhages within an area of retinal edema. Other signs of retinal edema in this case of diabetic retinopathy are the hard exudates. (See pp. 97 and 138.)

Plate 26. A cotton wool spot in an area of retinal hypoxia. When this occurs in diabetic retinopathy, the eye is considered to be in the preproliferative stage. (See pp. 102 and 139.)

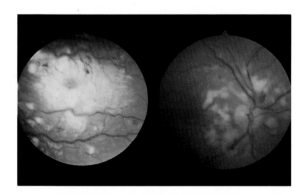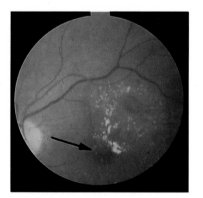

Plate 27. Cotton wool spots can also occur in other disease processes. The cotton wools in the eye on the left were secondary to systemic lupus, while those on the right were secondary to Purtcher's retinopathy. (See p. 102.) (*Purtcher's slide courtesy of C. Amos.*)

Plate 28. Hard exudates surround an area of edema and are encroaching into the macular area **(arrow).** (See pp. 105 and 138.)

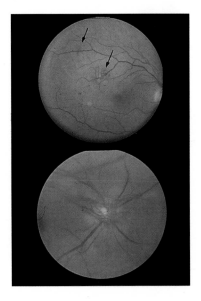

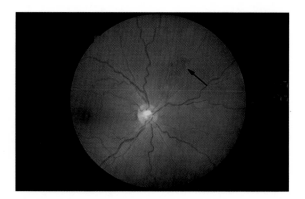

Plate 29. Top. Arrows point to two areas of neovascularization elsewhere in this case of proliferative diabetic retinopathy. The photo on the **bottom** demonstrates the haze over the optic nerve head with disc neovascularization. (See pp. 108 and 143.)

Plate 30. Acquired venous tortuosity and a small branch vein occlusion **(arrow).** The acquired tortuosity indicates overall retinal hypoxia. (See pp. 110 and 117.)

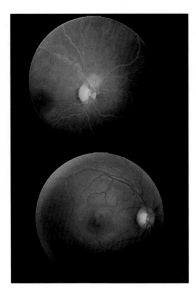

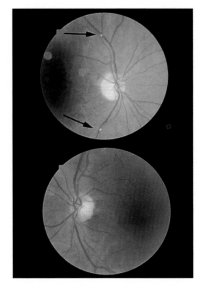

Plate 31. Top. Lipemic arteries and veins are indistinguishable in this case of severely elevated triglyceride levels. **Bottom.** The same patient with triglyceride levels under better control. (See p. 113.)

Plate 32. Top. Arrows point to emboli in this case. The emboli were secondary to severe cardiovascular and internal carotid disease. When comparing the disc to that in the **bottom** photo there is relative atrophy. This patient also had low-tension glaucoma. (See p. 113.)

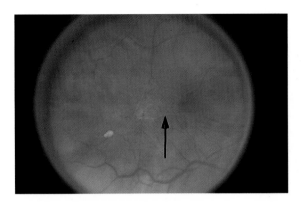

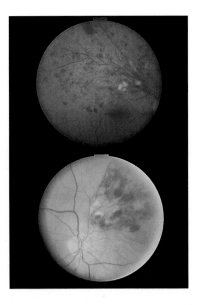

Plate 33. The arrow points to a "gathered pleat" variety of a preretinal membrane very near the macula. (See p. 116.)

Plate 34. Top. A classical branch retinal-vein occlusion with retinal edema encroaching into the macular area. Note the cotton wool spots indicating ischemia and the lipid deposits near the disc. **Bottom.** A branch retinal-vein occlusion affecting the nasal retina. (See p. 117.)

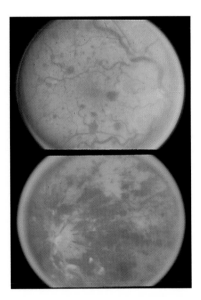

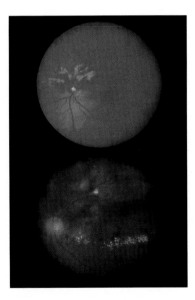

Plate 35. While both the top and bottom photos represent a central retinal-vein occlusion with reduced vision, the **bottom** is an ischemic variety with more of a tendency toward neovascular glaucoma, while the **top** is nonischemic. (See p. 123)

Plate 36. Top. An ischemic hemicentral retinal vein occlusion. Note the cotton wool spots. **Bottom.** The unfortunate sequelae to a hemicentral retinal vein occlusion—disc neovascularization. Also note the hard exudates at the preceding edge of the edema. (See p. 126.)

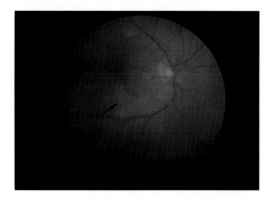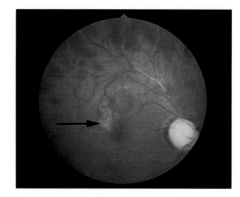

Plate 37. The arrow points to a zone of opaque retina secondary to a branch retinal artery occlusion. (See p. 129.)

Plate 38. The arrow points to a zone of opaque retina created by a branch retinal-artery occlusion within a branch retinal-vein occlusion. (See pp. 117 and 129.)

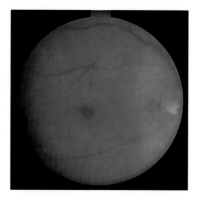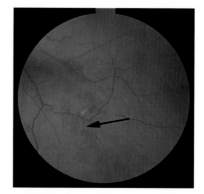

Plate 39. Opaque retina and severely compromised retinal-blood vessels in a case of central retinal-artery occlusion. (See p. 130.)

Plate 40. The arrow points to IRMA near a cotton wool spot in the eye of a patient with diabetes. Both signs indicate hypoxia and place this eye in the category of preproliferative diabetic retinopathy. (See p. 139.)

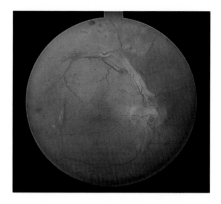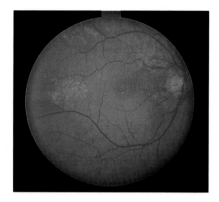

Plate 41. Fibrotic proliferation in severe proliferative diabetic retinopathy. (See p. 143.)

Plate 42. An example of several varieties of drusen in a single eye. While all of the drusen in this picture have a different appearance, they all have the same etiopathogenesis. (See p. 166.)

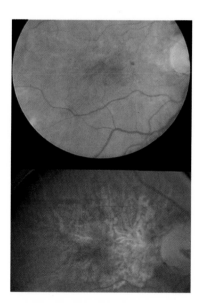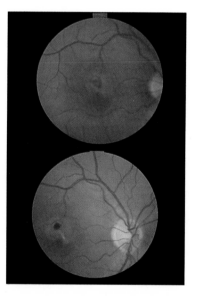

Plate 43. Two of the many variations of dry age-related maculopathy. All are characterized by changes in the RPE in an aged patient. (See pp. 166 and 170.)

Plate 44. Top. A grey-green choroidal neovascular net with a surrounding sensory retinal detachment. **Bottom.** The same eye one year later without treatment. Vision improved as the detachment resolved. The net developed characteristic RPE hyperplasia on the surface. (See p. 168.)

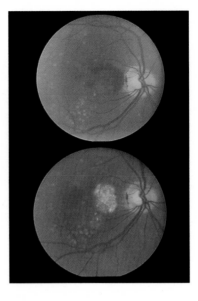

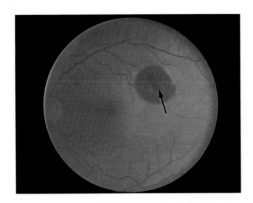

Plate 45. A grey green hemorrhage under the RPE **(arrow)** with a red subretinal hemorrhage overlying. (See pp. 99 and 168.)

Plate 46. Top. A subretinal hemorrhage secondary to a ruptured neovascular net near the edge of the disc. **Bottom.** Postphotocoagulative scarring of the lesion shown in the top photo. (See pp. 99 and 168.)

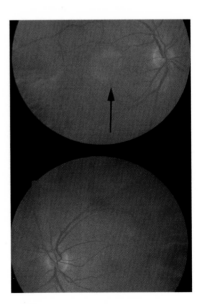

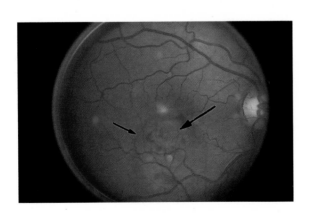

Plate 47. The subtlety of choroidal neovascular disease. The small arrow points to a sensory retinal elevation, while the large arrow points to the leaking choroidal neovascular net. (See p. 168.)

Plate 48. Top. The arrow points to a RPE detachment. This is often difficult to see but becomes obvious when comparing to the "normal" fellow eye **(bottom).** (See p. 168.)

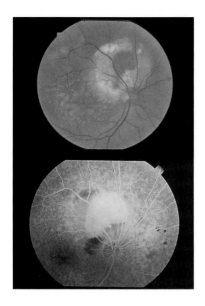

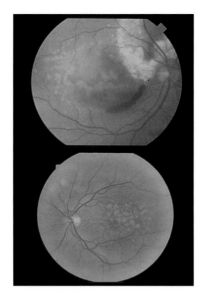

Plate 49. Top. The macula is characterized by soft drusen. Above the disc is a zone of hard exudates (Coat's response) surrounding a grey green zone. This zone proved to leak on fluorescein angiography **(bottom).** (See pp. 168 and 173.)

Plate 50. The neovascular disease in Plate 49 progressed to the hemorrhagic disease shown in the **top** photo. Severe vision reduction occurred. The **bottom** photo is of the fellow eye. There are numerous "soft drusen" thought to be RPE disease or detachment that is very conducive to choroidal neovascular disease. (See pp. 168 and 173.)

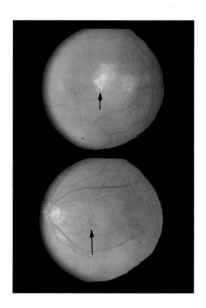

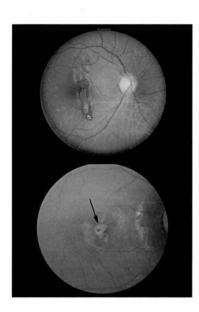

Plate 51. Wet age-related maculopathy. The arrow in the **top** photograph points to a disciform scar, while the arrow in the **bottom** photograph points to an evolving neovascular net. If there is a disciform scar in one eye, it is imperative to be especially careful in the fellow eye. (See p. 173.)

Plate 52. Top. A choroidal rupture following the contour of the disc. **Bottom.** An eye with multiple choroidal ruptures and a developing choroidal neovascular net **(arrow)** confirmed by fluorescein angiography. (See p. 174.)

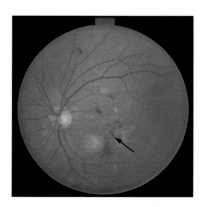

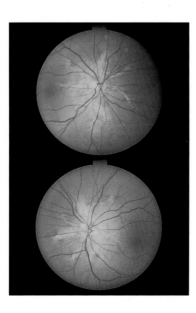

Plate 53. An arrow points to an area of neovascularization developing within a photocoagulation scar. The patient has diabetes with eye signs. (See p. 175.)

Plate 54. An example of the classical presentation of angioid streaks. (See pp. 20 and 179.)

Plate 55. ICSC. The arrow in the **top** photo points to a "discolored" zone that was elevated, creating metamorphopsia. The **bottom** photo demonstrates the leakage in the affected zone **(arrow).** (See p. 180.)

Plate 56. The **top** lamellar macular hole contrasts well within the **bottom** through-and-through macular hole. (See p. 183.)

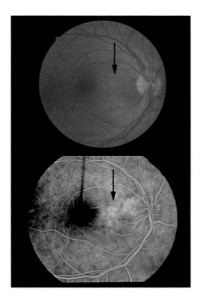
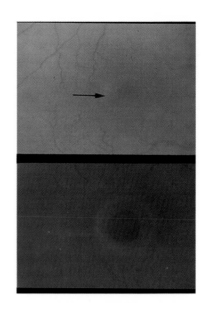

Plate 57. Top The arrows point to choroidal infiltrates—RPE disease—in a case of presumed ocular histoplasmosis. **Bottom.** The arrow points to a choroidal neovascular net in a case of presumed ocular histoplasmosis. Surrounding the "zone of leakage" are hemorrhages and exudates. (See pp. 20 and 186.)

Plate 58. Top. An area of RPE hypertrophy indicating a toxoplasmosis scar. **Bottom.** The same scar years later with an accompanying retinitis/vitritis **(arrow)**, indicating reactivation of the toxoplasmosis. (See p. 189.)

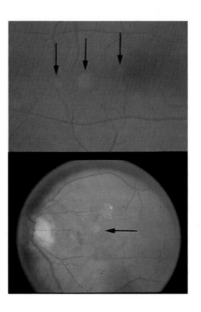
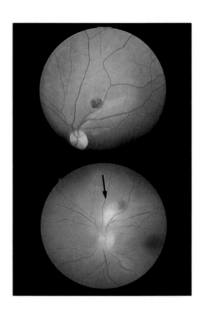

Plate 59. A toxocara granuloma. (See p. 193.) *(Courtesy R. Coshatt.)*

Plate 60. Top. The placoid lesions in the posterior pole characteristic of APMPPE. **Bottom.** The characteristic hypofluorescence of APMPPE on early strage fluorescein angiography. The same areas of hypofluorescence hyperfluoresce in the later stages of the fluorescein. (See p. 198.) *(Courtesy P. Ajamian.)*

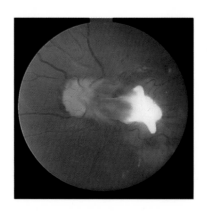
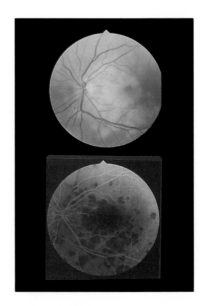

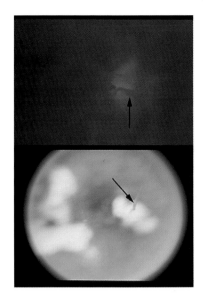

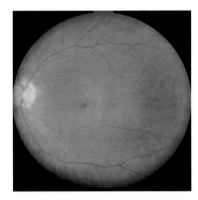

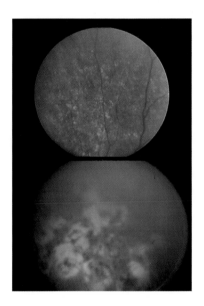

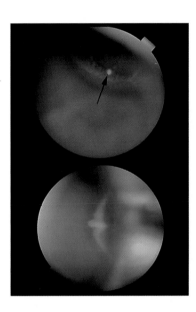

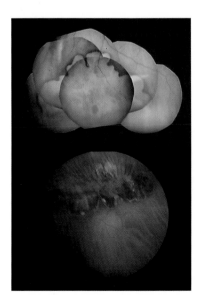

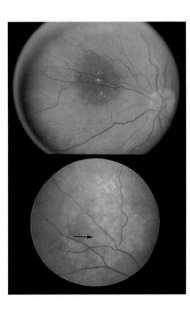

Plate 61. Top. The arrow points to the annular ring associated with a posterior vitreous detachment. **Bottom.** The arrow points to debris (condesate) in the vitreous associated with a postinflammatory chorioretinal scar. (See pp. 214 and 227.)

Plate 62. Congenital retinoschisis showing minimal rippling in the macular area. The rippling effect is the result of schisis of the nerve fiber layer. (See p. 218.)

Plate 63. Top. Peripheral retinal RPE disorganization associated with aging. The pigment often migrates and takes on a bone-spicule appearance similar to the "look" of retinitis pigmentosa. **Bottom.** Primary chorioretinal atrophy in the inferior equatorial retina associated with aging. (See p. 227.)

Plate 64. Top. The arrow points to a pearl of the ora serrata in an area of greyish peripheral cystoid degeneration. **Bottom.** A meridional fold on indentation. (See pp. 234 and 239.) *(Courtesy W. Townsend.)*

Plate 65. Top. A montage of a large congenital hypertrophy of the RPE. **Bottom.** A variation of a congenital hypertrophy of the RPE. (See p. 231.)

Plate 66. Top. A benign choroidal melanoma with overlying drusen. **Bottom.** A very suspicious lesion with elevation, drusen, and orange lipofusin pigmentation **(arrow).** This lesion should be considered malignant until proven otherwise. (See p. 232.)

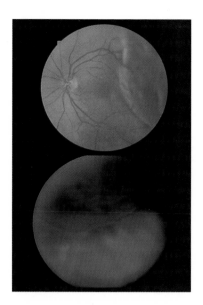
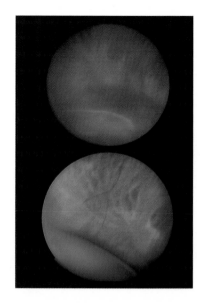

Plate 67. Top. A rhegmatogenous retinal detachment secondary to a retinal tear. **Bottom.** A nonrhegmatogenous retinal detachment secondary to an underlying malignant choroidal melanoma. (See pp. 233 and 258.)

Plate 68. Top. White without pressure not indented. **Bottom.** Indentation of the white without pressure. (See p. 235.) *(Courtesy W. Townsend.)*

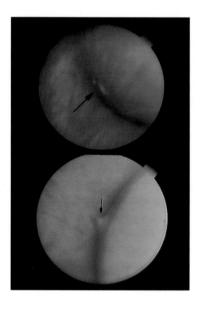
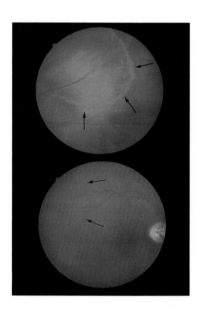

Plate 69. Top. A double cystic-retinal tuft **(arrow)** on indentation. **Bottom.** A zonular traction tuft on indentation. (See p. 238.) *(Courtesy W. Townsend.)*

Plate 70. Top. A bullous retinoschisis outlined by arrows. Note the dimming of underlying choroidal detail. **Bottom.** A bullous retinoschisis **(arrows)** progressing into the macular area. (See p. 241.)

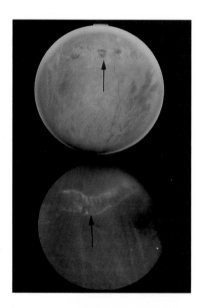
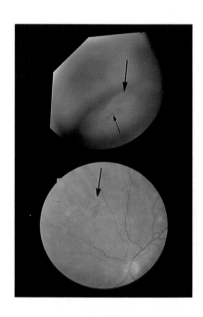

Plate 71. Top. Lattice degeneration **(arrow).** Only one of many variable ophthalmoscopic presentations. **Bottom.** Snail-track degeneration **(arrow),** a variant of lattice. (See pp. 244 and 246.) *(Courtesy M. Taroyan.)*

Plate 72. Top. Three small atrophic retinal holes on indentation **(small arrow)** with an overlying retinal cyst. *(Courtesy W. Townsend.)* **Bottom.** A large atrophic retinal hole in the posterior pole with a surround of edema. (See p. 249.)

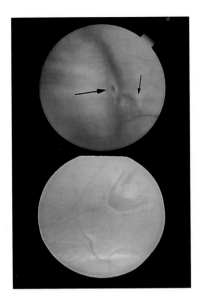

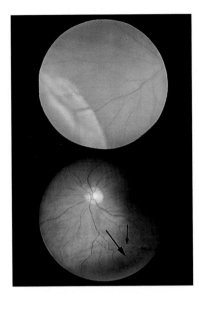

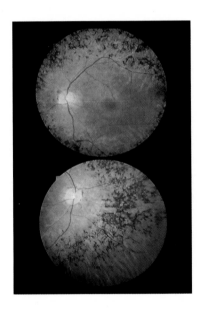

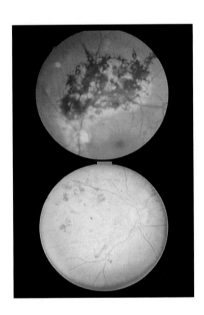

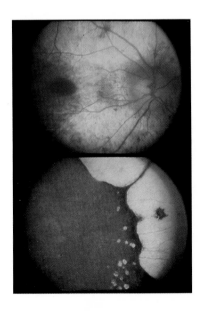

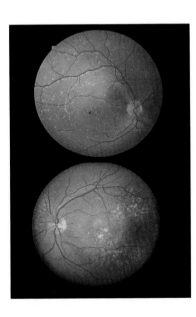

Plate 73. Top. A retinal tear (operculated hole) on indentation **(large arrow)** with an overlying plug of retinal tissue **(small arrow).** *(Courtesy W. Townsend.)* **Bottom.** A classical horseshoe retinal tear in the zone of retinal detachment. (See pp. 250 and 254.)

Plate 74. Top. A rhegmatogenous retinal detachment. **Bottom.** A rhegmatogenous retinal detachment evidenced by loss of choroidal detail. Also note the pigmented demarcation lines **(arrows).** (See p. 258.)

Plate 75. The classical bone spicule pigmentation and arterial attenuation present in retinitis pigmentosa. (See p. 274.)

Plate 76. Top. Pseudosector retinitis pigmentosa. This RPE hyperplasia is secondary to trauma. **Bottom.** Central or inverse retinitis pigmentosa with severe reduction in vision. (See p. 278.)

Plate 77. Top. An advanced case of choroideremia. **Bottom.** The scalloped borders and severe retinal/choroidal destruction asociated with gyrate dystrophy. (See pp. 281 and 283.) *(Courtesy R. Nowakowski.)*

Plate 78. Top. The fish-tail lesions associated with fundus flavimaculatus. Also note early macular changes. **Bottom.** In contrast is dominant drusen affecting the macula, with resultant early vision loss. (See pp. 285 and 290.)

Plate 79. Top. The flecks of fundus flavimaculatus with greyish yellow pigment **(arrow)** surrounding a normal-appearing fovea. A case of early Stargardt's disease. **Bottom.** Further deterioration in Stargardt's disease as evidenced by further RPE breakdown in the macular area. (See p. 285.)

Plate 80. Top. The macular area becomes ''slimed'' **(arrow)** with a surround of fish-tail flecks in Stargardt's disease. **Bottom.** The maculae is broken down further as Stargardt's disease progresses to decreased acuity. (See p. 285.)

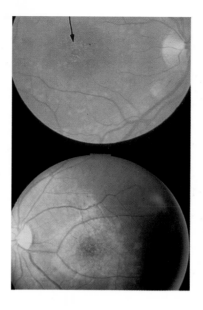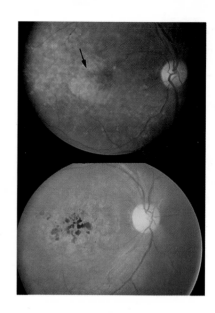

Plate 81. This set of photographs represents the confusion associated with hereditary retinal choroidal disease. There are certain characteristics of Stargardt's disease complicated by optic atrophy. Often diagnoses are evasive. (See p. 285.)

Plate 82. Variations of patterned anomalies of the RPE. (See p. 287.)

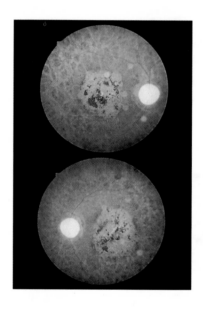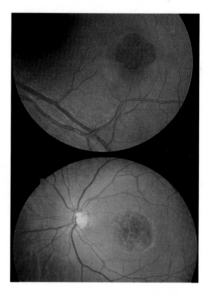

Plate 83. Top. The ''egg yolk'' pattern in the macula associated with mild vision reduction in vitelliform dystrophy. **Bottom.** Disorganization of the ''yolk'' associated with severe vision reduction in vitelliform dystrophy. (See p. 288.)

Plate 84. Top. The retinal hypopigmentation associated with albinism. **Bottom.** The ''normal''-appearing retina in achromatopsia. (See pp. 292 and 295.)

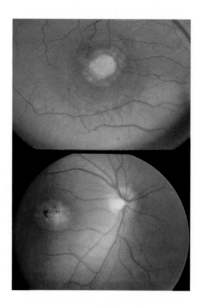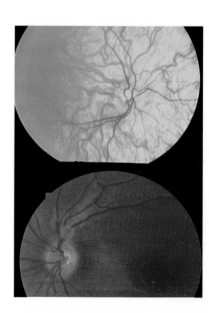

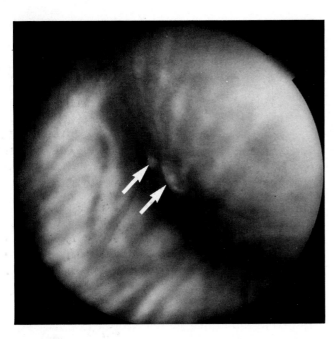

Figure 4–35. Arrows pointing to a double cystic vitreoretinal tuft on indentation. *(Photo courtesy W. Townsend.)*

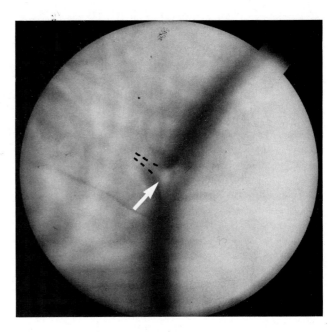

Figure 4–36. A zonular traction tuft on indentation. The dotted lines follow the traction. *(Photo courtesy W. Townsend.)*

can be seen from this schematic that should a PVD occur with the strong vitreoretinal traction tuft connections, there is a potential for a tear at the site of the tuft.

VITREORETINAL TUFTS—PEARLS

- Greyish tufts of tissue at the vitreoretinal interface between the equator and ora
- Often nasal within the vitreous base
- Noncystic tufts in 72 percent of population, cystic in 5 percent of population, and zonular in 15 percent of population
- Indentation may be needed to assess for retinal breaks
- Retinal tears may occur associated with vitreous liquefaction, syneresis, or detachment
- Management
  - Advise on signs/symptoms of retinal detachment.
  - Arrange retinology consultation with retinal breaks.
  - Monitor according to presence of other potentiators of retinal detachment.
  - Advise on importance of phosphenes.

Meridional Fold or Complex

Meridional folds (Figs. 4–37 and 4–38) are elevated. retinal tissue redundancies that develop in the area of the ora. **See color plate 64.** They may extend up to 4 DD posteriorly toward the equator and are perpendicular to the ora. They appear grey white and are best seen with scleral indentation. Meridional

folds occur in about 25 percent of the population with half of those being bilateral. Meridional folds occur in males more often than females. Multiple folds may present. Folds occur most often in the superior nasal quadrant, originating most frequently at dentate processes. Vitreoretinal traction may be present, running both anteriorly and posteriorly. Meridional folds are often associated with enclosed oral bays.

Meridional folds are altered retinal tissue composed of a proliferation of glial cells. The inner layer of the retina in these cases is degenerated and may have cystic-like changes. Retinal breaks may occur at the posterior edge of the fold secondary to traction. There is only a rare retinal detachment secondary to these folds.

Figure 4–37 demonstrates the genesis of a meridional fold with associated cystoid degeneration. It can be seen that meridional folds do occur at the ora serrata and set up potential for a retinal

TABLE 4–6. SIGNS AND SYMPTOMS OF EVOLVING RETINAL DETACHMENT

1. Any sudden onset of or increase in the number of *floaters*
2. Any sudden shower of small *floaters* (like gnats)
3. Any dramatic onset of *flashes of light* or a change in the pattern of flashes normally seen
4. Any sudden *change* in *vision*
5. Any *loss* of *side vision* when one eye is covered

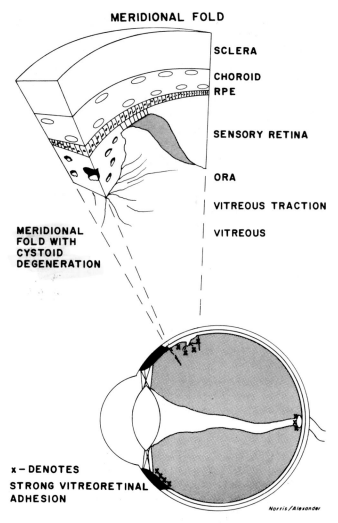

MERIDIONAL FOLD

SCLERA

CHOROID

RPE

SENSORY RETINA

ORA

VITREOUS TRACTION

VITREOUS

MERIDIONAL
FOLD WITH
CYSTOID
DEGENERATION

x — DENOTES
STRONG VITREORETINAL
ADHESION

Norris/Alexander

Figure 4–37. A schematic illustrating the clinicopathology of a meridional fold.

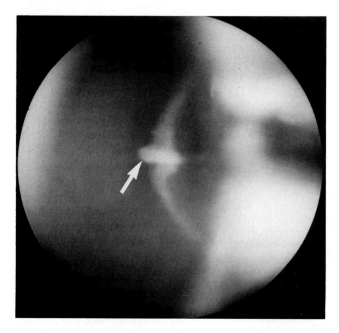

Figure 4–38. A meridional fold. *(Photo courtesy W. Townsend.)*

tear because of compromised retina as well as vitreous traction occurring in this area.

A clinical note should be made that a meridional complex is an enlarged dentate process and ciliary process aligned in the same meridian with a meridional fold extending from the dentate to the ciliary process. A peripheral retinal excavation may be located posterior to the complex. A peripheral retinal excavation is an area of thinned retina that is perpendicular to the ora and can occur as an isolated incident in 10 percent of the population. An excavation can mimic a retinal hole and must be indented to properly differentiate. Meridional complexes occur most commonly in the superior nasal quadrant in approximately 15 percent of the population. Because of the compromise of the retina, that is the retinal excavation, it is important to realize that there is potential for the development of a retinal tear in these particular conditions.

Management of patients with meridional folds consists of routine yearly follow-up examinations with assessment for tears. It is also important to make the patient aware of signs and symptoms of retinal detachment. A retinology consult is indicated for a retinal break.

MERIDIONAL FOLDS—PEARLS

- 0.5 to 4 DD greyish elevated tissue perpendicular to the ora
- Occur in about 25 percent of the population
- Most often in superior nasal quadrant
- Associated vitreoretinal traction may produce posterior border tears
- Meridional complexes in about 15 percent of population often associated with peripheral retinal excavations posterior to the complex
- Management
  - Routine yearly follow-up examinations
  - Patient education as to signs and symptoms of retinal detachment
  - Arrange retinology consultation for tears

Retinoschisis—Acquired

Introduction. Acquired retinoschisis (RS) is usually a bilateral (over 70 percent) condition with no particular predilection for sex that occurs with increasing frequency with age. RS occurs in about 4 percent of the population with about 7 percent occurrence over the age of 40 years. The change occurs most frequently in the inferior temporal quadrant, with a high percentage (over 70 percent) of the lesions attaining postequatorial borders. RS is most often asymptomatic but will show as a scotoma on field testing. It appears that a very low percentage (under 10 percent) of RS lesions demonstrate progression, expansion, development of retinal breaks, or progression toward retinal detachment. RS may develop in previously uninvolved areas of retina in an eye with RS.

Appearance. **See color plate 70.** Two forms of acquired RS (Figs. 4–39 and 4–40) have been described, flat (typical) and bullous (reticular). Typical, or flat, RS is believed to represent an advanced form of cystoid degeneration. Flat RS is usually confined to an area anterior to the equator and does not have associated retinal holes. The inner layer of a flat RS is typically smooth, thin, and has a beaten metallic appearance.

Bullous RS appears as a thin, transparent, ballooning forward of retinal tissue most often in the inferior temporal quadrant. The surface is very taut and typically does not move with eye movements. This is a direct contrast with rhegmatogenous retinal detachment that undulates freely with eye movements. There is about a 70 percent incidence of snowflakes or whitishlike bodies deposited on the surface of the RS. There is also an association with sclerotic or white-appearing vessels on the

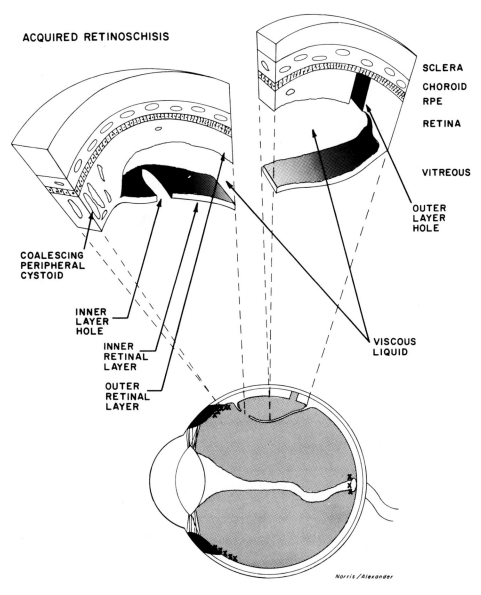

ACQUIRED RETINOSCHISIS

SCLERA
CHOROID
RPE
RETINA
VITREOUS
OUTER LAYER HOLE

COALESCING PERIPHERAL CYSTOID
INNER LAYER HOLE
INNER RETINAL LAYER
OUTER RETINAL LAYER
VISCOUS LIQUID

Norris/Alexander

x–DENOTES STRONG VITREORETINAL ADHESION

Figure 4–39. A schematic illustrating the clinicopathology of acquired RS.

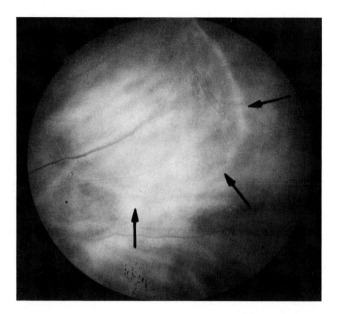

Figure 4–40. The arrows outline a zone of acquired RS.

surface of the RS. Under indirect kinds of illumination, the inner and outer layers of the RS may take on a honeycomb appearance, which helps significantly in the differential diagnosis from retinal detachment. The posterior leading edge of a RS may appear serrated but usually does not have a pigmented line of demarcation. The presence of a pigmented demarcation line is suggestive of the presence of a secondary detachment of the outer schisis layer, which has been stationary long enough to produce the change. There is always an area of cystoid degeneration between RS and the ora serrata. This zone may not present in cases of retinal detachment. With RS there are visible choroidal features, yet they are dim. This is an important differential diagnosis from retinal detachment in which choroidal features are significantly compromised. RS may develop breaks in the inner layer of the schisis, which are oval and clear. Retinal breaks in the outer layers of a RS are small and pink with rolled edges. Some clinicians refer to a group of small outer-layer breaks as frogs eggs. These breaks usually occur from the center to the posterior portion of the RS. A hemorrhage may occur at the edge of a RS or actually may bleed into the schisis cavity with a layered appearance.

A RS is actually a splitting of the sensory retina at the outer plexiform and inner nuclear layers. This is often associated with coalesced cystoid degeneration. The inner layer is usually very thin and may have snowflake deposition on the surface.

These snowflakes are considered by some to be condensed vitreous or remnants of glial pillars. The cavity of the RS is filled with hyaluronic acid, which is typically very viscous. This viscous fluid is responsible for making the RS so taut. This viscous fluid is also the reason that the RS does not undulate as does a retinal detachment. The cavity of a retinal detachment is filled with liquefied vitreous, which is not nearly as viscous in nature as hyaluronic acid.

Sixty percent of patients with RS have vitreous liquefaction. Over 25 percent of patients with RS have a break in at least one layer of the schisis and 40 percent of those patients have breaks in both layers. Visual field defects are present secondary to the RS but typically do not become evident until the RS progresses toward the posterior pole. Progression of a RS is very rare, with only about 13.5 percent of patients showing progression. If progression does occur, it is both circular in nature and moves toward the posterior pole. If a vitreous detachment occurs, progress stops because the traction on the schisis is actually relieved. Flashes and floaters can occur associated with the vitreous traction of a RS. As the schisis progresses toward the posterior pole there may be an associated cystoid maculopathy.

Prognosis and Management. In the management of RS it is important to note that up to 11 percent of patients with RS develop retinal detachment. It is important then to follow specific guidelines in the management of patients with RS and realize that bullous schisis has a significantly greater potential to procede to a schisis detachment than a flat schisis.

1. A patient with a RS without breaks should be observed semiannually for progression. He or she also should be made aware of the signs and symptoms of progression of RS as well as the signs and symptoms of retinal detachment.
2. A patient with RS that is progressing and that is threatening vision deserves a retinology consultation in spite of reports suggesting a very low incidence of vision loss even with progression. In these instances photocoagulation of the progressing border may result in flattening of the RS in about 50 percent of these cases. This is, however, very controversial.
3. A patient with RS with an inner-layer break anterior to the equator should be observed semiannually, as there is no particular potential to allow liquefied vitreous under the retina. Again, this patient should be made aware of the signs

and symptoms of progression of retinoschisis as well as the signs and symptoms of retinal detachment.

4. A patient with retinoschisis with outer-layer breaks should be referred to a retinologist. While the prevalence of retinal detachment in these cases is variable, there is some controversy as to whether or not these patients should be treated. It is well known that the viscous RS fluid usually does not leak in underneath the retina, but it must be remembered that it may. Where there is a controversy it is best to take the conservative approach to the management of these patients and to ask for a retinology consultation.

5. If there is a patient with RS with outer and inner layer breaks, this is an indication for immediate consultation with a retinologist.

6. A patient with RS with an associated progressive retinal detachment (schisis detachment) deserves an immediate retinology consultation for treatment with photocoagulation, cryotherapy, and/or possible scleral buckling. This is the *only* absolute indication for intervention.

7. A patient with a traction RS deserves a retinology consultation for proper management.

Figure 4–39, acquired bullous RS, demonstrates the actual splitting of the retinal tissue with viscous fluid in the resultant cavity. The schematic also demonstrates the presence of an inner-layer retinal hole and an outer-layer retinal hole. With an outer-layer retinal hole there is little chance of the development of a retinal detachment because the viscous fluid will not have a tendency to go into the hole and elevate the retina.

ACQUIRED RS CHARACTERISTICS—PEARLS

- Usually bilateral with increased incidence with aging
- Appears most often in inferior temporal quadrant, with over 70 percent attaining postequatorial borders
- Usually asymptomatic
- Flat RS is usually confined to area anterior to equator and is nonthreatening
- Bullous RS
  - Taut ballooning of tissue
  - 70 percent incidence of snowflake bodies on surface
  - Reticular (honeycomb) surface and dimmed choroidal detail
  - May have clear inner-layer breaks, small, pink, outer-layer breaks
  - Pigmented demarcation line strongly suggestive of schisis detachment

---

ACQUIRED RS MANAGEMENT—PEARLS

- If RS without breaks, observe every 6 months for progression and educate patient as to signs/symptoms of retinal detachment
- If RS with progression that is threatening vision, consult with a retinologist
- If RS with inner-layer break, observe every 6 months, and educate patient as to signs/symptoms of retinal detachment
- If RS with demonstrable outer layer breaks, ask for a retinology consultation
- If RS with inner and outer layer breaks, ask for a retinology consultation
- If RS with a progressive retinal detachment, ask for a retinology consultation

Snowflake Vitreoretinal Degeneration

Snowflake vitreoretinal degeneration is considered by some to be a genetically inherited anomaly that may have a relationship to retinitis pigmentosa. Some consider a snowflake vitreoretinal degeneration as a possible autosomal dominant inheritance pattern. Snowflake vitreoretinal degeneration seems to progress through four stages of development. In stage 1 occurring under the age of 15 years, there seems to be white without pressure throughout the peripheral retina. At stage 2, ages 15 to 25 years, yellow-white dots occur in the area of white without pressure, which appears slightly elevated. These yellow-white dots occur most frequently in the superior temporal quadrant. These dots may appear parallel to the equator in oval patches similar to the appearance of lattice degeneration. At stage 3, ages 25 to 50 years, there appears sheathing of the vessels in the affected area and RPE changes in the area of the snowflakes. Vitreous strands also appear at this particular stage, indicating concomitant vitreal changes. Often at this stage there is development of an early-onset cataract as well. At stage 4 there appears to be increased fundus pigmentation and chorioretinal atrophy. At this point cataracts progress to the point where visualization of the posterior pole becomes difficult. Visual field changes occur at this stage as well as low-amplitude scotopic b-wave electroretinogram changes and altered dark adaptation.

The layers involved in snowflake vitreoretinal degeneration include primarily the inner retinal layers. This presents from the ora to anterior to the equator. The condition progresses through stages and may develop retinal breaks. It is important that you educate the patient as to the genetics of the situation and make them aware of signs and symptoms of changes that occur as they progress through the stages. A referral for a retinal consultation is indicated at approximately stage 2 with consideration toward the signs and symptoms occurring in that stage.

SNOWFLAKE VITREORETINAL DEGENERATION—PEARLS

- Occurs in inner retinal layers—ora to equator
- Stage 1 (under 15 years)—WWOP throughout periphery
- Stage 2 (15–25 years)—yellow dots in oval patches in WWOP
- Stage 3 (25–50 years)—vessel sheathing and RPE changes with vitreous strands; possible early cataract and retinal break
- Stage 4 (over 50 years)—increased fundus pigmentation and chorioretinal atrophy with cataract and retinal break
- Management
  - Advise of signs/symptoms of retinal detachment
  - Arrange a retinology consultation on retinal breaks
  - Possible autosomal-dominant inheritance, therefore genetic counseling
  - Follow-up according to signs

Lattice Degeneration

Introduction. Lattice degeneration (Figs. 4–41 and 4–42) is also known as equatorial or circumferential retinal degeneration or perivascular lattice degeneration. Lattice degeneration affects the inner retinal layers appearing as a demarcated area of retinal atrophy with a tendency toward retinal breaks. Lattice degeneration appears often in young patients. Lattice degeneration is found typically in 6 to 10 percent of the general population and occurs bilaterally in approximately 50 percent of eyes. **See color plate 71.**

Appearance and Layers Involved. Lattice occurs most frequently in the superior and inferior retina, is usually 1 to 4 DD in length, and one half to 2 DD in width. The more posterior the lesion occurs, the wider the lesion. There is associated RPE hyperplasia in about 80 percent of the lesions, and yellowish flecks occur in about 80 percent of these lesions as well. The sclerosis of the white vessels, or fishboning, often attributed to these lesions increases in frequency with age. White without pressure may also occur along the borders of the lesions with a lacunae of liquefied vitreous overlying the lesion. Chorioretinal atrophy occurs quite

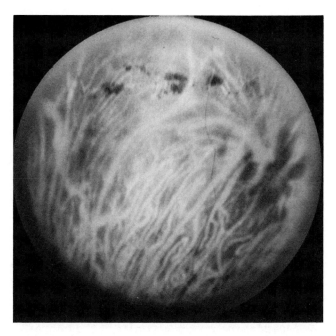

Figure 4–41. A typical presentation of lattice degeneration.

frequently inside the borders of the lesions. The various stages that are often associated with the development of lattice degeneration follow. *Stage 1:* The lattice degeneration presents as a greyish granular appearance of retinal thinning usually along a vessel. This can occur at a relatively young age in the equatorial region. *Stage 2:* At this stage the vessels become sheathed but are still patent. The vessels take on the fishbone appearance or sclerotic branching appearance often attributed to lattice degeneration. Also in this stage is the presentation of reactive retinal pigment epithelial hyperplasia.

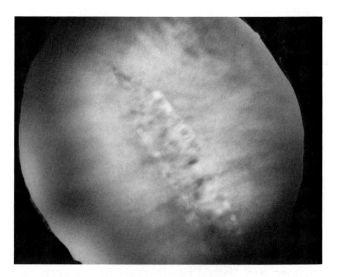

Figure 4–42. A variation of lattice degeneration known as snail-track degeneration.

Stage 3: At this stage there is an affectation of the larger vessels in the lattice degeneration. There is also an increase in pigment at this stage and an enlargement of the lesion. During this stage there may be the development of holes and tears. It is important to note that these holes are nothing more than the result of extreme thinning of the retinal tissue that occurs associated with lattice degeneration. The tears occur as a result of the vitreoretinal adhesions to these particularly thinned areas of the retina. The tears occur when there is a change in this vitreoretinal interface, such as that occurring with a posterior vitreous detachment. At this stage there is continual retinal thinning. Breaks inside of lattice degeneration are relatively common and present as round holes. These holes are reddish in color in contrast to the surrounding translucency of the lattice degeneration. If breaks occur outside the lesion, they are usually flat linear breaks or horseshoe tears at the posterior border of the lattice degeneration.

Lattice degeneration occurs as the result of loss of inner retinal layers down to the outer nuclear layer. There is overlying vitreal liquefaction plus vitreoretinal adhesions and often white without pressure at the borders of the lesion. The holes occur as a result of either continual degeneration of the retinal layers or the particular vitreoretinal adhesions that occur associated with these lesions.

Lattice degeneration is complex as far as prognosis is concerned. The more posterior the lattice, the more of a tendency to develop breaks. Breaks rarely develop in older, more heavily pigmented lesions. Twenty to thirty percent of eyes operated on for retinal detachment have lattice degeneration. If an eye has lattice degeneration, the chances of a retinal detachment are only about 0.3 percent to 0.5 percent. If an eye has lattice degeneration, the chance of atrophic retinal holes within that lesion is 18 to 30 percent. If an eye has lattice degeneration, the overall chance of retinal breaks in or around this lesion is approximately 25 percent. The frequency of retinal detachment associated with atrophic holes in lattice degeneration is 3 to 14 percent. These figures vary considerably in the literature. Retinal tears at the posterior edge of a lattice lesion occur in 1.4 percent of eyes with lattice degeneration. Table 4–7 lists the signs of progression of lattice-degeneration.

Prognosis and Management.
Management of lattice degeneration can be complex. It is very important to understand that all patients with lattice degeneration should be educated to the signs and symptoms of retinal detachment. The other considerations in the management of the patient with lat-

TABLE 4–7. SIGNS OF PROGRESSION OF LATTICE DEGENERATION

1. Enlargement of the lattice lesion
2. Appearance of holes or further thinning within the lattice lesion
3. Prominence of vitreous traction presenting at the border of the lesion, especially conducive to the development of linear tears at the posterior border
4. Alteration of the vitreous body in the form of liquefaction, shrinkage, and PVD

tice degeneration are the risk factors for retinal detachment. Table 4–8 lists specific risk factors in all peripheral retinal diseases that may contribute to the development of retinal detachment. Table 4–9 lists photopsia presenting as a clinical sign associated with retinal lesions.

With the risk factors for retinal detachment in mind, the practitioner can properly manage the patient with lattice degeneration. Lattice degeneration can be broken down to specific categories in regard to management. Following are these categories.

1. Lattice as the only sign or symptom—Examine this patient on a yearly basis and try to draw the size and location of the lesion. Also educate the patient as to signs and symptoms of retinal detachment. Scleral indentation is indicated when tears are suspected.
2. Lattice degeneration with symptoms of flashes and floaters—Examine this patient every 6 months, drawing the location and size of the lesion. Also educate the patient as to the signs and symptoms of retinal detachment. Scleral indentation is indicated.

TABLE 4–8. RISK FACTORS ASSOCIATED WITH THE DEVELOPMENT OF RETINAL DETACHMENT

1. Vitreous degeneration in the form of vitreous liquefaction or shrinkage
2. Younger patients have more of a tendency toward retinal detachments than older patients
3. Patients with myopia over 3 D have more of a tendency toward retinal detachment
4. Patients with a fellow eye with retinal detachment have a significantly higher rate of associated retinal detachment
5. Patients with a strong family history of retinal detachment have more of a tendency toward detachment
6. Patients with symptomatic breaks of the retina have a much higher frequency of associated retinal detachment
7. Patients with aphakia have a significantly higher rate of retinal detachments than phakic patients
8. Progression of retinal thinning or other signs in young patients has more of a tendency toward retinal detachments
9. The presence of significant vitreoretinal traction in elderly patients has more of a tendency toward retinal detachment

TABLE 4–9. PHOTOPSIA PRESENTING AS A CLINICAL SIGN ASSOCIATED WITH RETINAL LESIONS

Lattice alone	41%
Lattice with holes	31%
Snail track	10%
White with and without pressure	14%
Round holes	14%
Horseshoe tear	10%
Acute posterior vitreous detachment	14%

3. Lattice degeneration with associated asymptomatic atrophic holes but no associated risk factors—Examine this patient at 6-month intervals, drawing the size and location of the lattice lesion. Also educate the patient as to the signs and symptoms of retinal detachment.

4. Lattice degeneration with any of the accompanying risk factors—Request a retinology consultation.

5. Lattice with observed breaks at the margin of the lesion—Request a retinology consultation.

In addition to the commonly outlined features in the management of patients with lattice degeneration, the clinician must also consider environmental factors. An example of this would be a 15-year-old myopic football player with lattice degeneration and isolated asymptomatic atrophic holes. In this particular case a retinology consultation may be indicated for the possibility of intervention with cryopexy as a prophylactic measure. Certainly protective eyewear is indicated. Clinical judgment will dictate the best line of attack in these particular conditions. It is generally regarded that lattice degeneration with or without holes is a condition that should not be treated prophylactically unless the fellow eye has a retinal detachment. **See color plate 71.**

LATTICE DEGENERATION CHARACTERISTICS—PEARLS

- Usually occurs from the ora to equator in young patients, usually 1 to 4 DD long
- Bilateral in 50 percent most often in vertical meridians
- The more posterior the lesion, the wider the lesion
- Area of retinal thinning with overlying lacunae of liquefied vitreous
- RPE hyperplasia, yellow flecks, fishbone vessel sclerosis, chorioretinal atrophy within, surround of white without pressure commonly occurs in lattice
- High incidence of atrophic holes within the lesion

LATTICE DEGENERATION MANAGEMENT—PEARLS

- Lattice degeneration only—document lesion, indent when indicated, advise of signs/symptoms of retinal detachment, and examine in one year
- Lattice degeneration with symptoms—document lesion, indent for holes, advise of signs/symptoms of retinal detachment, and examine in six months
- Lattice degeneration with asymptomatic atrophic holes but no associated risk factors—document lesion, advise of signs/symptoms of retinal detachment, and examine in six months
- Lattice degeneration with risk factors for retinal detachment or signs of progression—retinology consultation
- Lattice degeneration with retinal breaks at the margin of the lesion—retinology consultation

---

Snail-Track Degeneration

Snail-track degeneration (Fig. 4–42) is also known as Scheckenspuren. Snail-track degeneration is in reality nothing more than lattice degeneration without the fishbone appearance to it. The lesion appears slick or slimy, like the trail left by a snail or slug. The layers involved are the same as lattice degeneration, with the exception that microglial cells containing lipoprotein material appear to be present. The prognosis and management of snail-track degeneration is essentially the same as lattice degeneration. Because of the retinal thinning and the overlying vitreous liquefaction, there is certainly the concern for the development of retinal holes and tears. **See color plate 71.**

Atrophic Retinal Holes

Appearance and Layers Involved. Atrophic retinal holes (Figs. 4–43 through 4–46) appear as pinpoint to 2-DD round, red lesions. These holes occur in about 2 to 3 percent of the general population. The redness of the lesion is nothing more than the retinal pigment epithelial/choroidal structure showing through an area that used to be occupied by retinal tissue. These atrophic retinal holes are often surrounded by a cuff of whitish edema or pigment. The whitish edema is nothing more than intraretinal edema or a subclinical sensory retinal detachment surrounding the lesion. The pigment associated with the lesion usually indicates that the lesion has been present for approximately 3 months. The pigment is reactive RPE hyperplasia. The whitish cuff indicates vitreoretinal

LATTICE DEGENERATION WITH ENCLOSED ATROPHIC HOLE

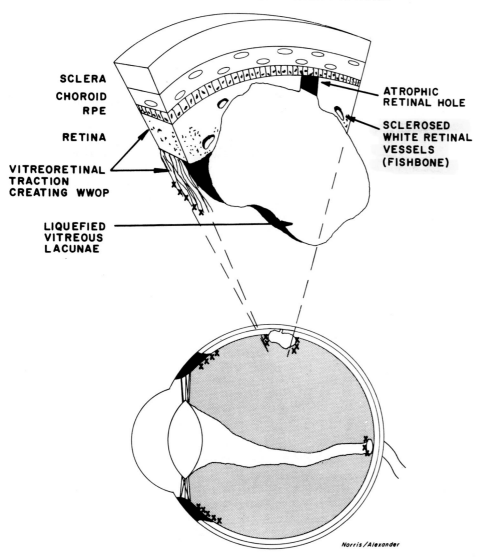

SCLERA
CHOROID
RPE

RETINA

VITREORETINAL
TRACTION
CREATING WWOP

LIQUEFIED
VITREOUS
LACUNAE

ATROPHIC
RETINAL HOLE

SCLEROSED
WHITE RETINAL
VESSELS
(FISHBONE)

Norris/Alexander

x—DENOTES STRONG VITREORETINAL
ADHESION

Figure 4–43. A schematic of the clinicopathology of lattice degeneration with an enclosed atrophic hole.

traction. When an atrophic hole is viewed with scleral indentation, the hole becomes volcanolike or fishmouth, that is, when the indentor is applied, the surround of the hole actually puckers. Atropic holes are seen in a variety of conditions, including peripheral cystoid degeneration, lattice degeneration, snail-track degeneration, pars planitis, and isolated within the retina. Atrophic holes are the most common of the retinal breaks (over 70 percent).

Atrophic retinal holes are round, full-thickness breaks in the retina due to progressive retinal thinning rather than true vitreoretinal traction. They are thought to be secondary to underlying vascular insufficiency that compromises the retina to the point where it actually develops breaks. Figures 4–

43 and 4–44 demonstrate the actual clinicopathology of atrophic retinal holes associated with lattice. You can see retinal thinning that is lattice degeneration. Overlying this thinning is a lacunae of liquified vitreous. In this area of retinal thinning, you will note that there is a punched-out or atrophic retinal hole down to the retinal pigment epithelium. It should be noted that in this particular case there is no associated retinal detachment, but there is vitreoretinal traction creating white without pressure at the edge of the lesion. It should also be noted in this schematic that there are sclerosed white retinal vessels giving the fishbone appearance to lattice degeneration. In the second schematic you can see that there is a localized retinal detachment at an atrophic hole in lattice. The only

LOCALIZED RETINAL DETACHMENT AT AN ATROPHIC HOLE IN LATTICE

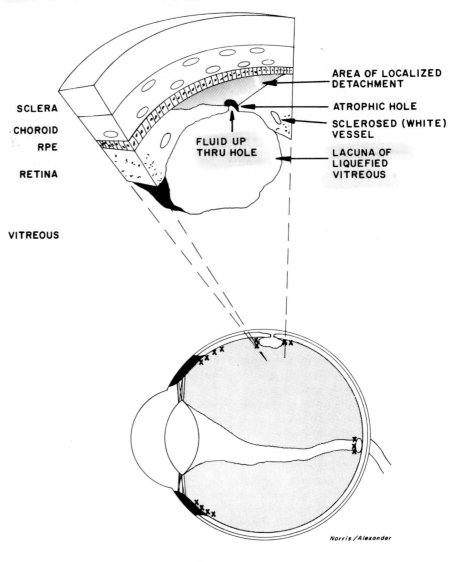

SCLERA

CHOROID

RPE

RETINA

VITREOUS

AREA OF LOCALIZED DETACHMENT

ATROPHIC HOLE

SCLEROSED (WHITE) VESSEL

LACUNA OF LIQUEFIED VITREOUS

FLUID UP THRU HOLE

Norris/Alexander

x — DENOTES STRONG VITREORETINAL ADHESION

Figure 4–44. A schematic of the clinicopathology of a localized retinal detachment at an atrophic hole within an area of lattice degeneration.

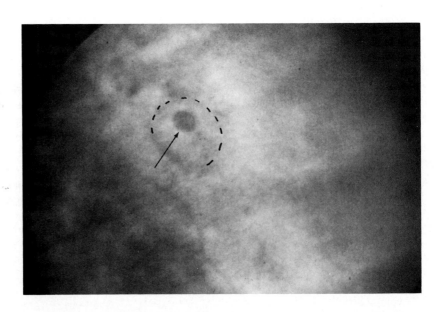

Figure 4–45. An atrophic retinal hole **(arrow)** with a surrounding subclinical detachment **(dotted).**

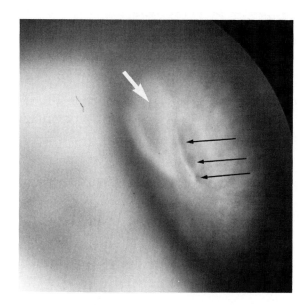

Figure 4–46. Three atrophic retinal holes **(black arrows)** near a retinal cyst **(white arrow)**. The area is indented. *(Photo courtesy W. Townsend.)*

difference between this lesion and the previous lesion is that the liquefied vitreous has gained access through the atrophic hole to the area between the retinal pigment epithelium and the sensory retina. This creates a localized retinal detachment that may progress to become a full rhegmatogenous retinal detachment.

Prognosis and Management. The atrophic retinal hole represents an access line for liquefied vitreous to seep underneath the sensory retina. When fluid accumulates between sensory retina and the retinal pigment epithelium, it is known as a sensory retinal detachment. However, it is known that only about 7 percent of atrophic holes develop progressive retinal detachment.

Management of patients with atrophic holes is as multifaceted as is lattice degeneration. Certainly all patients with atrophic holes should be educated as to the signs and symptoms of retinal detachment. Remember the risk factors relative to the development of retinal detachment when deciding on management strategies in patients with atrophic retinal holes. Management of atrophic holes can be broken into the following categories.

1. Patients with isolated asymptomatic atrophic holes—Monitor these patients on a yearly basis, and educate them as to the signs and symptoms of retinal detachment.
2. Patients with isolated asymptomatic atrophic holes with a cuff of edema or focal detachment less than 1 DD—Monitor these patients every 6 months, drawing the location and size of the lesion. Also educate these patients as to the signs

and symptoms of the development of retinal detachment.
3. Patients with isolated asymptomatic atrophic holes with a cuff edema larger than 1 DD— These patients deserve a retinal consult, as 30 percent of patients with atrophic holes with cuffs of edema over 2 DD progress to retinal detachment.
4. A patient with symptomatic atrophic retinal holes should have a retinal consultation in spite of the fact that the retinologist may not opt to treat at that particular point in time.
5. An atrophic hole with a flap tear indicates a strong vitreoretinal adhesion. Patients with strong vitreoretinal adhesions associated with atrophic holes should be considered at risk to develop a significant retinal tear with ensuing retinal detachment. These patients deserve a retinology consult.

All of these modes of management should be tempered with clinical judgment regarding associated risk factors for retinal detachment.
See color plate 72.

ATROPHIC RETINAL HOLES— CHARACTERISTICS—PEARLS

- Pinpoint to 2-DD round, red lesion, often with a surrounding cuff of retinal edema and/or RPE hyperplasia
- Usually ora to equator in a number of conditions of retinal thinning
- May be of vascular origin
- Represent full-thickness retinal breaks—an access line for liquefied vitreous under the sensory retina
- RPE hyperplasia indicates presence for 3 months
- Atrophic holes fish mouth on indentation

ATROPHIC RETINAL HOLES— MANAGEMENT—PEARLS

- Isolated asymptomatic atrophic holes—document, advise of signs/symptoms of retinal detachment, and examine in one year
- Isolated asymptomatic atrophic holes with cuff of edema or focal detachment less than 1 DD—document, advise of signs/symptoms of retinal detachment, and examine in 6 months
- Isolated asymptomatic atrophic holes with cuff of edema larger than 1 DD—retinology consultation indicated
- Isolated symptomatic atrophic holes—retinology consultation indicated
- Isolated atrophic holes with flap tear or demonstrable vitreoretinal adhesions—retinology consultation indicated

Operculated Retinal Hole

Appearance and Layers Involved. Operculated retinal holes (Figs. 4–47 and 4–48) typically occur from the equator to the ora serrata. These appear as round red holes with an overlying free-floating plug of retinal tissue attached to the vitreous. This free-floating plug is called the operculum and represents the vitreoretinal adhesion that has freed itself. The plug often appears smaller than the hole it came from because of atrophy of this retinal tissue secondary to removal from the nutritional supply of the retina. When an operculated retinal hole occurs, there may be an associated hemorrhage. This hemorrhage occurs when a retinal vessel is torn near the site of the break. Inside of the retinal holes may be yellowish bodies called pathological

drusen. These holes may be surrounded by white with pressure or white without pressure as well as a localized subclinical retinal detachment. As with an atrophic retinal hole, an operculated hole may develop a pigmented demarcation line. The operculated hole is similar in nature to the atrophic hole. The primary difference between an atrophic hole and an operculated hole is the associated plug of retinal tissue. In both conditions there is thinned atrophic retina that breaks down to the point where a hole occurs. **See color plate 73.**

Prognosis and Management. The operculated hole occurs as a result of an abnormal vitreoretinal adhesion that is tugged away by a change in the vitreous, often a vitreous detachment, creating a hole in the atrophic retinal tissue. The prognosis is

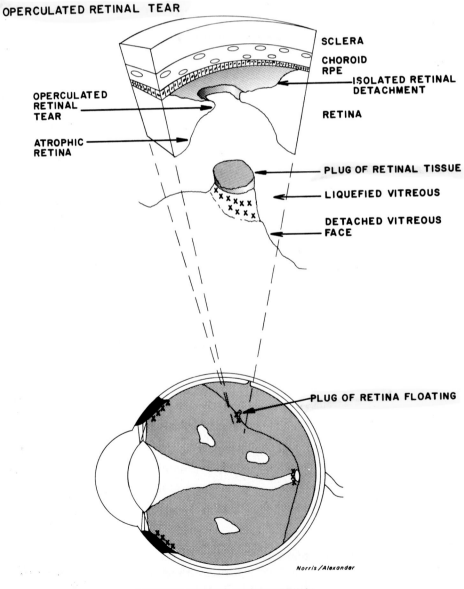

Figure 4–47. A schematic of the clinicopathology of an operculated retinal tear.

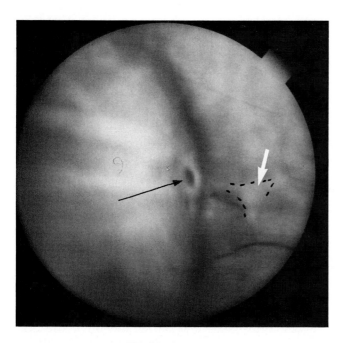

Figure 4–48. An operculated retinal hole on indentation **(black arrow)**. Note the surround of edema. The blurred plug is indicated by the white arrow. *(Photo courtesy W. Townsend.)*

ina. With this hole in the sensory retina there is potential for the liquefied vitreous to have access between the retinal pigment epithelium and the sensory retina, allowing for sensory retinal detachment.

OPERCULATED RETINAL HOLES— CHARACTERISTICS—PEARLS

- Result of an abnormal vitreoretinal adhesion being tugged forward
- Round, red holes with an overlying floating plug of tissue
- Occur between ora and equator
- Possible pathological drusen inside of holes
- May have associated hemorrhage and/or WWOP
- May have associated localized retinal detachment

OPERCULATED RETINAL HOLES— MANAGEMENT—PEARLS

- If asymptomatic single operculated hole—document, advise of signs/symptoms of retinal detachment, and examine yearly
- If asymptomatic multiple operculated holes—document, advise of signs/symptoms of retinal detachment, and examine every 6 months
- If symptomatic operculated hole, if in an aphakic eye, if there is a retinal detachment in the fellow eye, or if there is continued traction around the hole—retinology consultation is indicated
- If surround of edema exceeds 2 DD—retinology consultation is indicated

---

usually good with an operculated hole, as the abnormal vitreoretinal traction has been relieved.

Again, the management of a patient with an operculated retinal hole can be somewhat complex. It is important to educate the patient as to the signs and symptoms of retinal detachment. The variations in operculated retinal holes may be managed according to the following guidelines.

1. If a patient has an asymptomatic single operculated retinal hole, monitor the patient at yearly intervals, educating as to the signs and symptoms of retinal detachment. Indentation may be indicated.
2. If a patient has asymptomatic multiple operculated retinal holes, monitor this patient every 6 months, educating the patient as to the signs and symptoms of retinal detachment. Indentation may be indicated.
3. If the patient is symptomatic, aphakic, or there is a retinal detachment in the fellow eye or continued traction surrounding the operculated retinal tear, a retinology consultation is indicated.
4. Again, remember other risk factors regarding retinal detachment.
5. If surrounding cuff of edema exceeds 2 DD a retinology consult is indicated.

Figure 4–47 demonstrates the histopathology of operculated retinal tears. It can be seen that there is a plug of retinal tissue that is attached to the vitreous face. This vitreous face has fallen forward and has pulled the plug out of the ret-

Commotio Retinae

Introduction. Commotio retinae is the result of blunt trauma to the eye or surround, creating contrecoup shock waves that disturb the retina. Commotio retinae may occur anywhere in the retina. When it occurs in the posterior pole, it is often referred to as Berlin's edema.

Appearance and Layers Involved. Immediately after the trauma, the retina maintains its transparency. Within a few hours the traumatized area becomes opaque. The swelling and disorganization that creates this opaque appearance is believed to be confined to the outer retinal layers. The opaque retina blocks background choroidal fluorescence on fluorescein angiography. If the trauma is severe enough, choroidal rupture may occur.

The long-term appearance may vary from no observable changes, to reactive hyperplasia mixed with RPE atrophy, to traumatic macular holes, and to the remote possibility of choroidal neovascular development.

Signs and Symptoms. Symptoms depend upon the section of the retina that is involved. If the posterior pole is involved, visual acuity is reduced to variable levels. If the peripheral retina is affected, visual field defects will occur.

Prognosis and Management. Little can be done to hurry the course of the natural healing process of commotio retinae. The best that can be done is to carefully investigate for other vision-threatening signs associated with trauma that might be amendable to intervention.

COMMOTIO RETINAE—PEARLS

- Secondary to blunt trauma
- Opaque retina due to disorganization of the outer retinal layers
- May result in reactive RPE hyperplasia, RPE atrophy, macular holes, choroidal neovascular development
- May have reduced acuity or field defects
- Management
  - Educate the patient on signs/symptoms of retinal detachment
  - Monitor for the development of vision-threatening retinal changes associated with trauma

---

Pars Planitis

Introduction. Pars planitis is a chronic inflammatory disease of the peripheral retina that is characterized by remissions and exacerbations over 20 to 30 years. It has been reported to be the primary disease in between 7 to 8 percent of patients with uveitis. It is bilateral in 60 to 80 percent of patients and has no sexual predilection. The etiology of pars planitis is uncertain, although an autoimmune origin and a relationship to demyelinizing disease have been suggested.

The age of onset is thought to be in the childhood years, but this is obscure, as most patients are asymptomatic at this stage. The disease usually becomes apparent in young adulthood.

Appearance and Layers Involved. Initially, dirty, yellowish exudates aggregate near small-sheathed vessels in the extreme periphery. These early "snowbanks" lie on the retina and move easily into the vitreous as cells and flare in the retrolental space. This process occurs most frequently in the inferior retina. Should the process continue, the globular exudates coalesce and may form a large plaque (snowbank) covering the ora serrata. This plaque has fuzzy, raised edges when active and appears to be membranous with a hard covering when inactive. The fibrovascular membrane

may eventually develop neovascularization in the anterior chamber; yellowish gelatinous exudates may also deposit over the trabecular meshwork and iris surface.

Signs and Symptoms. The patient with pars planitis may enter with complaints of hazy vision or floaters from the cells and flare in the retrolental space. The patient may also complain of reduced visual acuity secondary to the cystoid macular edema. Remissions and exacerbations are characteristic. There is the remote relationship of pars planitis to demyelinizing disease.

Prognosis and Management. Pars planitis is a chronic disease that runs a prolonged course. Since the condition is inflammatory, corticosteroids in the form of sub-Tenon-injections or oral forms are indicated to "control" the development of the snowbanks and to minimize the cystoid macular edema. Improvement is slow, and often the best that can be expected is to hold the process down while it runs the course. Because of the prolonged use of corticosteroids, posterior subcapsular cataracts develop in many patients. Glaucoma is another complication. The associated cystoid macular edema is the cause of reduced acuity in many patients. Other complications include band keratopathy and vitreoretinal changes that can precipitate RS, retinal detachment, and hemorrhage.

The patient should be on routine follow-up care and should be educated as to the signs of exacerbation. Careful investigation should be performed for associated retinal breaks. Up to 80 percent of patients with pars planitis have very good visual prognosis with no intervention whatsoever. There is, however, the occasional need for surgical intervention.

PARS PLANITIS—PEARLS

- Chronic inflammatory process—bilateral in 60 to 80 percent
- Early age of onset
- Symptoms are hazy vision, with possible vision reduction secondary to cystoid macular edema
- Dirty yellow exudates appear in periphery near sheathed vessels
- Exudates may coalesce to form snowbanks that may break off into vitreous—may form large plaque
- Complications include cataracts, glaucoma, retinal problems
- Management
  - Control vision-threatening inflammatory process with corticosteroids
  - Provide routine follow-up care and patient education
  - Possible need for vitrectomy

PERIPHERAL RETINAL CHANGES THAT POSE A DIRECT THREAT TO VISION

Linear Retinal Tear
See color plate 73.

Appearance and Layers Involved. A linear retinal tear may also appear as a horseshoe tear (Figs. 4–49 and 4–50). A linear retinal tear appears red, surrounded by atrophic grey retinal tissue. This retinal tissue may also be edematous in the early phases of the tear. The flap of retinal tissue that has detached typically shrinks over time because of lack of nutritional blood supply. This shrinkage or atrophy is similar to that occurring in the retinal plug of an operculated retinal tear. A linear tear may be in the shape of a horseshoe with the apex

usually but not always pointing toward the posterior pole. These tears usually occur near the posterior border of the vitreous base, around lattice, around retinal tufts, around snowflake degeneration, and around white without pressure. Horseshoe tears are the direct result of an abnormally strong vitreoretinal adhesion. This vitreoretinal adhesion occurs in an area of atrophic retina. When vitreous collapse occurs, the strong vitreoretinal adhesion pulls on the already compromised atrophic retina creating a tear. Should a retinal vessel be involved in the tear, there may be an associated hemorrhage. Also, there may be retinal tissue bridging the gap of the tear as well as vitreoretinal traction bands. As with many other tears, holes and other alterations in retinal tissue, RPE hyperplasia may occur over a period of time. The genesis

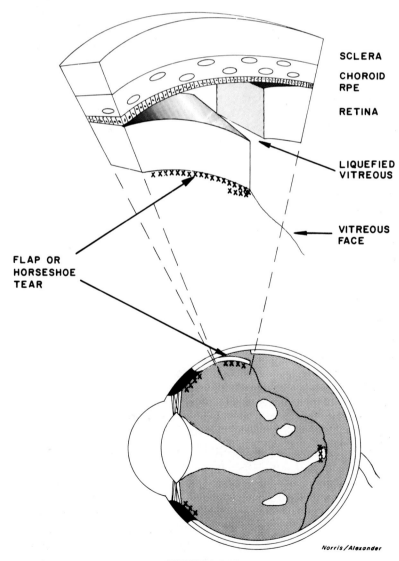

HORSESHOE OR FLAP RETINAL TEAR

SCLERA
CHOROID
RPE
RETINA
LIQUEFIED VITREOUS
VITREOUS FACE
FLAP OR HORSESHOE TEAR

Norris/Alexander

x—DENOTES STRONG VITREORETINAL ADHESION

Figure 4–49. A schematic of the clinicopathology of a linear or horseshoe retinal tear.

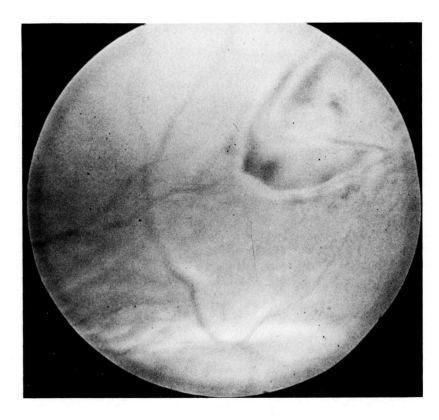

Figure 4–50. A horseshoe retinal tear within a retinal detachment.

of the horseshoe or flat retinal tear is demonstrated in Figure 4–49. **See color plate 73.**

It should be noted that traction remains after the tear, allowing for further development of retinal detachment. Linear retinal tears usually occur superiorly, creating even more difficulty because of gravity pulling on the retinal tissue. Linear retinal tears occur most commonly in situations where the retina is thin, where there is trauma, or where there is a condition associated with vitreous degeneration. It occurs most commonly in patients over 40 years of age, in those with myopia, in patients with lattice degeneration, in patients with aphakia, and often secondary to trauma.

Prognosis and Management. Linear retinal tears are the leading cause of rhegmatogenous retinal detachment. There is approximately a 30 percent chance of retinal detachment associated with a horseshoe or flap retinal tear. Management of patients with retinal tears of any kind in any location is immediate consultation with a retinologist. Judgment regarding therapeutic intervention is at the discretion of the retinal surgeon.

LINEAR RETINAL TEAR—PEARLS

- A tear in the retina is red, with a surround of grey retinal tissue
- The detached flap shrinks over time
- If in the shape of a horseshoe, the apex usually points toward posterior pole
- Result of strong vitreoretinal adhesion in an area of thin retina
- Thirty percent chance of retinal detachment—retinology consultation is indicated

---

Prophylactic Therapy

Which retinal conditions discussed thus far have indications for intraventive prophylactic therapy? We have discussed flap tears, operculated tears, round holes, lattice degeneration with or without holes, and outer layer holes in RS. All of these pose a potential threat for the development of retinal detachment. In general, all eyes with breaks in the retina or thinned retina should be treated if the fellow eye has retinal detachment. Patients with aphakia need consideration for prophylactic therapy should a flap tear or an operculated tear occur. Patients with symptomatic breaks or tears should be considered for treatment should that tear be a flap tear or an operculated tear. Patients that are asymptomatic should have only flap tears treated prophylactically. There is some controversy regarding outer-layer holes in RS which are best managed by a retinology consultation for consideration for prophylactic therapy.

Retinal Dialysis

Appearance and Layers Involved. Retinal dialysis (Fig. 4–51) is a retinal tear occurring near the ora serrata. A retinal dialysis may be spontaneous in young patients and in these instances are bilateral, occurring in the inferior temporal quadrant. More commonly, retinal dialysis is associated with trauma, occurring most often in the superior nasal quadrant. Retinal dialysis appears as any other tear

or hole in the retina. The hole or tear in a dialysis is red with greyish retina surrounding it. This greyish retina is either atrophic or edematous, depending upon elapsed time. The dialysis is often only observable in early stages with scleral indentation. It is therefore important to carefully investigate the oral area in patients who have suffered recent trauma. Retinal dialysis is usually asymptomatic and usually involves less than 90 degrees of the peripheral retina. There is no particular vitreous connection in the genesis of retinal dialysis except an occasional concurrent vitreous hemorrhage.

Prognosis and Management. In either the spontaneous or the traumatic retinal dialysis there

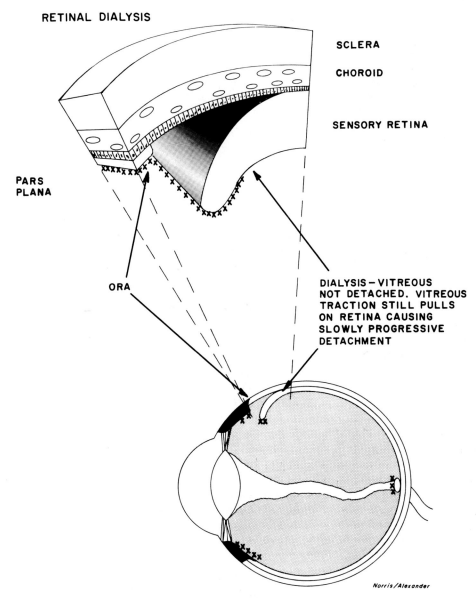

RETINAL DIALYSIS

SCLERA

CHOROID

SENSORY RETINA

PARS PLANA

ORA

DIALYSIS – VITREOUS NOT DETACHED. VITREOUS TRACTION STILL PULLS ON RETINA CAUSING SLOWLY PROGRESSIVE DETACHMENT

Norris/Alexander

x – DENOTES STRONG VITREORETINAL ADHESION

Figure 4–51. A schematic of the clinicopathology of a retinal dialysis.

can be the slow progression toward retinal detachment because of the fact that strong vitreoretinal adhesions remain attached to the sensory retina. The strong vitreoretinal adhesions are subject to continued pull and stress by the vitreous. Because there is a relatively slow progression toward retinal detachment, retinal dialysis may have multiple demarcation lines. In traumatic retinal dialysis, there may be a significant delay in the development of a retinal dialysis. It is safe to say that with retinal dialysis one may assume eventual retinal detachment. Management for retinal dialysis is a retinology consultation. Some of these may be treated with cryopexy; some of them may necessitate the employment of a scleral buckle.

Figure 4–51 demonstrates a retinal dialysis, which is nothing more than a retinal tear or detachment at the ora serrata. It is important to note that the vitreous is not detached in these instances and that the strong vitreoretinal traction at the base of the vitreous still remains. This can cause a continual pull on the retina with the genesis of a slowly progressive retinal detachment.

RETINAL DIALYSIS—PEARLS

- Red retinal tear at the ora less than 90 degrees
- Usually asymptomatic, often involving trauma
- Need to indent cases of trauma to pick up early retinal dialysis
- If spontaneous in the young, they are bilateral
- Slow progression toward retinal detachment—retinology consultation is indicated.

Giant Retinal Tear

Appearance and Layers Involved. A giant retinal tear (Figs. 4–52 and 4–53) is a form of retinal dialysis that involves over 90 degrees of the peripheral retina. It typically occurs four times as frequently in males as females and is associated with myopia over 8 D. Giant retinal tears are also very symptomatic. Seventy percent of giant retinal tears are idiopathic. Twenty percent of giant retinal tears are traumatic, and 10 percent occur in the areas of chorioretinal degeneration. There is usually considerable vitreous liquefaction in the patient with a giant retinal tear. There is often abnormal traction causing the retina to fold back on itself similar to a taco shell. This is called a bucket-handle detachment if the ciliary body is also detached.

A giant retinal tear may occur along the posterior margin of white without pressure, in extensive areas of lattice degeneration, and in areas of previous cryopexy therapy or photocoagulated retina. Giant retinal tears often occur at the ora serrata involving the ciliary body epithelium. A giant retinal tear is a sensory retinal detachment with vitreoretinal traction at the rolled edge of the tear.

Prognosis and Management. The prognosis for a giant retinal tear is very poor. There is invariable progression toward retinal detachment. Of more importance is the fellow eye. Over twelve percent of fellow eyes to giant retinal tears has giant breaks as well. Nearly twelve percent of fellow eyes has retinal tears, about 10 percent of fellow eyes has retinal holes, 0.4 percent has retinal dialysis, and nearly 16 percent of fellow eyes to giant retinal tears has retinal detachment.

Giant retinal tears have a very poor surgical prognosis. However, the sooner the tear is discovered the better the prognosis. An immediate retinology consultation is indicated. It is also important to be aware of the associated complications in the fellow eye. The overall prognosis is worsened postsurgically by the high incidence of proliferative vitreoretinopathy. The giant retinal tear is shown in schematic cross-section demonstrating persistence of vitreal traction and progression of the retinal detachment.

GIANT RETINAL TEAR—PEARLS

- Retinal tear at ora greater than 90 degrees with retina folding over onto itself—Taco
- Four times more frequent in males
- Usually associated with myopia over 8 D
- Seventy percent idiopathic, 20 percent associated with trauma, 10 percent associated with chorioretinal degeneration
- Considerable vitreoretinal traction at edge of tear leading to invariable retinal detachment
- Fellow eyes have
  - 12.8 percent giant tears
  - 11.9 percent retinal tears
  - 10.2 percent retinal holes
  - 15.9 percent retinal detachment
- Retinology consultation is indicated

Retinal Detachment

Retinal detachment is the result of breaks in the peripheral retina. The clinician must realize that there is a very weak bond between the sensory retina and the RPE. There is a strong bond between RPE and Bruch's membrane. As such, most retinal detachments occur between the RPE and the sensory retina. It is also very important to realize that the immediate cause of rhegmatogenous retinal detach-

GIANT RETINAL TEAR

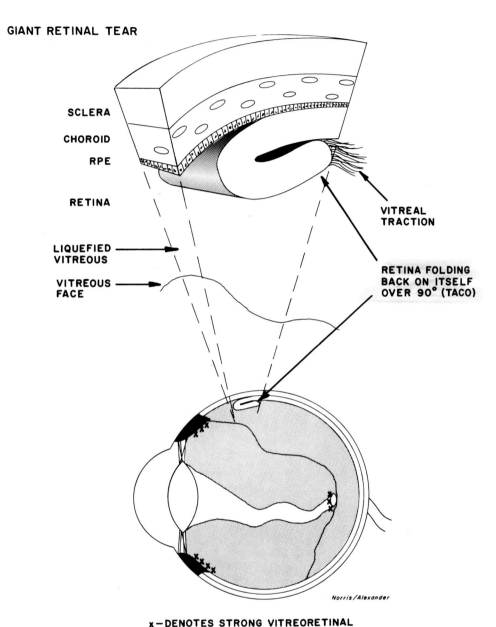

SCLERA
CHOROID
RPE
RETINA
LIQUEFIED VITREOUS
VITREOUS FACE

VITREAL TRACTION

RETINA FOLDING BACK ON ITSELF OVER 90° (TACO)

Norris/Alexander

x — DENOTES STRONG VITREORETINAL ADHESION

Figure 4–52. A schematic illustrating the clinicopathology of a giant retinal tear.

ment is vitreoretinal traction in areas of atrophic or thinned retina. In the area of thinned retina, a hole or a tear is created for the ingress of liquefied vitreous between the sensory retina and retinal pigment epithelium. This ingress of liquefied vitreous in addition to the continued vitreoretinal traction is the beginning of the retinal detachment. One of the symptomatic results of the retinal detachment is the presence of floaters and flashes of light. The majority of retinal detachments are symptomatic. Often the patient will have floaters in the anterior vitreous resulting from liberated red blood cells and pigment granules when the break occurs. This is known as tobacco dust or Shaffer's sign. Any sign of floaters or flashes should be considered in-

dicative of a retinal detachment until proven otherwise. Peripheral field loss occurs with retinal detachment and is a very important sign.

Rhegmatogenous Retinal Detachment

Introduction. A rhegmatogenous retinal detachment is the result of a retinal break. Retinal detachment occurs in 8.9 to 12.9 per 100,000 of the phakic population. Retinal detachment occurrence peaks between ages 50 and 60 years. Only 1 to 3 percent of patients with high myopia develop retinal detachment. Between 1.7 and 5 percent of aphakic patients develop retinal detachment, 50 percent of

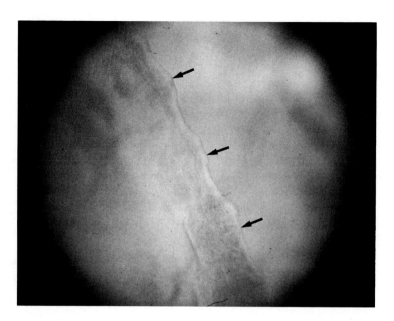

Figure 4–53. The edge of a giant retinal tear.

those occurring 1 year postsurgically. A full 50 percent of retinal detachments occur from retinal tears with continuing traction. Thirty percent of retinal detachments are associated with lattice degeneration, while 20 percent of retinal detachments are associated with holes or retinal dialysis.

See color plates 67 and 74.

Appearance and Layers Involved. A retinal detachment (Figs. 4–54 through 4–56) appears as an undulating elevation that is semitransparent. This elevation contains retinal vessels and is well-known to obscure underlying choroidal detail. A shallow retinal detachment is more difficult to see, and often the clinician must use the scleral indenter to discover this subtlety. Billowing folds of retina indicate a significant accumulation of subretinal fluid. Progression of a retinal detachment is determined by location, the size and number of breaks in the retina, and the strength of the remaining vitreoretinal adhesions **(Table 4–10).** If a retinal detachment remains stationary for about 3 months, a pigment hyperplasia line develops at its posterior border. This is known as a demarcation line or a high-water line. Demarcation lines occur more frequently in inferior retinal detachments because of the slower progression. Superior retinal detachments will occur at a faster rate because of the involvement of gravity. Demarcation lines may be multiple in appearance. A long-standing retinal detachment is taut because of proliferation of glial and connective tissues on its surface. Contraction of these tissues can produce folds, but undulation

with movement is minimized. Pigment may accumulate, and eventually the retinal tissue becomes necrotic. Massive preretinal proliferation may occur but it is more commonly characteristic of postsurgical retinal detachment complications.

The retinal detachment is due to abnormal vitreoretinal traction, causing a break in compromised sensory retina. This break allows access of liquefied vitreous into the subretinal space. Continuing traction with increased liquefied vitreous in the space will allow for a progression in the development of the retinal detachment. Figure 4–54, a rhegmatogenous retinal detachment with the demarcation line, demonstrates the liquefied vitreous in the subsensory retinal space. This figure also demonstrates the reactive hyperplasia creating the demarcation line.

Prognosis and Management. Traumatic retinal detachment usually occurs in young males and may be two years in evolution. If nontraumatic, the cause is usually a retinal break, and the detachment will progress to include the macula at a relatively rapid rate. It must be remembered that the longer the macula is detached, the poorer the prognosis.

There are indicators of the duration of a retinal detachment. These could be useful in determining the general prognosis of a patient. It should be remembered that when a retinal detachment has been present in the upper quadrant for over 4 weeks, the subretinal fluid often sinks into the lower half of the fundus where large balloons of

RHEGMATOGENOUS R. D. WITH DEMARCATION LINE

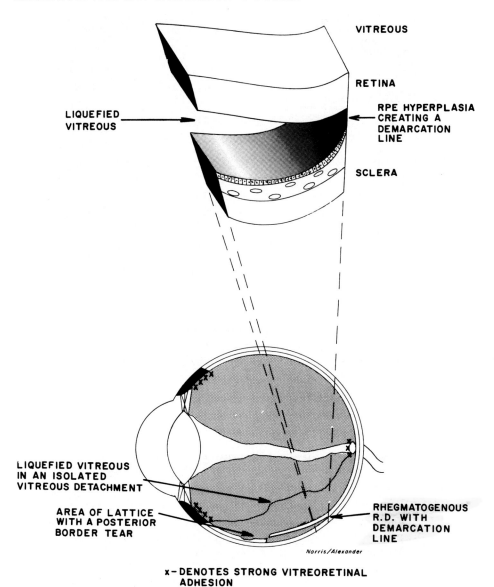

VITREOUS

RETINA

RPE HYPERPLASIA
CREATING A
DEMARCATION
LINE

LIQUEFIED
VITREOUS

SCLERA

LIQUEFIED VITREOUS
IN AN ISOLATED
VITREOUS DETACHMENT

AREA OF LATTICE
WITH A POSTERIOR
BORDER TEAR

RHEGMATOGENOUS
R.D. WITH
DEMARCATION
LINE

Norris/Alexander

x – DENOTES STRONG VITREORETINAL
ADHESION

Figure 4–54. A schematic illustrating the clinicopathology of a rhegmatogenous retinal detachment with a pigmented demarcation line.

detachment present. Another indicator of the duration is the demarcation line. A pigmented demarcation line usually takes approximately 3 months to form. Other pigmentary changes also occur over a longer period of time. Marked retinal atrophy or thinned retina results from a long-standing retinal detachment. The longer the retina is detached, the more prone this retina is toward the development of intraretinal cysts and fixed retinal folds. Also it should be noted that shifting subretinal fluid indicates a retina that has been detached for a while with small breaks in that area of detached retina. Another sign of duration of the retinal detachment is the presence of intraretinal yellowish exudates. These exudates appear in an area of detached ret-

ina after a prolonged period. These yellowish intraretinal exudates disappear once the retina is reattached. Management of retinal detachment in all cases consists of an immediate retinology consultation.

A brief note should be made regarding nonrhegmatogenous retinal detachments. The nonrhegmatogenous retinal detachment, by definition, has no retinal break. This may occur overlying a choroidal tumor and often is a sign of a space-occupying lesion. Other nonrhegmatogenous retinal detachments include those associated with optic nerve head anomalies such as optic pits and/or colobomas and conditions such as idiopathic central serous choroidopathy. The underlying fluid in a

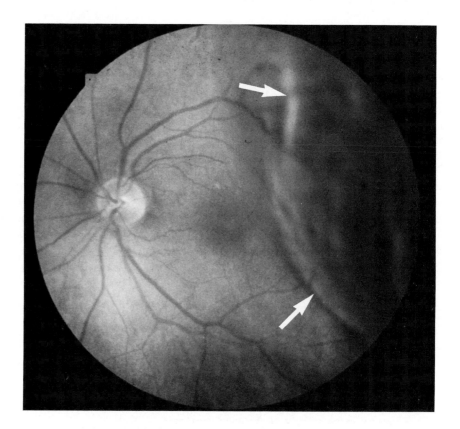

Figure 4–55. A fresh retinal detachment with the progressing border approaching the macula.

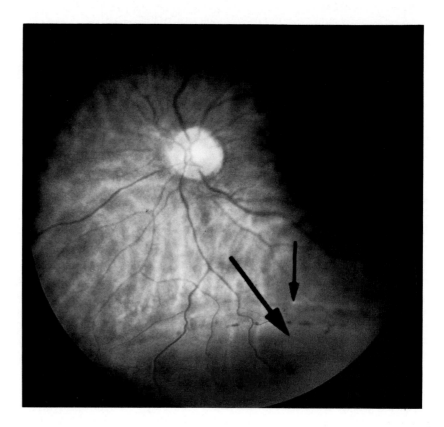

Figure 4–56. An old retinal detachment with dual(**arrows**)-pigmented demarcation lines.

TABLE 4–10. INDICATORS OF DURATION OF RETINAL DETACHMENT

1. Pigmented demarcation line—3 months
2. Taut surface and connective tissue on surface—long-standing
3. Balloons of subretinal fluid inferior—4 weeks in superior retina
4. Thinned retina—long-standing
5. Intraretinal cysts and fixed retinal folds—long-standing
6. Shifting subretinal fluid—long-standing with breaks in detached retina
7. Intraretinal exudates—long-standing

nonrhegmatogenous retinal detachment is very viscous. Therefore there are a minimum number of folds, and undulation on movement is minimal to absent. This make the makes the nonrhegmatogenous retinal detachment very difficult to discover on routine eye examinations.

Table 4–11 summarizes the major characteristics, prognoses, and management for all of the disorders discussed in this section.

RHEGMATOGENOUS RETINAL DETACHMENT—PEARLS

- Strong vitreoretinal adhesion in area of thin or weak retina allowing for a tear or hole, creating a tunnel for liquefied vitreous under the sensory retina
- Vitreous breaks mucopolysaccharide bonds liberating RPE and allowing for sensory retinal separation
- Key diagnostic sign is obscuration of underlying choroidal detail
- Must use indentation to discover shallow retinal detachment
- Appears as semitransparent undulating elevation when fresh
- Billowing folds of retina indicate a lot of subretinal fluid
- Management is a retinology consultation if fresh

Epilogue—Is Prophylactic Therapy the Answer to Prevention of Retinal Detachment?

Prophylactic therapy has long been a controversial issue. There were times in recent history when prophylactic therapy was applied to every lattice lesion. It is important to know whether or not prophylactic therapy is beneficial in our patient population.

The first question to ask is: Is prophylactic therapy harmless? There are complications associated with prophylactic therapy. Macular pucker (preretinal membranes) occurs in up to 3 percent of patients with prophylactic photocoagulation therapy and 1 to 2 percent of patients with prophylactic cryopexy therapy. Also it is important to realize that retinal detachment occurs anyway in 1.9 to 13.7 percent of eyes treated prophylactically. This significant range of complications is totally dependent upon the report cited.

The next question to ask is: "Is prophylactic therapy beneficial?" There has been no specific reduction in the incidence of retinal detachment reported with prophylactic therapy to lattice degeneration. There has, however, been a reduction in associated retinal detachment from 11 percent to 3 percent in prophylactically treated fellow eyes to retinal detachment. Prophylactic therapy of potentiators of detachment in fellow eyes to a retinal detachment is definitely indicated. It is proven that prophylactic therapy is beneficial in the treatment of symptomatic horseshoe retinal tears and operculated holes with continual vitreous traction. There is no statistical proof that asymptomatic breaks benefit from prophylactic therapy except, again, in fellow eyes to retinal detachment and aphakic eyes fellow to retinal detachment. Logic dictates that it is best to treat asymptomatic breaks prior to cataract surgery or in patients subject to repeated head trauma. Primary care involves diagnosis of the problem. When the question of therapeutic intervention becomes an issue, the retinologist should make the decision.

TABLE 4–11. THE RETINA BEYOND THE POSTERIOR POLE

	Primary Location Signs/Symptoms	Layers Involved	Prognosis	Management
Peripheral senile pigmentary degeneration	Ora to equator. Over age of 40 years. Granular pigment may be spicule; may cuff venules.	Choriocapillaris through sensory retina	No effect on vision	No treatment. Routine eye examinations
Primary chorioretinal atrophy	Usually inferior near ora; depigmented pale punched out areas that may coalesce	Choriocapillaris atrophy with overlying RPE and sensory loss	No effect on vision	No treatment. Routine eye examinations
Postinflammatory chorioretinal scar	Anywhere, any size; white to yellow areas (round or oval) with RPE reaction; may have overlying vitreous condensation	Choroid, choriocapillaris, RPE, retina, vitreous	Breaks may develop in areas of vitreoretinal traction. Toxoplasmosis may reactivate.	Educate regarding signs and symptoms retinal detachment or if toxoplasmosis, Recheck yearly.
Peripheral cystoid degeneration—typical	Usually within one half DD from ora; in all patients over 8 years; hazy grey band with enclosed hazy red dots	Cystoid changes in sensory retina	Benign but may form inner layer holes; possible precursor to RS	No treatment. Routine eye examinations
Peripheral cystoid degeneration—reticular	Usually posterior to but continuous with typical cystoid	Cystoid spaces in NFL that eventually extend to inner plexiform layer	Benign	Routine eye examinations
RPE window defect	Anywhere, any size; white to yellow; round, sharp-edged areas	RPE	Benign	Routine eye examinations
Congenital hypertrophy of RPE "Halo Nevus"	Anywhere, any size; dark grey to black; often with an area of depigmentation surrounding; chorioretinal atrophy within	RPE, choriocapillaris	Benign. May produce scotoma	Routine eye examinations
RPE Hyperplasia	Anywhere, any size; reaction to retinal insult	RPE	Benign	Routine eye examinations
Benign choroidal melanoma	Anywhere, usually under 5 DD; flat slate grey with indistinct margins; may have overlying drusen and/or serous detachment	RPE	Usually benign	Must follow at six-month intervals to establish no change
Malignant choroidal melanoma	Anywhere, usually over 5 DD; mottled, elevated whitish to grey-green mass; may have overlying lipofusin, retinal detachment, melanoma bodies	Originate in choroid but may extend to vitreous	Poor. Potential for metastasis	Cancer evaluation; irradiation; careful enucleation

Condition	Clinical appearance	Histology	Significance	Management
White without pressure	From the ora posterior to the equator; transluscent grey retinal tissue bounded posteriorly by a reddish-brown line; may occur near areas of retinal thinning (e.g., lattice)	NFL and sensory retina with unusual vitreoretinal adherence	White without pressure with lattice, scalloped borders, and PVD can lead to breaks	Follow yearly. Follow twice a year if threat of breaks. Signs/symptoms retinal detachment; retinology consult if breaks develop
Oral pearls	Single white spheres in oral area	RPE/Bruch's equivalent to retinal drusen	Benign	Routine eye examinations
Enclosed oral bay	Near ora—horizontal brownish depressions surrounded by sensory retina	Nonpigmented epithelium of pars surrounded by retina	15%–20% develop breaks	Routine eye examinations; yearly examinations if break occurs; signs/symptoms retinal detachment
Pars plana cysts	At ora; one fourth to 3 DD cysts that are oval to oblong	Separation of pigmented and nonpigmented epithelium of pars (schisis)	Benign	Routine eye examinations, patient education
Vitreoretinal tufts	Ora to equator; greyish-white tissue with vitreoretinal connection	Proliferated glial cells on top of retina	Usually benign but may cause tears with vitreal degeneration	Evaluate tufts. Regard other potentiators of retinal detachment. Signs/symptoms of retinal detachment; retinology consult if breaks develop
Meridional folds	At ora. Grey-white redundant tissue often with traction lines running posteriorly and anteriorly	Proliferated glial cells near ora	Usually benign but may be an associated retinal break secondary to traction	Follow at yearly intervals for signs of a break. Signs/symptoms retinal detachment; retinology consult for tears
Acquired RS	Flat or bullous, with ballooning anterior to equator that does not undulate with eye movement; often snowflakes on surface; which is honeycomb; may have inner holes (oval white) or outer holes (pink with rolled edges)	Splitting of sensory retina at outer plexiform/inner nuclear layer; cavity filled with hyaluronic acid	25% have breaks with 40% in both eyes; possible progression to posterior pole; rare development of progressive detachment	1. RS without breaks—see semiannually 2. RS with progression—retinology consult 3. RS with inner breaks—see semiannually 4. RS with outer breaks—retinology consult 5. RS with retinal detachment—retinology consult 6 Signs/symptoms RD
Snowflake vitreoretinal degeneration	Ora to equator; yellow-white dots in oval patches in white without pressure; sheathing of vessels, pigment, and early cataracts	Inner retinal layers	Possible breaks and retinal detachment	Retinology consult at signs of breaks; Signs/symptoms RD

continued

TABLE 4–11. THE RETINA BEYOND THE POSTERIOR POLE (cont.)

	Primary Location Signs/Symptoms	Layers Involved	Prognosis	Management
Lattice degeneration (snail track similar without fishbone vessels)	Ora to equator—wider toward equator; an oval area of retinal atrophy often surrounded by white without pressure with an overlying lacuna of liquefied vitreous; often RPE hyperplasia, yellow flecks, sclerosed vessels, and atrophic holes	Loss of inner retinal layers down to ONL; vitreal liquefaction	Atrophic holes—18% to 30%; retinal detachment—0.3% to 0.5%; retinal detachment from atrophic hole—3% to 14%; retinal tears at edge—1.4%	1. Lattice only—yearly examination 2. Symptomatic lattice—six-month examination 3. Lattice with holes—six-month examination 4. Lattice with risk factors or signs of progression—retinology consult 5. Signs/symptoms of retinal detachment
Atrophic retinal holes	Ora to equator in many atrophic retinal conditions. Round red lesion with surrounding cuff of edema. Pigment surround may occur	A full-thickness retinal break	7% chance of RD	1. Isolated asymptomatic—yearly examination 2. Isolated with edema cuff of 1 DD—six-month examination 3. Isolated with edema cuff > 1 DD—retinology consult 4. Symptomatic or risk factors—retinology consult 5. With flap—retinology consult 6. Signs/symptoms of retinal detachment
Operculated retinal hole	Equator to ora; round, red holes with overlying plug of retinal tissue; may be associated bleed; may have localized white without pressure and/or retinal detachment	Full-thickness loss of retina from abnormal vitreoretinal adhesion	Usually benign except in high-risk eyes	1. Asymptomatic—yearly examination 2. Asymptomatic multiple—six-month examination 3. Symptomatic, aphakia, retinal detachment in fellow, vitreous traction around hole—retinology consult 4. Signs/symptoms of retinal detachment
Linear retinal tear	Red surrounded by atrophic grey retinal tissue; may be horseshoe-shaped with apex pointing posterior; may see vitreoretinal traction bands	Vitreoretinal adhesion tearing away sensory retina	30% chance of retinal detachment	Retinology consult
Retinal dialysis	At ora less than 90 degrees; Red tear at ora with atrophic retinal tissue posterior	Sensory retinal tear	Delayed or slowly progressing retinal detachment	Retinology consult

| Giant retinal tear | A retinal tear at the ora greater than 90 degrees. The retina folds over on itself because of continued traction—taco | Sensory retinal detachment with traction at rolled edge of tear | Invariable retinal detachment. Fellow eye potential: Giant tears—12.8% Tears—11.9% Holes—10.2% Retinal detachment—15.9% | Immediate retinology consult |

REFERENCES

Alexander LJ, Jones WL, Potter J: *Retina Retina Retina.* Primary Eye Care, Philadelphia, 1985.

Benson WE: *Retinal Detachment. Diagnosis and Management.* Hagerstown, Md, Harper and Row, 1980.

Benson WE, Morse PH, Nantawan P: Late complications following cryotherapy of lattice degeneration. *Am J Ophthalmol* 1977;84:514–516.

Benson WE: Prophylactic therapy of retinal breaks. *Surv Ophthalmol* 1977;22:41–47.

Byer NE: Changes in and prognosis of lattice degeneration of the retina. *Trans Am Acad Ophthalmol Otolaryngol* 1974;78:114–125.

Byer NE: Lattice degeneration of the retina. *Surv Ophthalmol* 1979;23:213–248.

Byer NE: Prognosis of asymptomatic retinal breaks. *Arch Ophthalmol* 1974;92:208–210.

Byer NE: The natural history of asymptomatic retinal breaks. *Ophthalmology* 1982;89:1033–1039.

Byer NE: Long-term natural history study of senile retinoschisis with implications for management. *Ophthalmology* 1986;93:1127–1137.

Colyear BH, Pischel DK: Clinical tears in the retina without detachment. *Am J Ophthalmol* 1956;41:773–792.

Cox MS, Schepens CL, Freeman HM: Traumatic retinal detachment due to ocular contusion. *Arch Ophthalmol* 1965;76:678–685.

Davidorf FH, Pajka JT, Makley TA, Kartha MA: Radiotherapy for choroidal melanoma. An 18-year experience with radon. *Arch Ophthalmol* 1987;105:352–355.

DeJuan E, McCuen BW, Machemer R: The use of retinal tacks in the repair of complicated retinal detachments. *Am J Ophthalmol* 1986;102:20–24.

Davis MD: Natural history of retinal breaks without detachment. *Arch Ophthalmol* 1974;92:183–194.

Dumas J, Schepens CL: Chorioretinal lesions predisposing to retinal breaks. *Am J Ophthalmol* 1966;61:620–630.

Eagling EM, Roper-Hall MJ: *Eye Injuries. An Illustrated Guide.* Philadelphia, Lippincott, 1986.

Foos RY: Senile retinoschisis. *Trans Am Acad Ophthalmol* 1970;74:33.

Freeman HM: Fellow eyes of giant retinal tears. *Trans Am Ophthalmol Soc* 1978;76:343–382.

Glaser BM: Treatment of giant retinal tears combined with proliferative vitreoretinopathy. *Ophthalmology* 1986;93:1193–1197.

Glaser BM, Cardin A, Biscoe B: Proliferative vitreoretinopathy. The mechanism of development of vitreoretinal traction. *Ophthalmology* 1987;94:327–337.

Haas BD, Jakobiec FA, Iwamoto T, et al: Diffuse choroidal melanoma in a child. A lesion extending the spectrum of melanocytic hamartomas. *Ophthalmology* 1986;93:1632–1638.

Hamilton AM, Taylor W: Significance of pigment granules in the vitreous. *Br J Ophthalmol* 1972;56:700–702.

Hanson A: Norrie's disease. *Am J Ophthalmol* 1968;66:306–332.

Hines JL, Jones WC: Peripheral microcystoid retinal degeneration and retinoschisis. *J Am Optom Assoc* 1982;53:541–545.

Hirokawa H, Takahashi M, Trempe CL: Vitreous changes in peripheral uveitis. *Arch Ophthalmol* 1985;103:1704–1707.

Hunter JE: Retinal white without pressure. Review and relative incidence. *Am J Optom Physiol Opt* 1982;59:293–296.

Jones WL, Reidy RW: *Atlas of the Peripheral Fundus.* Butterworth, Boston, 1985.

Kanski JJ: *Retinal Detachment. A Colour Manual of Diagnosis and Treatment.* Butterworths, Boston, 1986.

Mafee MF, Goldberg MF: Persistent hyperplastic primary vitreous (PHPV): role of computed tomography and magnetic resonance. *Radiol Clin North Am* 1987;25:683–692.

Merin S, Feilers, Hyams S, Ivry M: The fate of the fellow eye in retinal detachment. *Am J Ophthalmol* 1971;71:477–481.

Minardi JC, Bettencourt DE: Optometric diagnosis and management of lattice degeneration. *S J Optom* 1985;4:17–25.

Nagpal KC, Goldberg MF, Asdourian G, et al: Dark without-pressure fundus lesions. *Br J Ophthalmol* 1975;59:476–479.

O'Malley PO, Allen RA, Strattsma BR, O'Malley CC. Pavingstone degeneration of the retina. *Arch Ophthalmol* 1965;73:169–182.

Robertson DM, Norton EWD: Long-term follow-up of treated retinal breaks. *Am J Ophthalmol* 1973;75:395–404.

Rutnin U, Schepens CL: Fundus appearance in normal eyes. *Am J Ophthalmol* 1967;64:840–859, 1040–1062, 1063–1078.

Shulka M, Ahuja OP: Photopsia—due to retinal disease. *Ind J Ophthalmol* 1982;30:91–93.

Schepens CL: *Retinal Detachment and Allied Diseases.* Philadelphia, Saunders, 1983, vols 1 and 2.

Sigelman J: Vitreous base classification of retinal tears: Clinical application. *Surv Ophthalmol* 1980;25:59–74.

Sigelman J: *Retinal Diseases. Pathogenesis, Laser Therapy and Surgery.* Boston, Little, Brown, 1984.

Spalton DJ, Hitchings RA, Hunter PA: *Atlas of Clinical Ophthalmology.* London, Gower Publishing, 1984.

Spencer LM, Foos RY: Paravascular vitreo-retinal attachment: Role in retinal tears. *Arch Ophthalmol* 1970;84:557–564.

Straatsma BR, Zeegen PD, Foos RY, Feman SS, Lattice degeneration of the retina. *Am J Ophthalmol* 1974;77:619–649.

Tasman W, Shields JA: *Disorders of the Peripheral Fundus.* Hagerstown, MD, Harper and Row, 1980.

Transactions of the New Orleans Academy of Ophthalmology Symposium on Medical and Surgical Disease of the Retina and Vitreous. St. Louis, Mosby, 1985.

Watzke RC: The ophthalmoscopic sign of "white with pressure." *Arch Ophthalmol* 1961;66:812–823.

Zimmerman LE, Spence WH: The pathologic anatomy of retinoschisis with a report of two cases diagnosed clinically as malignant melanoma. *Arch Ophthalmol* 1960;63:10–19.

5

Hereditary Retinal—Choroidal Diseases

A CLINICAL GUIDE TO UNDERSTANDING VISUAL ELECTRODIAGNOSIS

In addition to standard differential diagnostic testing techniques such as visual acuities, visual fields, color vision testing, and objective observation technique, the clinician has visual electrodiagnosis to assist in differential diagnosis of hereditary retinal and choroidal diseases. Visual electrodiagnosis is a complex issue and is covered in great detail in several texts. The reader should refer to those texts for more detail. *This section is intended to briefly explain electrodiagnostic tests and to relate these tests to hereditary retinal and choroidal disease.* The intent is to sensitize the clinician to the indications for electrodiagnostic testing procedures and to provide the clinician with an understanding of the results and how the results apply to the patient.

The Electroretinogram

The electroretinogram (ERG) is a measurement of the electrical response of the eye to a flash of light. The test is nonspecific, as the stimulus is presented throughout the retina by ganzfeld illumination. In spite of nonspecificity, the ERG is of value in diagnosing ocular disease in which rods or cones are altered in a generalized fashion. The rod-cone dystrophy, retinitis pigmentosa, is the best example of a generalized disease process that affects the ERG.

The Test. The ERG is performed on a patient whose eyes have been maximally dilated. The patient must be light adapted for the photopic ERG and dark adapted for a scotopic ERG. A ground electrode (earclip) is attached to the earlobe that has been appropriately cleaned to enhance contact. A skin electrode is then attached to either the mastoid process or the forehead, after the area has been appropriately cleaned. The skin electrode is the reference against the potential created when the retina is stimulated by light. A contact lens electrode is then placed on the patient's anesthetized cornea, and the fellow eye is occluded. All of the electrode leads are then attached to a preamplifier, and the impedance of the system is checked. The patient then places the chin on a chin rest in a ganzfeld (hemispherical) bowl that assures uniform distribution of the light flash so that the retina is uniformly stimulated. Flashes of light are presented at specified intervals, and the system averages the eye's response, creating a waveform on the oscilloscope. This waveform and its alterations offer a means of analyzing components of retinal function. The ERG is then repeated on the fellow eye. After dark adaptation, the process is repreated to generate a scotopic ERG.

The Waveform. Figure 5–1 illustrates a typical waveform that is generated during an ERG. The figure legend describes the various components as well as which components are attributed to which retinal components. While variable and complex, the a-b amplitude is the most frequently measured component and is reduced in diseases such as rod-cone dystrophy.

One extremely useful variation of the ERG is the flicker ERG. The patient is set up in the same manner, and a flashing light of increasing frequency creates a measured response. The macular cones can respond to a flicker of around 30 Hz, while the peripheral rods and cones will cease to function at around 20 Hz. The flicker ERG will therefore be especially useful in patients suspected of having macular cone dysfunction.

The Electro-oculogram

The electro-oculogram (EOG) is a measure of the electrical potential generated by the retinal pigment epithelium (RPE/photoreceptor complex. The measure of this potential is achieved by setting up a

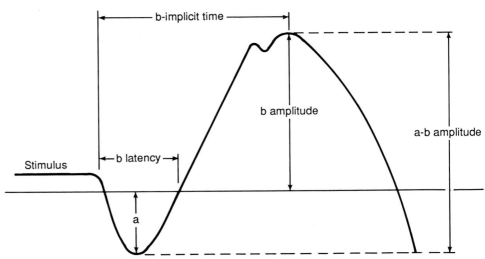

NOTE:
- a-b amplitude (major interest) is measured in uv.
- Average 80-150 uv photopic 300-500 uv scotopic with high intensity flash (photopic is usually 30% of scotopic).
- Average b implicit is 30 ms photopic and 50 ms scotopic.

WAVEFORM	RETINAL COMPONENT	ALTERED IN
Photopic A	Cones	Cone dystrophies
Scotopic A	Rods	Congenital stationary night blindness
Photopic B	Inner nuclear layer (cones)	
Scotopic B	Inner nuclear layer (rods)	
Flicker ERG	Macular cones	Cone dystrophies (macular degeneration)

Figure 5–1. The components of the photopic clinical ERG.

system to measure the electrical potential difference between the "voltage positive" cornea as it is related to the posterior pole. A comparison is then made between the potential difference in the dark and the potential difference in the light. If there is disease of the retinal pigment epithelium, this light peak-dark-trough ratio is reduced. The light rise in the potential is generated by light stimulation of the photoreceptor/RPE complex (ie, electrical activity is created by light). It is important to note, however, that midretinal layers must also be functioning properly.

The Test. It is not necessary that the patient be maximally dilated for the performance of an EOG. Electrodes must be placed on the medial and lateral canthi of the patient's eyes after the areas have been appropriately cleansed. An earclip electrode is then placed to serve as a ground. A correction may be worn if necessary. The electrode leads are then attached to a preamplifier and the impedance is checked. The patient then places the chin in the chin rest of the ganzfeld and is instructed to look from right to left as the targets alternate flashes.

The test takes approximately 30 minutes, including a brief training period. Recordings are typically made for about 15 seconds of each minute. The test is started with the lights on and is run for about 10 minutes. The lights are then turned off, and the test is run for 10 minutes in the dark. The lights are then turned on again, and the test is run for the final 10 minutes. The test generates light and dark amplitudes.

The Waveform. The ratio of the amplitudes is called the Arden ratio and is around 2/1 in normals and is less than 1.6/1 in abnormal conditions. Figure 5–2 illustrates a typical EOG waveform showing light and dark amplitudes. The EOG test will be altered in diseases such as vitelliform dystrophy and the latter stages of retinitis pigmentosa. The EOG is most specific for vitelliform dystrophy.

The Visually Evoked Cortical Potential

The visually evoked cortical potential (VECP, or VEP), also known as visually evoked response (VER), is a measure of the very small electrical potential at the visual cortex when the eye is stimulated by either flashes of light or more defined, alternating, checkerboard patterns on a television monitor at a fixed distance. When using the alternative checkerboard patterns at a fixed distance, an indirect measure of foveal acuity is being determined. The patient should always wear the best possible refraction for performance of this test.

Since the waveform is dependent on an intact visual pathway from the cornea to the cortex, it is possible that the waveform could be altered by dis-

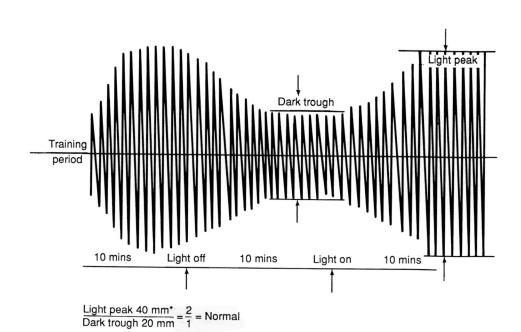

$$\frac{\text{Light peak 40 mm*}}{\text{Dark trough 20 mm}} = \frac{2}{1} = \text{Normal}$$

NOTE:
*Example only

Figure 5–2. The components of the clinical EOG.

ease anywhere in this pathway. The results are therefore nonspecific.

The Test. Initially a skin electrode (reference) is placed on the mastoid process or forehead, and a ground electrode is attached to the earlobe after the skin has been properly prepared. Another skin electrode is placed about 1 1/2 cm above the inion overlying the visual cortex. The electrode leads are then attached to the preamplifier, and the impedance of the system is checked. Most commercial systems are produced for neurology and will create an upside-down waveform unless the reference and active electrode leads are switched at the preamp. The patient then views a point on a television monitor from a fixed distance (1 m) with best corrected vision. The response to an alternating checkerboard pattern is then recorded according to the established protocol. It is often necessary to run through several alternative patterns to create a large enough summated waveform to be clinically useful. The amplitude of the waveform can be increased to a point by enlarging the size of the checkerboard squares.

The difficulty in measuring the VEP arises because the amplitude of the wave is so small, and it must be amplified by summation. The extraneous electrical noise from the brain and the environment must also be filtered to create a usable waveform.

The only way to overcome the problems of recording usable waveforms is the use of a computer system to selectively filter the noise and to summate the multiple waveform. Fortunately technology has decreased the cost and size of the equipment necessary to accomplish the job.

Another stimulus may be used in pediatric patients and in nonattentive or noncommunicative patients. A flash stimulus or a light emitting diode (LED) flash in goggles will create a waveform. The LED goggles may even be used with the eyes closed.

The Waveform. Figure 5–3 illustrates a typical VEP waveform. As with ERG and EOG, interpretation is subject to many factors. All of these tests are but a part of the diagnostic puzzle. It may be said that a reduction in amplitude indicates a reduction in acuity levels. This interpretation is not absolute, however, as there are reports of "normal" VEP patterns in patients who are legally blind. Interpretations and advice must be given with caution so as not to be misinterpreted. Interpretation of the implicit time is also of value, as delays indicate altered nerve fiber conductivity, as one would expect in cases of demyelinizing diseases. A change in target contrast, which decreases waveform amplitude, is also a sensitive test for eyes with nerve-fiber conduction defects.

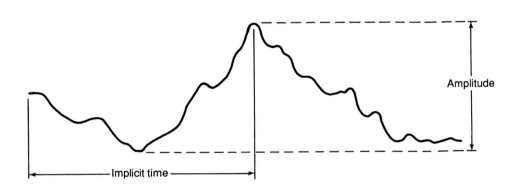

EXPECTEDS:

	TARGET/CHECK SIZE		
	7.5' arc	15' arc	30' arc
Implicit time	115 ms	100 ms	30 ms
Amplitude	5 uv	12 uv	10 uv

Figure 5–3. The components of the typical VECP waveform.

A CLINICAL GUIDE TO UNDERSTANDING GENETICS

The purpose of this section is to familiarize the clinician with inheritance patterns and application of these patterns to patient management. The topic of genetics is far too complex to address in a text about posterior segment disease, but it is hoped that armed with these basics, the clinician will at least be able to generate a pedigree and know when genetic counseling is necessary. Definition of basic terminology is necessary to the understanding of clinical genetics. Table 5–1 provides a *brief* definition of some of these terms.

Genetic disorders can be classified into three basic categories: single-gene disorders, chromosome disorders, and multifactorial disorders. Single-gene disorders are the result of mutations that may be on one or both pairs of chromosomes. The single-gene disorders occur at the frequency of 1 in 2,000. Chromosome disorders are due to excesses or deficiencies of chromosomes or segments of chromosomes. Down syndrome is an example of a chromosome disorder. The frequency of chromosome disorders is 7 in 1,000 live births and accounts for about 50 percent of first trimester abortions. Multifactorial disorders result from a combination of many small variations that together create a major defect. These disorders recur in families, but usually no specific pedigree pattern can be established.

Because of the complexity of hereditary retinal disease, the establishment of a good family history (pedigree) when considering specific conditions is crucial. The family history can assist in diagnosis. The pedigree can give *some* guidance as to whether the condition is genetic and can assist the clinician in educating the patient as to prognosis and as to the likelihood of passing the condition to future generations.

Generating a Pedigree

Generating a pedigree involves nothing more than establishing a very basic family tree to look for specific characteristics. A step-by-step procedure will be presented below to examine a hypothetical 38-year-old male complaining of night blindness of recent onset. Figure 5–4 defines the symbols that will be used in pedigree analysis.

TABLE 5–1. DEFINITIONS OF BASIC GENETIC TERMINOLOGY

Alleles—Alternate forms of a gene located at corresponding points on homologous chromosomes

Autosome—Any chromosome other than the sex (X or Y) chromosome. Man has 22 pairs of autosomes and one pair of sex chromosomes, or a diploid total of 46

Carrier—A phenotypically normal person who is heterozygous for a normal gene and an abnormal gene

Chromosome—A structure composed of DNA and protein located in the nucleus of all cells and that functions as the genetic blueprint of the person
- **Hemizygous**—A term that applies to the genes on the X chromosome in a male. Males have only one X; therefore males are hemizygous with respect to X-linked genes
- **Heterozygous**—A term that applies to an individual with two different alleles on corresponding points on homologous chromosomes, that is, one allele is normal
- **Homozygous**—A term that refers to an individual with identical alleles at corresponding loci on homologous chromosomes

Congenital—Present at birth, may or may not be genetically determined

Consanguinity—Mates being genetically related, literally by blood lines

Dominant(gene)—A gene that may produce an expression of its phenotype in a single dose

Expressivity—The degree to which a trait is manifested; may vary from mild to severe

Familial—Refers to any trait that is more commonly expressed in relatives of an affected individual than in the general population

Gene—A segment of a DNA molecule that codes the synthesis of a polypeptide chain or RNA molecule

Genotype—The genetic constitution; more specifically, the alleles present at one locus

Homologous chromosomes—A pair of chromosomes, one from each parent, having the same gene loci in the same order

Multiplex—Refers to a pedigree in which there is more than one case of a particular disease

Pedigree—A variety of a family tree established to study genetic characteristics

Penetrance—The frequency of expression of a gene or pair of genes

Phenotype—The physical expression of genetic characteristics (genotype)

Proband (propositus)—The index case if they are affected; the case from which the pedigree is generated

Recessive (gene)—A gene that is only expressed phenotypically if homozygous. Identical alleles must be present at the same loci

Sibs (siblings)—Brothers or sisters

Simplex—Refers to no known family history

Trait—A transmitted genetic condition

X-linked—Genes on the X-chromosome or traits determined by such genes

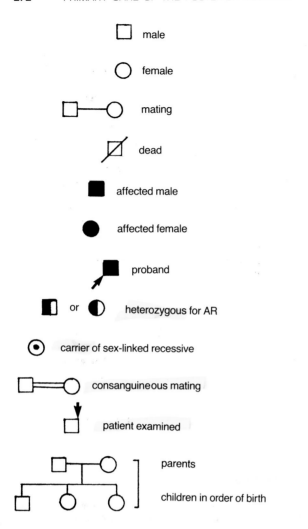

Figure 5–4. Standardized symbols used in the generation of a pedigree.

Step 1. Ask your patient with night blindness to list his brothers and sisters in descending order of birth and to state if any of them are affected with night blindness or if they are deceased. He has a sister, aged 57 years, who is night blind, a brother, aged 43 years, who is not night blind, and a sister who died at the age of 19 years in an automobile accident.

Draw:

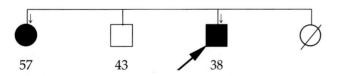

57   43   38

Step 2. Ask if parents or aunts or uncles were affected with night blindness, and draw them on the tree. The father is night blind, the mother is not. The paternal aunt is not

affected, and the maternal aunt and uncle are not affected.

Draw:

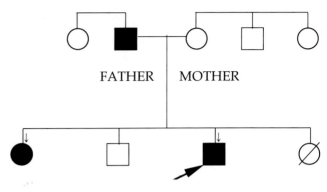

FATHER   MOTHER

Step 3. Ask if grandparents were affected with night blindness, and add them to the tree. The maternal grandparents were not night blind but are deceased. The paternal grandfather is not night blind, but the grandmother was night blind and is now deceased.

Draw:

   I. Grandparents
  II. Parents
 III. Siblings

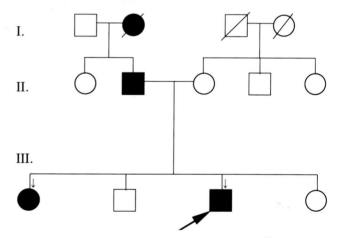

While simplistic, this exercise represents the basics for generating a pedigree. There are many variations that occur in a pedigree because of variability in phenotypic expression of the gene. Figures 5–5 through 5–8 and Table 5–2 represent the classical pedigree presentations that are encountered in hereditary ocular disease. When referring to these, the clinician should recall that variability of expression and spontaneous mutation can "break all the rules" in effective pedigree analysis. In fact, the rules are usually broken.

Characteristics

1. The trait appears in every generation. Exceptions arise because of mutations and/or variability of expression or penetrance.
2. The children of an affected person have a 50 percent risk of inheriting the trait.
3. Unaffected family members will not transmit the trait through family lines.
4. There is no sexual predilection for transfer of the trait; i.e., males and females are affected equally.

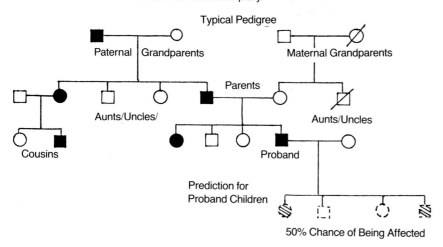

Figure 5–5. Characteristics of AD inheritance patterns.

Ocular Problems Suspected of AD Inheritance

Amyloidosis
Aniridia
Axenfeld Syndrome
Angiomatosis Retinae
CENTRAL AREOLAR CHOROIDAL DYSTROPHY
Corneal Dystrophies
CONE-ROD DYSTROPHIES

DOMINANT DRUSEN
Marfan Syndrome
Neurofibromatosis
NIGHT BLINDNESS (Congenital Stationary)
RETINOBLASTOMA
RETINITIS PIGMENTOSA
STARGARDT'S
VITELLIFORM DYSTROPHY

THE HEREDITARY RETINAL–CHOROIDAL DISEASES

Hereditary retinal–choroidal diseases will be grouped according to affected peripheral or night vision and affected central vision or color vision. This concept makes application of low-vision devices a bit easier to understand. There are cases where crossover occurs, such as macular involvement in retinitis pigmentosa. The descriptions will be clinical and truncated, as the complexity of each process exceeds the boundaries of primary care.

DISEASES AFFECTING PERIPHERAL OR NIGHT VISION

Retinitis Pigmentosa

Introduction. Retinitis pigmentosa (RP) (Fig. 5–9) is the most common of the hereditary retinal dystrophies. As with so many other ocular conditions,

the "itis" suffix is misleading, as inflammation is not a consideration in this condition. The incidence of RP varies with definition but is considered to occur between 1 per 2000 to 1 per 7000. RP appears to respect no racial boundaries but does occur slightly more frequently in males.

Heredity plays an important role in RP, but many epidemiological studies point to the difficulty of geneological analysis. Reports also suggest that the traditional definition of RP as consisting of a group of simple mendelian traits does not account for the true distribution of patients. Most clinicians do, however, continue to group RP patients into categories of autosomal recessive, autosomal dominant, and X-linked inheritance patterns. Unfortunately nature is not quite so simplistic, as over 50 percent of cases of RP are simplex (no family history) or are multiplex (affected siblings only). There is considerable disagreement regarding the sporadic appearance of RP, as many clinicians believe this to be a representation of the autosomal recessive form. The percentages of distribution of the

Characteristics
1. The phenotypic presentation occurs only in homozygotes who have received the recessive gene from both parents. Affected persons have carrier parents.
2. The trait characteristically appears (often unexpectedly) in siblings but not in the parents.
3. The risk of the trait occurring in the siblings of the proband is 1 in 4; that is, there is a 25 percent risk.
4. There is no sexual predilection for transfer of the trait; i.e., males and females are equally affected.
5. The parents of an affected child may be consanguineous; i.e., blood line relatives.

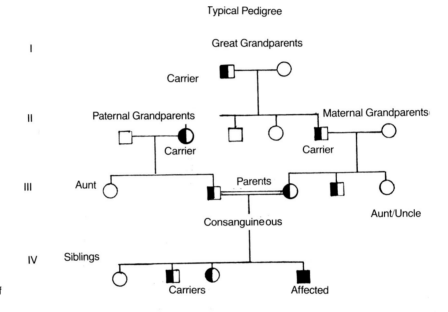

Figure 5–6. A. Characteristics of AR inheritance patterns.

various forms of RP hereditary patterns are useless, as there is tremendous variation reported in the literature. As a general rule, however, autosomal recessive forms are considered the most prevalent, followed by autosomal dominant and X-linked forms. There is also the suggestion that snowflake vitreo retinal degeneration is a variant of RP.

Appearance and Layers Involved. In general, hereditary dystrophies are secondary to defects in the genetic code that result in abnormal protein. It appears that the defect in RP is related to a disturbance in the disk membrane renewal process in the outer segments of the photoreceptor cells. The disk membranes are shed in the normal renewal process, and it is the responsibility of the RPE to mediate the disposal of the membranes. When this system is interrupted, the normal process is altered, allowing for accumulation of debris (lipofuscin) and alteration of photoreceptor function. There is also the occurrence of gliosis, neuronal loss, photoreceptor loss, choriocapillaris occlusion, and invasion of the retina to the internal limiting membrane by the RPE cells. Table 5–3 lists syndromes

associated with RP. It appears that in addition to creating dysfunction of the photoreceptors, the RPE alteration creates an alteration of the blood-retinal barrier leading to leakage and potential macular edema seen in the later stages of RP.

The ophthalmoscopic picture of RP is considered typical, but this author has observed many variations (Fig. 5–10). Among the first signs of RP is attenuation of the arterioles. Bone spicule pigmentation occurs in the midperiphery, presenting early as fine pigment mottling surrounded by moth-eaten areas of atrophy. As the disease progresses there is a clumping of pigment with an affinity for perivascular accumulation. (Note: Variations in presentation occur such as RP sine pigmento or without pigment.) **See color plate 75.** Also later in the process there is pallor of the nerve head secondary to poor vascular perfusion and gliosis and development of cystoid macular edema. The appearance of cystoid macular edema is thought to be as high as 70 percent.

Additional ocular findings in RP include disc drusen, cells in the vitreous accompanied by degeneration, posterior subcapsular cataracts (a high

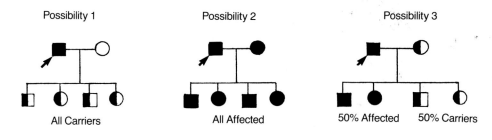

Predicting the Offspring of AR Affected

Possibility 1	Possibility 2	Possibility 3
All Carriers	All Affected	50% Affected 50% Carriers

All Unaffected

Ocular Problems Suspected of AR Inheritance

Choroidal Sclerosis	GYRATE ATROPHY
CONGENITAL CONE DYSFUNCTION	LAURENCE-MOON-BIEDL
CONE-ROD DYSTROPHY	Oguchi Disease
Corneal Dystrophy	RETINITIS PIGMENTOSA
FUNDUS FLAVIMACULATUS	STARGARDT'S
	USHER'S SYNDROME

Figure 5–6 (Continued). B. Predicting the offspring of AR affected and ocular problems suspected of AR inheritance.

percentage appearing in patients under the age of 40 years), tapetal macular reflex, and macular mottling and choroidal neovascularization.

Signs and Symptoms.
The most common initial symptom of RP is night blindness. The age of onset of night blindness, including age ranges, is summarized in Table 5–4. Associated with night blindness is difficulty with mobility secondary to peripheral vision loss. This is especially apparent as the environment darkens.

Visual field findings include midperipheral annular scotomas that enlarge to occupy the 10- to 40-degree meridians. Should the macula not become involved, a central 5 to 10-degree tubular field remains. Electrodiagnostic testing demonstrates variability with the hereditary "type" of RP but can be said to present an abnormal ERG and EOG. Dark adaptometry testing will as well demonstrate abnormalities.

In the later stages, fluorescein angiography will demonstrate areas of atrophy as well as an alteration of the blood retinal barrier in the form of cystoid macular edema. There is an association of RP to myopia, and X-linked carriers often have the presence of astigmatism over 1.50 diopters.

Prognosis and Management.
As with all hereditary dystrophies, the best management is genetic counseling to advise of the risk and to attempt to prevent the occurrence. Management of the symptoms is best achieved by low-vision consultation. Low-vision management has evolved to a very sophisticated level. Provision of infrared blocking-sun lenses is recommended.

One aspect of the disease, the appearance of cystoid macular edema, which is a direct threat to the remaining central vision, can be actively treated. It has been shown that grid photocoagulation can actually minimize the risk of severe vision loss over the short term in cystoid macular edema in RP. Laser is also of benefit when neovascularization complicates RP.

There has been some disagreement in the past regarding the advisability of cataract extraction in patients with RP. It has been shown, however, that cataract extraction or intraocular lens (IOL) implantation had no negative effects on prognosis when

Characteristics
1. Sex-linked inheritance may be related to X or Y but X-linked has the only clinical significance. The Y chromosome is essential for male sex determination.
   Male XY   Female XX
2. The incidence of the trait is higher in males than females.
3. The trait is never transmitted directly from father to son.
4. The trait is transmitted from an affected male through all his daughters (carriers) to 50 percent of their sons.
5. The trait may be transmitted through carrier females.
6. Carriers may show variable phenotypic expression of the trait.

Typical Pedigree X-Linked Recessive

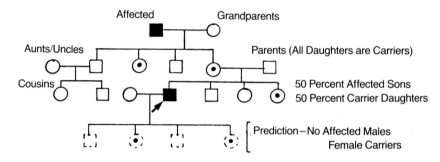

Figure 5–7. Characteristics of X-linked recessive inheritance patterns.

Ocular Problems Suspected of X-Linked Inheritance
OCULAR ALBINISM   RETINITIS PIGMENTOSA
Juvenile Retinoschisis   CONGENITAL CONE DYSFUNCTION

Characteristics
1. Affected males have no normal daughters.
2. Affected females are more common than affected males but they are heterozygous therefore have variable expression.
3. The trait is never transmitted directly from father to son.
4. Affected heterozygous females transmit the trait to 50 percent of children of either sex.
5. Affected homozygous females transmit the trait to all their children.
6. Heterozygous and homozygous females transmit the trait exactly like an autosomal dominant trait.
7. There are no "carriers."

Typical Pedigree–X-Linked Dominant

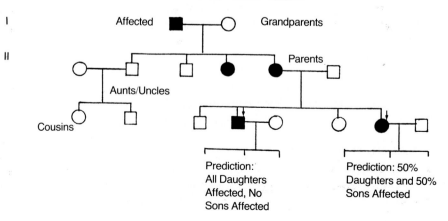

Figure 5–8. Characteristics of X-linked dominant inheritance patterns.

TABLE 5–2. EXPECTEDS ON X-LINKED RECESSIVE MATING

Mating Types	Phenotype Offspring
Normal male = normal female	All normal
Normal male = recessive heterozygous female	Daughters—50% normal 50% carriers
	Sons—50% normal 50% affected
Normal male = recessive homozygous female	Daughters—100% carriers
	Sons—100% affected
Affected male = normal female	Daughters—100% carriers
	Sons—100% normal
Affected Male = recessive heterozygous female	Daughters—50% normal 50% carriers
	Sons—50% normal 50% affected
Affected male = recessive homozygous female	All affected

performed skillfully. Unfortunately, predicting prognosis for patients is as difficult as all other aspects of RP.

It appears that the AD patients with RP maintain excellent vision until after childbearing years, with a slow visual deterioration after that. AR patients maintain reasonable vision until their 30s, and a few have significant early central loss. The X-linked patients usually present an early rapid loss of acuity. Simplex varieties of RP are characterized by unpredictability, but many have good vision past childbearing years. Night blindness and eventual severity of RP are not well correlated. Because of the relatively slow progression of the disease, the patients are often able to adapt well to their handicap as the disease progresses.

RETINITIS PIGMENTOSA—PEARLS

- Variable inheritance pattern: AR, AD, X-linked, simplex, multiplex
- Mean age of onset 9 to 19 years
- Disturbance in RPE metabolism
- Arteriolar attenuation, moth-eaten midperiphery, bone spicule accumulation, pallor of nerve head, cystoid macular edema
- Posterior subcapsular cataracts
- Night blindness, photophobia, restricted fields, abnormal electrodiagnosis
- Management
  - Possible grid macular photocoagulation
  - Pedigree analysis, rule out associated systemic diseases
  - Genetic counseling
  - Low-vision rehabilitation

Brief Notes About RP Variants

Retinitis Sine Pigmento

While often recognized as a distinct entity, retinitis pigmentosa sine pigmento is probably a variation of RP in which the alterations of the RPE are so

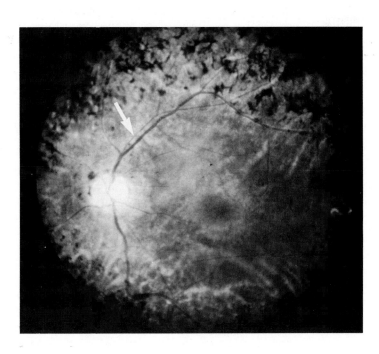

Figure 5–9. An example of bone-spicule pigment accumulation and arterial attenuation **(arrow)** in retinitis pigmentosa.

TABLE 5–3. SYNDROMES ASSOCIATED WITH RETINITIS PIGMENTOSA

Syndrome	Inheritance	Associated Findings
Usher's	AR, AD	Hearing loss
Hallgren's	AR	Ataxia, mental retardation, nystagmus, deafness
Refsum's	AR	Ataxia, polyneuropathy, deafness
Laurence-Moon-Bardet-Biedl	AR	Obesity, mental retardation, polydactyly, syndactyly, hypogenitalism
Pelizaeus-Merzbacher	X-linked, AR, AD	Head tremors, nystagmus, ataxia, mental retardation
Bassen-Kornzweig	AR	Celiac disease (diarrhea), spinocerebellar ataxia

Abbreviations: AR, autosomal recessive; AD, autosomal dominant.

subtle that they are clinically unrecognizable. This may actually just be an early stage in the full-blown development of RP, as longitudinal observations will often present development of the classical picture. The standard symptoms and clinical signs are present, with prognosis and management similar to RP.

Sector Retinitis Pigmentosa

See color plate 76.

Sector RP is a variant of RP that is usually bilateral and symmetrical, involving both inferior quadrants. The remainder of the retina appears normal but actually has RPE changes demonstrable with fluorescein angiography and threshold field testing. Vessels are attenuated in the affected area. The ERG is usually subnormal but not as altered as the ERG in circumferential RP. Progression of sector RP is slow, with function remaining intact until the ages of 50 to 60 years. Sector RP has been reported as AR and AD. Retinal trauma and inflammation

can mimic sector RP because of reactive RPE hyperplasia occurring in the affected areas (Fig. 5–11).

Unilateral Retinitis Pigmentosa

Unilateral retinitis pigmentosa is probably extremely rare. The appearance usually is a manifestation of trauma or inflammation. When there is a bona fide case of unilateral RP, the patient is often asymptomatic until the macula becomes involved. Prognosis is similar to bilateral RP, but management problems are minimized. Genetic counseling is necessary.

Inverse Retinitis Pigmentosa

See color plate 76.

Inverse RP (Fig. 5–12) is thought to occur in an AR inheritance pattern. Inverse or central RP is manifested by clumped pigmentary changes around the macular area rather than the periphery. Visual function is compromised, as it is in typical RP, with central vision loss often the result. Vessel attenuation (VA) and disc pallor occur. Choroidal atrophy occurs and is obvious on fluorescein angiography. Color vision loss and central scotomas are the rule, and the ERG photopic wave is altered. Prognosis is poor because of severe central vision loss. Effective treatment modalities are currently unavailable. Pedigree generation and genetic counseling are absolutely necessary.

Leber's Congenital Amaurosis (Congenital Pigmentary Dystrophy)

Leber's congenital amaurosis is a cause of blindness in the first year of life. The condition is usually AR. The child presents with reduced vision, searching nystagmus, and, at times, photophobia in the first year. The patient also has a tendency to poke at his eyes (digito-ocular sign). The patient of-

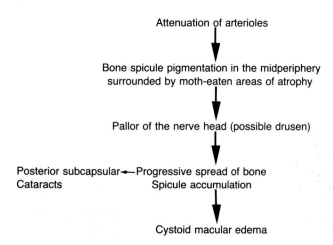

Figure 5–10. A flow chart illustrating the ocular changes associated with retinitis pigmentosa.

TABLE 5–4. APPROXIMATE AGE OF ONSET FOR VARIOUS HEREDITARY FORMS OF RETINITIS PIGMENTOSA

	Autosomal Recessive	Autosomal Dominant	X-linked	Simplex	Multiplex
Mean age of onset	16 yr	19 yr	9 yr	20 yr	16 yr
Range in years	0–54 yr	0–57 yr	3–18 yr	0–71 yr	0–67 yr
95% symptomatic by age	40 yr	50 yr	18 yr		

ten has accompanying neurological disorders, mental retardation, and other ocular findings. Pupils are poorly reactive, and the retina may appear as classic RP with optic atrophy. The ERG is either minimally present or nonrecordable in the patient. Prognosis is poor. Pedigree analysis and genetic counseling are crucial.

Retinitis Punctata Albescens

Progressive-Type Albipunctate Dystrophy

Progressive albipunctate dystrophy presents as discrete whitish dots deep in the retina that do not progress to confluence. They are spread throughout the retina but are concentrated near the posterior pole. RPE hyperplasia may accompany the dots, as may disc pallor and vessel attenuation. The clinical signs and symptoms are similar to RP, but progress is slower, with maintenance of good vision into and beyond the fifth decade. Pedigree analysis and genetic counseling are important. Progressive albipunctate dystrophy is usually AR.

Stationary-Type Fundus Albipunctatus Degeneration

Fundus albipunctatus degeneration presents as dull white dots scattered throughout the retina but concentrated in the midperiphery and perimacular zone. Vessels are not attenuated, and the optic disc is normal. Nonprogressive night blindness is characteristic, and vision is usually excellent. These patients often have alterations in dark adaptation and abnormal ERGs. Pedigree analysis and genetic counseling are indicated. Fundus albipunctatus degeneration is usually AR **(See Table 5–5).**

Congenital Stationary Night Blindness

Introduction. Congenital stationary night blindness (CSNB) may be transmitted in AR, AD, or X-linked forms. CSNB is characterized by night blindness, mild acuity reduction, and a normal retina. As the name implies, the night blindness, while severe at times, is stationary.

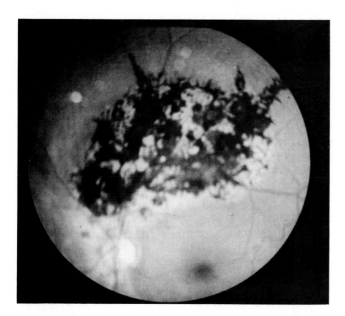

Figure 5–11. An example of a misdiagnosis of sector retinitis pigmentosa. This is an example of reactive RPE hyperplasia secondary to trauma.

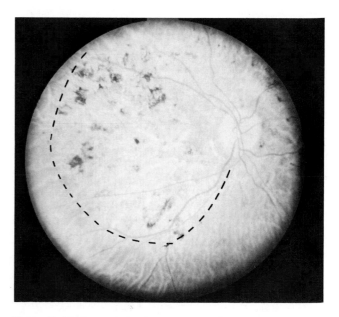

Figure 5–12. An example of inverse or central retinitis pigmentosa. The dotted line outlines the RPE clumping in the macular area.

TABLE 5–5. COMPARISON OF HEREDITARY WHITE-DOTS-IN-THE-RETINA SYNDROMES

	Heredity	Symptoms	Fundus Picture	ERG	EOG	Progression/Final Visual Acuity
Progressive albipunctate dystrophy (RP-like)	AR	Night blindness, field constriction	Small white dots concentrated in posterior pole but also into periphery, nonconfluent	Abnormal	Abnormal	Maintains visual acuity until fifth decade, but is slowly progressive
Fundus albipunctatus degeneration	AR	Night blindness	Dull white dots concentrated in midperiphery and perimacular zone	Normal to abnormal	Normal to abnormal	Nonprogressive with good final visual acuity
Dominant drusen	AD	Metamorphopsia and decreased central vision	White dots in or near macula that increase in size and become confluent, leading to a macular plaque or wet maculopathy	Normal to abnormal	Abnormal in late stages	Progressive, leading to variable acuity reduction
Fundus flavimaculatus	AR	None to mild vision reduction	Yellow-white fish-tail flecks in posterior pole; progression toward macula	Normal to abnormal	Normal to abnormal	Mild progression, but macula may become atrophic
Stargardt's	AR	Vision loss, color vision loss	Slimed oval macular zone leading to beaten bronze; surround of fundus flavimaculatus	Normal to abnormal	Normal to abnormal	Severe progression

AR, autosomal recessive; AD, autosomal dominant

Appearance and Layers Involved. The retina appears essentially normal, but the macular reflex is lost when the vision is reduced. It has been proposed that the defect involves the light-activated enzymatic processes involved in normal rod functioning or a defect in the synaptic transfer of the message.

Signs and Symptoms. Night blindness is the primary symptom. When AR or X-linked, vision may be reduced to 20/30 to 20/50. Nystagmus and severely reduced acuity may also present. Myopia is omnipresent in AR and X-linked forms. There appear to be two distinctive patient responses to electrodiagnostic testing. In one form there is a markedly reduced-to-absent rod response in scotopic conditions, abnormal photopic findings during ERG, and an abnormal EOG. In another form there is a normal scotopic a-wave and a severely reduced b-wave, while the photopic ERG is normal and the EOG is normal. Color vision is usually normal, and visual fields are constricted in mesopic conditions. Dark adaptation is also affected.

Prognosis and Management. CSNB is considered to be a stationary condition. In the AR and X-linked forms, central vision may be affected but not severely reduced. Pedigree analysis and genetic counseling are important in CSNB. Support through low-vision consultion is important when indicated.

CONGENITAL STATIONARY NIGHT BLINDNESS—PEARLS

- Variable inheritance pattern: AR, AD, X-linked
- Normal-appearing retina but loss of foveal reflex
- Night blindness, possible mild vision reduction, possible nystagmus
- Variable electrodiagnostic findings, field constriction in low light
- Management
  - Pedigree analysis
  - Genetic counseling
  - Low-vision rehabilitation when necessary

A Variant of CSNB— Oguchi's Disease

Oguchi's disease is a variety of CSNB associated with discoloration of the retina that is reversed to normalcy by 2 to 3 hours of dark adaptation (Mizuo's sign). Under light adaptation the retina has a yellow-grey tint that may extend to the equator. Retinal and choroidal vessels are difficult to differentiate, as their color is altered. Clinical findings are similar to CSNB, with only mild reduction of

acuity (20/40) likely. Fluorescein angiography demonstrates hyperfluorescence under light adaptation. The condition appears to be secondary to structural alterations between the retina and RPE and within the outer segments of the rods and cones. The condition is inherited in an AR fashion, with consanguinity common. Genetic counseling is in order.

Choroideremia

Introduction. Choroideremia (Figs. 5–13 and 5–14) is an X-linked recessive dystrophy with initial symptoms of night blindness presenting in the first to second decades. This disease is usually manifest as diffuse atrophy of the entire choroid and RPE in males and as aborted atrophy that is usually stationary in female carriers.

Appearance and Layers Involved. See color Plate 77. The first changes in the fundus consist of fine RPE stippling in the midperiphery in the affected male. The RPE disorganization then spreads in both directions, with the oldest areas developing choriocapillaris and choroidal atrophy. Eventually bare sclera shows through and simulates gyrate atrophy. In the later stages optic atrophy and vessel attenuation may occur. Female carriers will often show areas of RPE disorganization in the midperiphery and at times in the macular area.

While genetic mapping has been accomplished, the underlying biochemical/structural retinal choridal alteration has not been elucidated.

Signs and Symptoms. In the first to second decades the affected male patient presents with night blindness and peripheral field constrictions. The erosion of the visual field progresses through life with central vision often affected by ages 50 to 60 years. As in other progressive choroidal dystrophies, visual fields, electrodiagnostic testing, and dark adaptometry are altered.

Prognosis and Management. Prognosis for males affected with choroideremia is grim. Loss of central vision is almost inevitable in later life. Female carriers have an excellent prognosis.

Fortunately, affected males have a slow progression of choroideremia and as such are usually prepared for the loss of central vision. Rehabilitation with low-vision aids is difficult at this stage, as central and peripheral vision are compromised. Genetic counseling after pedigree generation is imperative, as prevention is the only known cure.

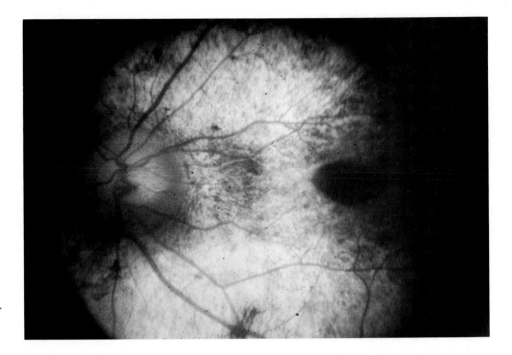

Figure 5–13. A photograph illustrating the devastation of choroidal structure in choroideremia.

CHOROIDEREMIA—PEARLS

- Inherited as X-linked
- Starts as RPE stippling in midperiphery followed by choriocapillaris/choroidal atrophy in these areas, which spreads
- May have macular atrophy
- Night blind, field constriction, loss of central vision, altered electrodiagnosis
- Management
  - Pedigree analysis
  - Genetic counseling
  - Low-vision rehabilitation

Gyrate Dystrophy of the Choroid and Retina

Introduction. Gyrate dystrophy of the choroid and retina (Figs. 5–15 and 5–16) is an autosomal recessive, progressive dystrophy usually associated with hyperornithinemia and deficient ornithine ketoacid aminotransferase activity. The enzyme levels in affected individuals are very low to absent and are reduced in carriers. This association is not absolute but is typical. Serum lysine levels are usually low. Plasma ornithine levels are often 10 to 20 times elevated over normal levels. Age of onset is typically 15 to 45 years.

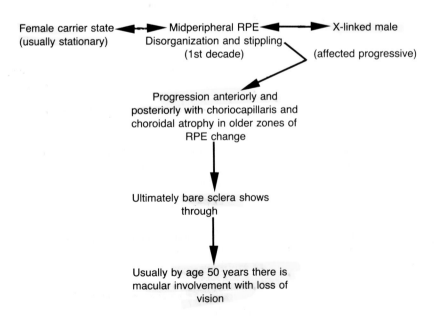

Female carrier state ←→ Midperipheral RPE ←→ X-linked male
(usually stationary)   Disorganization and stippling   (affected progressive)
                              (1st decade)

Progression anteriorly and posteriorly with choriocapillaris and choroidal atrophy in older zones of RPE change

Ultimately bare sclera shows through

Usually by age 50 years there is macular involvement with loss of vision

Figure 5–14. A flow chart depicting the ocular changes associated with the progression of choroideremia.

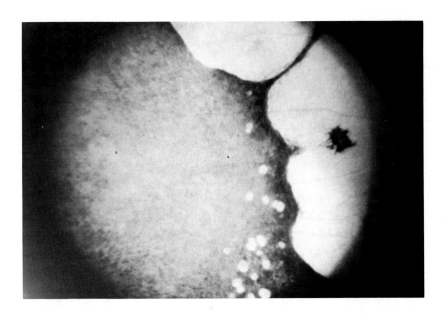

Figure 5–15. A photograph illustrating the destruction of the RPE and choroid with scalloped borders associated with gyrate dystrophy. (Photo courtesy of R. Nowakowski.)

Appearance and Layers Involved. **See color plate 77.** Initial fundus changes occur in the midperiphery in patients with gyrate dystrophy. There is atrophy of the RPE and choroid with bare sclera showing through. The areas of atrophy coalesce and assume scalloped borders. The RPE clumps, and the borders progress posteriorly. At times, central zones of atrophy may develop and expand to meet the peripheral zone. The transition between the atrophic zones and the normal islands of retina are abrupt, contrasting with the appearance of choroideremia. Late in the disease, optic atrophy and vessel attenuation occur.

Signs and Symptoms. Myopia is present in 80 percent to 100 percent of cases of gyrate dystrophy in the first decade, with night blindness occurring with the presentation of midperipheral RPE changes in the second decade. Peripheral field loss occurs with progression of atrophy. Posterior subcapsular cataracts occur in about 40 percent of cases, requiring extraction by the third to fourth

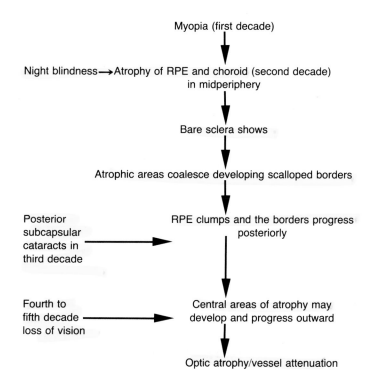

Myopia (first decade)

Night blindness → Atrophy of RPE and choroid (second decade) in midperiphery

Bare sclera shows

Atrophic areas coalesce developing scalloped borders

Posterior subcapsular cataracts in third decade → RPE clumps and the borders progress posteriorly

Fourth to fifth decade loss of vision → Central areas of atrophy may develop and progress outward

Optic atrophy/vessel attenuation

Figure 5–16. A flow chart illustrating the progression of ocular changes associated with gyrate dystrophy.

TABLE 5–6. HEREDITARY RETINAL/CHOROIDAL DISEASE PRIMARILY AFFECTING PERIPHERAL AND NIGHT VISION

	Heredity	Mean Age Onset	Progressive/ Stationary	Signs/ Symptoms	ERG	EOG	Fundus Appearance	Visual Fields
RP	AR, AD, X-linked, simplex, multiplex	9–19 years	Progressive but variable	Night blind, restricted fields, loss of central vision possible, photophobia	Abnormal	Abnormal	Attenuation of arterioles, midperipheral moth-eaten appearance, midperipheral bone spicules, disc pallor, cystoid macular edema (variations exist)	Spreading ring scotomas from 30°–50°
CSNB	AR, AD, X-linked	Congenital	Stationary	Night blind, possible mild vision reduction, possible nystagmus	Variable but often abnormal	Variable but often abnormal	Normal, but may have loss of foveal reflex	Constricted in mesopic conditions
Choroideremia	X-linked males	First to second decade	Slowly progressive	Night blind, eventual loss of central vision	Altered	Altered	RPE stippling in midperiphery spreading, eventual choriocapillaris/ choroid atrophy in areas of stippling, macular atrophy	Peripheral field constriction
Gyrate dystrophy	AR	First to second decade	Progressive	Night blind, loss of central vision, myopia	Abnormal	Abnormal	RPE atrophy and choroidal atrophy in midperiphery with scalloped borders progressing anteriorly and posteriorly, possible central atrophy	Peripheral field constriction

AR, autosomal recessive; AD, autosomal dominant

decade. Electrodiagnostic testing and dark adaptometry show abnormalities consistent with degree of destruction. Neurological signs may occur in the form of seizure disorders.

Prognosis and Management. Macular changes result in loss of central vision in the fourth to fifth decade. Since gyrate dystrophy is related to accumulation of serum ornithine levels, it is thought that reductions in these levels may positively affect outcome. These levels can be modified by diet. Arginine-deficient diets may reduce serum ornithine levels. Oral pyridoxine (vitamine B_6) may also reduce serum ornithine levels. There is some evidence that if serum ornithine levels are maintained between 55 and 355 μM, that the dystrophy does not progress as fast but will not regress. Genetic counseling is mandatory in cases of gyrate dystrophy. Vision rehabilitation is difficult once central vision is compromised.

Table 5–6 summarizes the characteristics of hereditary choroidal/retinal disease primarily affecting peripheral and night vision.

GYRATE DYSTROPHY—PEARLS

- Inherited as AR
- Starts as RPE atrophy and choroidal atrophy in mid-periphery, with scalloped borders progressing inward and outward
- Development of central zones of atrophy
- Myopia
- Night blindness, loss of central vision, field constriction
- Management
    - Diet Modification?
    - Pedigree analysis
    - Genetic counseling
    - Low-vision rehabilitation?

DISEASES AFFECTING CENTRAL VISION AND AFFECTED COLOR VISION

Stargardt's Disease and Fundus Flavimaculatus (FF)

Introduction. Stargardt's disease (Figs. 5–17 through 5–21) is the name applied to fundus flavimaculatus when atrophic macular lesions occur early in life along with the yellow flecks of fundus flavimaculatus. Most cases of Stargardt's are considered to be AR, although dominant cases have

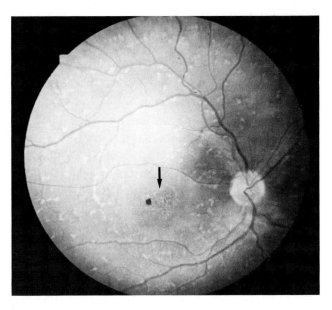

Figure 5–17. A patient with the characteristic fish-tail flecks of fundus flavimaculatus surrounding the early macular changes **(arrow)** of Stargardt's disease.

been reported. The yellowish white flecks of isolated fundus flavimaculatus start to appear in the first to second decades and progress toward the macula, creating mild vision reduction. Should the macula then become atrophic, severe loss of vision occurs. **See color plates 78 through 81.**

Appearance and Layers Involved. In the initial stages of Stargardt's there are minimal fundus changes, in spite of vision reduction. The first fun-

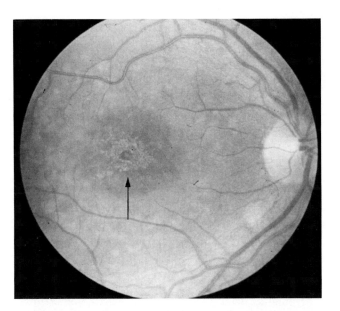

Figure 5–18. A patient with mild fundus flavimaculatus changes surrounding the pigmentary changes in the macula **(arrow)** in Stargardt's disease.

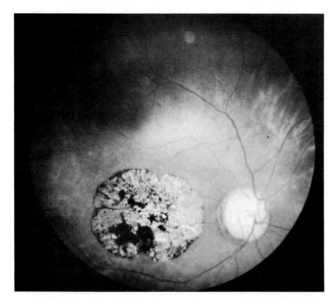

Figure 5–19. An illustration of severe atrophy of the macular area in Stargardt's disease with minimal fundus flavimaculatus changes.

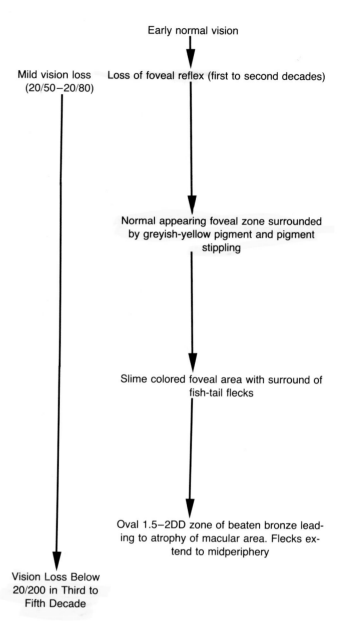

Figure 5–21. A flow chart illustrating the progression of Stargardt's disease and fundus flavimaculatus.

dus sign is loss of the foveal reflex. This progresses to an area of normal-appearing central retina surrounded by a zone of greyish yellow depigmentation and pigment stippling. The foveal area then progresses to develop a slime-covered appearance with yellow flecks (called pisciform or fish tail) developing deep in the retina peripheral to the macula. Eventually a horizontal oval area (2 disc diameters (DD) by 1.5 DD) of atrophic RPE appears as "beaten bronze" or metallic in nature, with a surround of flecks. As the lesion continues to develop,

further atrophy of the macular area occurs, and the flecks extend to the midperiphery. It is of interest that the flecks may precede the macular atrophy, may be coincident with the macular atrophy, or may follow the macular atrophy. From a clinicopathological standpoint, there is an enlargement of RPE cells in the zones of the flecks and a total disappearance of the cones, rods, and RPE cells in the circumfoveal zone.

Signs and Symptoms. With Stargardt's, decreased vision usually presents in the first to second decades in a patient with prior normal vision. The condition may be mistaken for a conversion re-

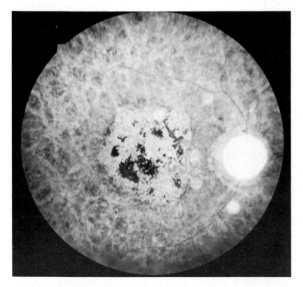

Figure 5–20. Severe macular atrophic changes surrounded by significant RPE changes associated with fundus flavimaculatus.

action. Photophobia may be an early complaint. As the condition progresses, vision drops significantly.

Color vision defects present early because of cone loss but are usually not as severe as those in cone dystrophy. Fluorescein angiography will demonstrate hypofluorescence in "young" flecks, but hyperfluorescence is the rule as atrophy progresses. The ERG is usually normal to slightly abnormal, and the EOG is variable, depending on the extent of fleck formation resulting from RPE disease. Visual fields demonstrate central scotoma.

Prognosis and Management. Alone, fundus flavimaculatus creates a reduction in acuity to the 20/50 to 20/80 zone, but macular involvement results in vision below 20/200. The probability of maintaining vision of 20/40 in at least one eye in Stargardt's is over 50 percent by the age of 19 years, over 30 percent by the age of 29 years, and over 20 percent by the age of 39 years. Once acuity drops below 20/40, it appears that vision then deteriorates rapidly to 20/200. Low-vision rehabilitation can offer help to the patient with Stargardt's, and genetic counseling is an absolute necessity.

STARGARDT'S/FUNDUS FLAVIMACULATUS

- Inherited as AR
- Starts as loss of foveal reflex, then zone of normal retina at macula surrounded by RPE changes
- Fovea then becomes slimed, leading to 2 DD oval beaten-bronze zone
- Fundus flavimaculatus surrounds macular area
- Color vision loss, vision loss, central scotoma, normal to abnormal electrodiagnosis
- Management
    - Pedigree analysis
    - Genetic counseling
    - Low vision

Patterned Anomalies of the RPE

Introduction. Patterned anomalies of the RPE are probably dystrophies, but there is controversy as to the exact etiology. These anomalies appear as variations of three entities: (1) Sjögren's reticular pigment epithelial dystrophy, (2) macroreticular pattern dystrophy, and (3) butterfly dystrophy. These dystrophies affect the macular area and are usually inherited in an AD pattern. The onset of signs is usually in the first to third decades. The signs are usually bilateral and somewhat symmetrical.

Appearance and Layers Involved. See color plate 82. In the reticular form of patterned anomalies of the macula, pigmented lines form that radiate from the fovea. This may be preceded by fine granular pigment dispersed in the macular area. The lines join to form a "fishnet" appearance with "knots" at overlap points. The fishnet extends to the equator. In the butterfly form (Fig. 5–22), the pigmentary changes are more solid and appear as butterfly wings or as an iron cross overlying the macula. The macroreticular form is a variation of the fishnet form. The remainder of the retina usually appears normal.

Many variations of the dystrophies exist. The diagnosis is made by establishing a pedigree. Different members in the pedigree may present totally different fundus pictures. Patients have minimal acuity loss in most cases in spite of a dramatic macular picture.

One case has been reported in which the patient had butterfly dystrophy in one eye and vitelliform in the other, suggesting a common etiopathogenesis.

Signs and Symptoms. Symptoms usually do not match the appearance of the macula. Visual acuity is usually in the 20/20 to 20/50 range, while scant reports show visual reduction to be severe. Color vision and central scotomas are consistent with acuity reduction. Fluorescein angiography demonstrates hypofluorescence in areas of increased pigmentation and hyperfluorescence in areas of RPE atrophy. The ERG is normal, but the EOG is variable, depending on RPE dysfunction.

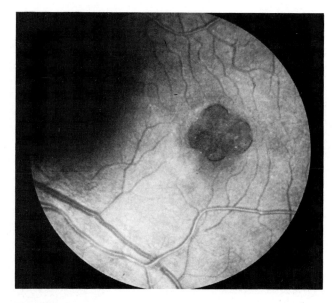

Figure 5–22. An example of a patterned anomaly of the RPE. The shape is often in the form of butterfly wings or an iron cross.

Prognosis and Management. Prognosis is good, with most cases having vision loss limited to the 20/50 level. The best refraction should be provided, and genetic counseling is advised. In cases with associated late-stage atrophic stages, vision may be reduced, necessitating low-vision rehabilitation.

PATTERNED DYSTROPHIES—PEARLS

- Inherited as autosomal dominant
- Reticular, macroreticular, butterfly types—bilateral and symmetrical
- Reticular—fishnet of pigment with knots at crossings to equator
- Butterfly—solid RPE changes at macula as butterfly wings
- Mild reduction in acuity usually, but may be severe
- Management
  - Pedigree analysis
  - Genetic counseling
  - Provision of best possible prescription

Vitelliform Dystrophy (Best's Disease)

Introduction. Vitelliform dystrophy is an inherited macular disorder characterized by an early onset "egg yolk" appearance in the macula (Figs. 5–23 through 5–25). Vitelliform dystrophy is considered to be autosomal dominant, with variable penetrance and variable expressivity. Heterozygous carriers (no penetrance) can be detected by an abnormal EOG. Presentation of the lesion is usually between the ages of 4 years to 10 years, with minimal reduction in acuity initially.

Appearance and Layers Involved. **See color plate 83.** Stages of progression characterize the fundus appearance of vitelliform dystrophy. Even before there is any fundus change, an abnormal EOG may be recorded. The disease is usually bilateral, but there is often asymmetry. The classically described "egg yolk" (Fig. 5–23) usually appears between the ages of 4 years and 10 years. The "egg yolk" is a yellow mound surrounded by a darker border and is thought to be the result of an abnormal accumulation of materials in the RPE cells. The vitelliform lesion is usually centered on the fovea and is often one half to 5 DD in size. Variations of centricity will occur. Tremendous variation occurs in the actual presentation of the yellow deposits and can make recognition difficult. The "egg yolk" often remains stable for years with only a mild reduction in visual acuity (20/30 to 20/50). With age the yolk may disappear only to reappear. The yolk material may also disintegrate, leaving a "scrambled egg" appearance (Fig. 5–24). Leakage, rupture, or hemorrhage may occur, resulting in vision loss. The cyst may also liquefy at the later stage, resulting in a layering effect within the cyst, giving what is described as the pseudohypopyon stage. With rupture of the "egg yolk" cyst, there is retinal infiltration and scarring, resulting in vision reduction below 20/100.

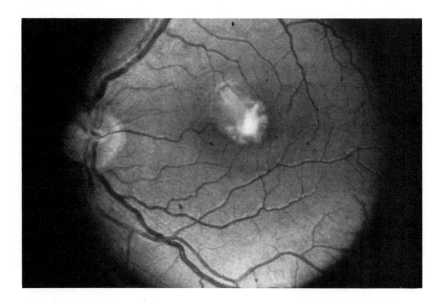

Figure 5–23. The "egg yolk" pattern in the macula associated with vitelliform dystrophy.

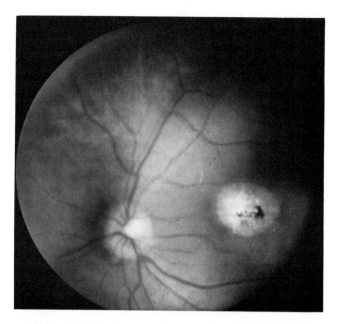

Figure 5–24. The "egg yolk" pattern has been scrambled, resulting in vision reduction in this case of vitelliform dystrophy.

Signs and Symptoms. Vitelliform dystrophy is a disease that has a fundus appearance much more dramatic than the resultant acuity loss until the later stages. Fundus changes occur in the first to second decades, with only a slight reduction in acuity. Vision is usually maintained at a fairly good level until later life.

Fluorescein angiography demonstrates hypofluorescence early within the areas of yellow material accumulation. As the RPE breaks down, hyperfluorescence will occur. Should leakage or neovascularization occur, fluorescein angiography will reflect these changes. The ERG will be normal to minimally abnormal, while the EOG is always abnormal. The EOG is the definitive test even in heterozygous carriers. Color vision will be compromised concordant with vision loss. Central scotomas will vary depending on the stage of the disease.

Prognosis and Management. While visual acuity remains in the minimally compromised zone (20/30 to 20/50) for many years, with degeneration of the vitelliform lesion vision drops to below 20/100. Complications such as hemorrhage and neovascularization can also result in decreased visual acuity.

Pedigree analysis and genetic counseling are important in this autosomal dominant disease. This is one condition in which a heterozygous carrier can be determined by EOG in spite of the lack of funduscopic changes.

From a clinicopathological standpoint, it is thought that the RPE is the focus of the disease process. Material (possibly lipofusion) accumulates in the RPE cells, resulting in malfunction, atrophy, and eventual loss of photoreceptor function. The abnormal EOG characteristic of vitelliform dystrophy supports the hypothesis of a widespread RPE disease.

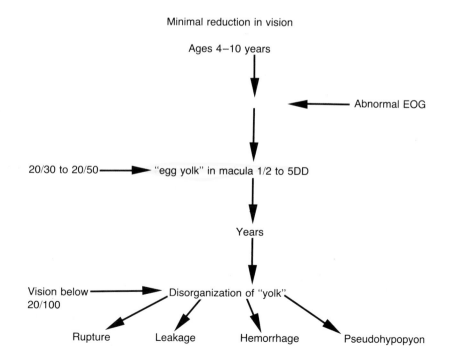

Figure 5–25. A flow chart illustrating the development of ocular changes in vitelliform dystrophy.

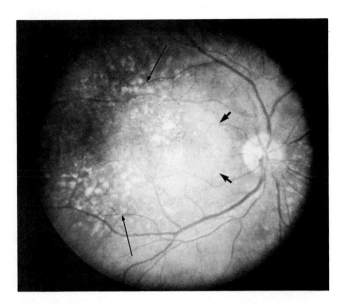

Figure 5–26. In this photograph the small broad arrows outline the area of RPE degeneration in the macular area associated with dominant drusen. The small thin arrows point to the large dominant drusen.

VITELLIFORM DYSTROPHY—PEARLS

- Inherited as autosomal dominant with variability
- Fundus signs start as 1/2 to 5DD egg yolk in macula that scrambles over many years
- Yolk may rupture, leak, hemorrhage, create pseudo-hypopyon
- Key sign is abnormal EOG even before vision loss
- Vision loss later with central scotoma
- Management
  - Pedigree analysis
  - Genetic counseling
  - Low-vision rehabilitation

Dominant Drusen (Doyne's Honeycomb Dystrophy)

Introduction. Dominant drusen is a condition that is inherited in an autosomal dominant pattern with variable penetrance and variable expressivity. The drusen usually present in the posterior pole and are contrasted with "senile type" drusen that result from age-related degeneration of the RPE. Dominant drusen present within the first three decades and progress to include the macular area, resulting in decreased vision by the fifth to sixth decade.

Appearance and Layers Involved. Initially, the dominant drusen appear as irregular white dots in or near the macula at the layer of the RPE (Figs. 5–26 and 5–27). With age, the drusen increase in number and enlarge. The drusen decrease in size as they become more remote to the macula. In addition to enlarging, the drusen become more confluent and often develop associated RPE hyperplasia. Eventually the drusen calcify, and the RPE atrophies, resulting in a white plaque in the macular zone. **See color plate 78.**

As the RPE/Bruch's barrier is compromised, there is the strong possibility of the development of sensory retina and/or RPE detachments, choroidal neovascularization, and/or disciform maculopathy.

From a clinicopathological standpoint, dominant drusen result from a faulty RPE. There appears to be an inherited faulty metabolic process in the RPE. Deposition of acid mucopolysaccharide and cerebroside develops as the result of the RPE dystrophy. The RPE cells then become grossly ab-

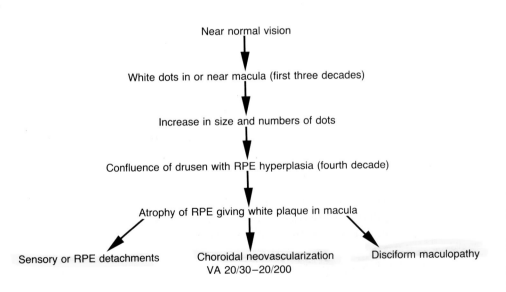

Figure 5–27. A flow chart illustrating the stages of development in dominant drusen.

Near normal vision

White dots in or near macula (first three decades)

Increase in size and numbers of dots

Confluence of drusen with RPE hyperplasia (fourth decade)

Atrophy of RPE giving white plaque in macula

Sensory or RPE detachments

Choroidal neovascularization VA 20/30–20/200

Disciform maculopathy

normal, creating compromise of the blood retinal barrier and the overlying photoreceptors.

Signs and Symptoms. The symptoms of dominant drusen are metamorphopsia and loss of central vision and usually do not present until after the fourth decade. Final acuity can vary between 20/30 to worse than 20/200. Color vision is affected, and central scotomas present as drusen accumulate. Fluorescein angiography best demonstrates the loss of RPE by gross areas of hyperfluorescence. The ERG is normal to minimally abnormal, and the EOG is subnormal in the later stages but not as dramatic as in vitelliform dystrophy. Should choroidal neovascularization occur, signs and symptoms associated with that process will present.

Prognosis and Management. Final visual acuity is unpredictable in cases of dominant drusen because of incomplete penetrance and variable expressivity. Should choroidal neovascularization develop, prognosis becomes more grim. At this point intervention with laser photocoagulation should be considered.

Pedigree analysis, genetic counseling, and low-vision consultation when appropriate are indicated in patients with dominant drusen.

DOMINANT DRUSEN—PEARLS

- Inherited as autosomal dominant with variability
- White dots in or near macula that enlarge, become confluent, and may form a plaque in macula
- May also precipitate "wet" maculopathy
- Vision loss, central scotomas, metamorphopsia
- Management
  - Pedigree analysis
  - Genetic counseling
  - Low-vision rehabilitation
  - Laser intervention in "wet" maculopathies

Central Areolar Choroidal Dystrophy

Introduction. Central areolar choroidal dystrophy (CACD) has been described as having both an AD and AR inheritance pattern. There is considerable confusion regarding this condition, as clinical presentation is dramatically variable. At times, only the choriocapillaris is involved, while other cases show involvement deep into the choroid. CACD rarely occurs before the age of 30 years and usually presents after the age of 40 years.

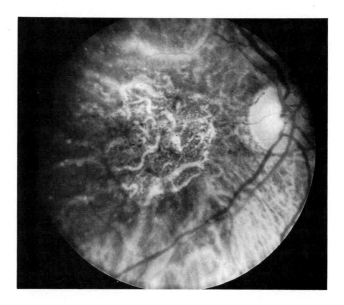

Figure 5–28. A photograph illustrating one stage in the development of an areolar choroidal dystrophy. Note atrophy of the RPE, choriocapillaris, and choroid in the macular area.

Appearance and Layers Involved. The earliest fundus changes that present in CACD are areas of RPE stippling in and around the macula (Figs. 5–28 and 5–29). These areas progress to atrophy of the RPE and choriocapillaris in a sharply outlined zone in the fovea or around it. The RPE may clump, but this is rare. The further atrophy of the deeper vessels may occur, and the lesion may enlarge and expand with time. The atrophic area is excavated with stereoscopic observation. Optic disc atrophy and vessel attenuation have been reported but only in isolated cases. The fundus appearance is usually bilateral and symmetrical. From a clinicopathological standpoint, it appears that chorio-

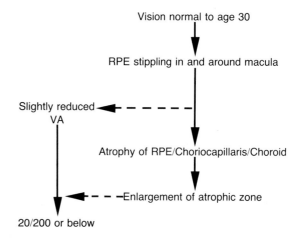

Figure 5–29. A flow chart illustrating the stages of development of central areolar choroidal dystrophy.

capillaris atrophy exists with subsequent RPE loss and sensory retinal atrophy.

Signs and Symptoms. The primary symptom of CACD is reduced vision presenting from age 30 to 40 years, with a slow progression to 20/200 or below with further aging. Color vision loss and central scotomas are related to degree of destruction. Fluorescein angiography shows hyperfluorescence early in the disease, with eventual loss of choriocapillaris flow. The ERG and EOG is normal to minimally abnormal.

Prognosis and Management. The patient with CACD has a poor prognosis for visual acuity, as eventually acuity drops to below 20/200. The peripheral vision is, however, retained, which improves the changes of rehabilitation with low-vision devices. Genetic counseling is again in order.

CENTRAL AREOLAR CHOROIDAL DYSTROPHY—PEARLS

- Inherited as AD and AR
- Starts as RPE stippling in and around macula with continued atrophy of RPE/choriocapillaris/choroid
- Reduced acuity, pericentral and central scotomas
- Management
  - Pedigree analysis
  - Genetic counseling
  - Low-vision rehabilitation

Notes on a Variant—Total Choroidal Vascular Atrophy

Total choroidal vascular atrophy (TVCA) is inherited in an AD manner. TVCA begins at birth with a large area of choroidal atrophy in the temporal retina. Over the next 10 to 15 years the lesion enlarges, with finger projections to the equator. Next, the process begins in the nasal retina until the entire fundus is involved to the equator. The entire retina to the equator, except for small strips extending inferior and superior from the disc, is involved by the third or fourth decades of life. Since the condition begins at birth, nystagmus may be a sign. Genetic counseling is in order, and low vision rehabilitation has minimal success.

Rod Monochromatism (Stationary Congenital Cone Dystrophy; Complete Achromatopsia)

Introduction. Rod monochromatism is the most common and most visually debilitating of the stationary congenital cone dystrophies. The condition is inherited in an AR manner, with an incidence of about 3 per 100,000. Rod monochromatism is also known as complete achromatopsia.

Appearance and Layers Involved. See color plate 84. In the case of rod monochromatism, the fundus is usually normal in appearance (Fig. 5–30). Foveal reflexes may be absent, and mild pigment stippling may occur. This is a disease in which there is either a congenital absence of cones or the presence of abnormal photoreceptors.

Signs and Symptoms. Signs and symptoms are the key to the diagnosis in rod monochromatism. Photophobia is a key symptom. Pendular nystagmus is present. Decreased vision is invariable, usually to below 20/200. Color vision tests are abnormal, and the photopic ERG is decreased. The scotopic ERG is normal to only slightly abnormal. Fluorescein angiography is normal, and visual fields are often unattainable because of the nystagmus.

Prognosis and Management. Symptoms improve with age, and nystagmus may often minimize. The condition is stationary. Low-vision rehabilitation is in order, and dark glasses may be prescribed to minimize the photophobia. Pedigree analyses and genetic counseling are recommended.

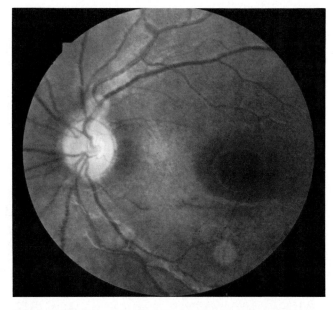

Figure 5–30. A photograph of the fundus of a patient known to have rod monochromatism. This photo illustrates that there are no readily demonstrable retinal/choroidal changes by ophthalmoscopy.

Clinical Note on a Variant— Incomplete Rod Monochromatism

In incomplete rod monochromatism, visual acuity is in the 20/40 to 20/100 range, with less severe photophobia and nystagmus. The ERG may demonstrate a minimal waveform, and color vision may be present.

Progressive Cone Dystrophies (Incomplete Achromatopsia)

Introduction. Progressive cone dystrophies are characterized by severe color vision problems that are inconsistent with the corresponding loss in vision. Heredity is considered AD, but recessive and X-linked forms have also been reported. The condition is considered to be congenital.

Appearance and Layers Involved. The most common type of fundus lesion is the "bull's eye" zone of atrophic RPE surrounding a central homogenous darker zone in the macula (Fig. 5–31). In the AR varieties there may be a diffuse pigment stippling in the posterior pole with pigment clumps. The RPE may, at times, atrophy along with the choroid. Optic atrophy and vessel attenuation are also findings in this condition.

Retinal changes may occur away from the macula in the form of flecks similar to fundus flavimaculatus or bone-spicule clumping similar to RP.

Clinicopathological findings in progressive cone dystrophy are rare. It appears that there is a loss of the outer nuclear layer of rods and cones with RPE changes.

Signs and Symptoms. Patients with progressive cone dystrophy usually have vision reduced to 20/60 to 20/100 in the first to second decades of life with a prior history of "near normal" vision. Photophobia is often severe, and a fine micronystagmus may be present that is only visible with slit lamp or by fine oscillations of the fundus view with direct ophthalmoscopy. When central vision falls to 20/40 to 20/60, marked color-vision abnormalities occur. Central scotomas are invariable. Myopia and astigmatism also appear to be common findings.

The fluorescein angiography demonstrates a classical "bull's eye" hyperfluorescent ring that may actually demonstrate some fine areas of leakage. The photopic ERG is abnormal, and the scotopic ERG is normal to slightly abnormal. In a certain subgroup there is a supernormal scotopic ERG that occurs with a flash of moderate intensity. The EOG may be abnormal if midperipheral RPE demonstrates dystrophic changes. It should be noted that the detection of a photopic ERG, however small, is a sign that dysfunction is incomplete and that the prognosis is slightly improved.

Prognosis and Management. In progressive cone dystrophies, vision usually decreases to 20/200 or worse over several years and then stabilizes. Photophobia is a problem that can be managed by dark glasses. Low-vision rehabilitation is very useful in progressive cone dystrophy. Pedigree analysis and genetic counseling are of utmost importance.

Table 5–7 summarizes the characteristics of hereditary retinal/choroidal disease primarily affecting central and color vision.

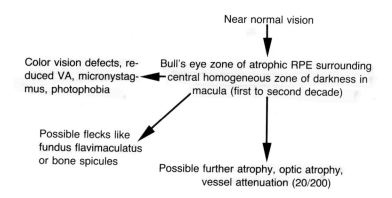

Figure 5–31. A flow chart illustrating the stages in the development of progressive cone dystrophy.

TABLE 5–7. HEREDITARY RETINAL/CHOROIDAL DISEASE PRIMARILY AFFECTING CENTRAL AND COLOR VISION

	Heredity	Mean Age Onset	Progressive/ Stationary	Signs/ Symptoms	ERG	EOG	Fundus Appearance	Visual Fields
Stargardt's	AR	First to second decades	Progressive	Color vision loss, vision loss	Normal to abnormal	Normal to abnormal	Loss of foveal reflex, then zone of normal retina surrounded by RPE changes; slimed fovea then progresses to 2-DD oval beaten bronze, fundus flavimaculatus surrounds macula	Central scotoma
Vitelliform dystrophy (Best's)	AD with variability	First decade	Progressive	Color vision loss, vision loss	Normal to abnormal	Abnormal[a]	½DD–5DD "egg yolk" in macula; may scramble giving rupture, hemorrhage, pseudohypopyon	Central scotoma
Dominant drusen (Doyne's)	AD with variability	First three decades	Progressive	Vision loss, metamorphopsia	Normal to abnormal	Abnormal in late stages	White dots in or near macula that increase in size and become confluent; macular plaque or wet maculopathy	Central scotoma
CACD	AD, AR	Third to fifth decades	Progressive	Vision loss	Normal to abnormal	Normal to abnormal	RPE stippling in and around macula, then atrophy of RPE/ choriocapillaris in macula	Pericentral and central scotomas
Rod monochromatism	AR	Congenital	Stationary	Photophobia, nystagmus, vision loss, color vision loss	Abnormal	Normal to abnormal	Normal fundus with possible loss of foveal reflex	N/A
Progressive cone dystrophy	AD, possible AR, X-linked	First to second decade	Progressive	Photophobia, micronystagmus, color vision loss, reduced VA	Abnormal	Normal to abnormal	Bull's eye zone of RPE atrophy surrounding dark macula, possible disc pallor and vessel attenuation and further macular atrophy	N/A

[a]Definitive diagnostic test

AR, autosomal recessive; AD, autosomal dominant

PROGRESSIVE CONE DYSTROPHIES—PEARLS

- Inherited as AD but possible AR and X-linked
- Bull's eye zone of atrophic RPE surrounding central homogeneous dark macula
- Possible further macular atrophy, optic atrophy, vessel attenuation, possible midperiphery flecks/spicules
- Photophobia, micronystagmus, color vision loss, reduced vision, altered electrodiagnosis
- Management
  - Pedigree analysis
  - Genetic counseling
  - Low-vision rehabilitation
  - Sun lenses for photophobia

Albinism

General. Albinism is a broad term that refers to a group of genetically determined disorders of the melanin pigmentary system. Albinism is characterized by congenital hypopigmentation of the hair, skin, and eyes. Ocular characteristics include nystagmus, foveal hypoplasia, photophobia, and reduced visual acuity. Albinoidism refers to conditions of hypopigmentation with normal visual acuity and no nystagmus. Oculocutaneous albinism is characterized by hypopigmentation of the hair, skin, and eyes and is inherited as AR in all but one AD form. Ocular albinism is characterized by hypopigmentation (Fig. 5–32) limited to ocular structures and inherited as an X-linked and AR manner. The prevalence of albinism is estimated at approximately one in 20,000 worldwide.

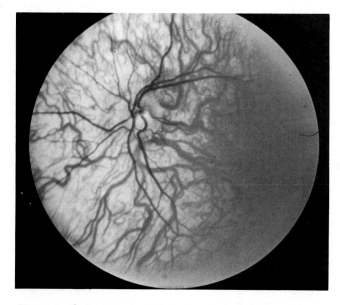

Figure 5–32. A photograph illustrating the fundus hypopigmentation characteristic of albinism and its effects on the ocular system.

Appearance and Layers Involved, Signs and Symptoms. See color plate 84. **Appearance of the types of oculocutaneous and ocular albinism vary considerably and are best described by Tables 5–8 and 5–9.** Characteristics common in all forms of albinism include (1) nystagmus present at birth that may lessen as the child grows older; (2) reduced visual acuity; (3) foveal hypoplasia (absence of foveal reflex); (4) iris translucency by globe transillumination and/or slit lamp retroillumination; (5) fundus hypopigmentation; (6) a high incidence of strabismus; (7) normal color vision; (8) photophobia; (9) tendencies toward cancerous and precancerous skin lesions; (10) high refractive errors; and (11) supernormal ERG and EOG due to light scatter.

Albinoidism is differentiated from oculocutaneous albinism (OCA) and ocular albinism (OA) by the absence of nystagmus and photophobia and usually by the lack of reduced vision. There is a generalized hypopigmentation of the skin or skin and eyes, without the foveal hypoplasia. Albinoidism is often associated with deafness.

The genesis of the basic defects surround a defect in melanogenesis before birth. This appears to be related to an abnormality in tyrosinase, which is a copper-containing enzyme. Without the presence of melanin in the pigment cells, there develops an anomalous routing of neurons to the brain from the eye as well as an anomaly in the development of the fovea (foveal hypoplasia). Similar developmental anomalies occur in the auditory system. With foveal hypoplasia, there is reduced vision and nystagmus. In most humans, 45 percent to 50 percent of optic nerve fibers remain uncrossed at the chiasm, that is, temporal retinal nerve fibers remain uncrossed. In the albino the majority of nerve fibers originating in the temporal retina decussate at the chiasm, resulting in a transfer of abnormal field representations to the visual cortex. This crossing results in abnormal hemifield VEP responses and creates a situation in which there is a poor anatomical substrate for the development of efficient binocular vision. This decussation of temporal fibers does not appear to occur in patients without nystagmus.

Prognosis and Management. Since OCA and OA are congenital, resulting in nystagmus, the clinician must deal with reduced vision from the onset. The nystagmus and reduced vision tend to improve with age, but the basic problem of a visual handicap always exists.

The clinician is responsible for providing the best possible refraction. It should be emphasized that near vision is often better than distance vision because of the convergence-induced reduction of

TABLE 5–8. VARIATIONS IN OCA

	Inheritance	Skin	Hair	Eyes	Vision	Eye Signs/Symptoms	Systemic Problems
Tyrosinase-negative OCA	AR	Pink, no freckles	Snow white	Iris translucency, foveal hypoplasia	20/200	Severe photophobia, nystagmus, strabismus	
Platinum OCA	AR	Pink	Cream/Platinum	Iris translucency, foveal hypoplasia, possible small amount pigment in iris	20/200–20/400	Photophobia, nystagmus, strabismus	
Yellow mutant OCA	AR	Whites—cream to yellow with capacity to tan; blacks—dark cream with nevi	Whites—yellow to red hair; blacks—dark yellow to red hair	Early iris translucency with pigment accumulation in a cartwheel by age 3 years, foveal hypoplasia, reduced fundus pigment	Improves with age but still reduced 20/200	Mild photophobia, mild nystagmus	
Tyrosinase-positive OCA, pigment accumulates with age	AR	Pink at birth but freckles, nevi, and tanning with age	White at birth but yellow to tan with age	Iris translucency is variable with cartwheel pattern, foveal hypoplasia, reduced fundus pigment	20/60–20/120	Mild photophobia, mild nystagmus	
Hermansky-Pudlak syndrome	AR—Puerto Ricans	Variable	Variable	Iris translucency, foveal hypoplasia	20/100–20/300	Nystagmus, photophobia	Hemorrhagic diathesis, lung disease
Chédiak-Higashi syndrome	AR	Creamy white with patches of slate grey	Light brown with metallic sheen	Variable with reduced pigment, foveal hypoplasia	Variable reduction	Variable nystagmus and photophobia	Susceptibility to gram-positive infection, malignancies
Rufous (red) OCA	AR	Red	White to black	Mild to absent iris translucency, fovea, hypoplasia	Variable reduction	Nystagmus (66%), photophobia	
AD OCA	AD	Pink but variable	White but variable	Marked iris translucency, foveal hypoplasia	Variable reduction	Nystagmus, photophobia	

AR, autosomal recessive; AD, autosomal dominant

TABLE 5–9. VARIATIONS IN OA

	Inheritance	Skin	Hair	Eyes	Vision	Eye Signs/Symptoms	Systemic Problems
X-linked OA	X-linked affected males	Normal but lighter than sibs, spots of hypopigment	Normal but lighter than sibs	Iris translucency, foveal hypoplasia, reduced fundus pigment, not apparent in blacks	20/80 or less	Photophobia, nystagmus strabismus	
	Heterozygous females	Normal	Normal	Hypopigmented and hyperpigmented spots in fundus, iris translucency	Usually normal	Usually none	
Forsius-Eriksson syndrome	X-linked affected males	Normal	Normal	Iris translucency, foveal hypoplasia, reduced fundus pigment	Reduced but variable	Protan color blind, nystagmus, astigmatism, axial myopia, photophobia	
AR OA	AR	Normal but lighter than sibs	Normal but lighter than sibs	Iris translucency, foveal hypoplasia, reduced fundus pigment	Reduced but variable	Nystagmus, photophobia	
OA–lentigenes—deafness	AD	Normal	Normal	Iris translucency, foveal hypoplasia, reduced fundus pigment	Reduced	Nystagmus, photophobia	Cutaneous lentigenes, deafness, imbalance

AR, autosomal recessive; AD, autosomal dominant

nystagmus. As with many patients with nystagmus, *the use of a reading addition at all ages may improve performance.* The photophobia accompanying OCA and OA may be managed by using tinted sun lenses or prescription sun lenses.

From a systemic standpoint, it is important to advise the patient regarding dermatological protection against cancerous and precancerous U-V induced lesions as well as to alert to life-threatening syndromes that may be associated with albinism. Pedigree analysis and genetic counseling are also indicated in all cases of albinism.

ALBINISM—PEARLS

- Inherited as AR, AD, X-linked
- Oculocutaneous albinism appears as hypopigmented hair, skin, and eyes with foveal hypoplasia; patients have nystagmus, photophobia, and reduced vision
- Ocular albinism appears as normal colored hair and skin but with hypopigmented eyes with foveal hypoplasia; patients have nystagmus, photophobia, and variably reduced vision
- Albinoidism refers to hypopigmentation of skin or skin and eyes without foveal hypoplasia or reduced vision
- Management
  - Pedigree analysis
  - Genetic counseling
  - Provision of best prescription and tinted lenses
  - Possible reading addition
  - Protect against skin cancer
  - Rule out systemic diseases

REFERENCES

Albert DM, Pruett RC, Craft JL: Transmission microscopic observations of vitreous abnormalities in retinitis pigmentosa. *Am J Ophthalmol* 1986; 101:665–672.

Alexander LJ: Diseases of the retina, Barlett JD, Jaanus SD (eds): in *Clinical Ocular Pharmacology.* Boston, Buttersworth, 1984.

Alexander KR, Fishman GA: Supernormal scotopic ERG in cone dystrophy. *Br J Ophthalmol* 1984; 68:69–78.

Auerbach E, Merin S: Achromatopsia with amblyopia. A clinical and electroretinographic study of 39 cases. *Doc Ophthalmol* 1974; 37:79–117.

Bastiaensen LA, Hoefnagels KL: Patterned anomalies of the retinal pigment epithelium: Dystrophy or syndrome. *Doc Ophthalmol* 1983; 55:17–29.

Bloome MA, Garcia CA: *Manual of Retinal and Choroidal Dystrophies.* New York, Appleton-Century-Crofts, 1982.

Carr RE: Congenital stationary night blindness. *Trans Am Ophthalmol Soc* 1977;72:498.

Carr RE, Siegel IM: *Visual Electrodiagnostic Testing. A Practical Guide for the Clinician.* Baltimore, Williams & Wilkins, 1972.

Cibis GW, Morey M, Harris DJ: Dominantly inherited macular dystrophy with flecks (Stargardt's). *Arch Ophthalmol* 1980;98:1785–1789.

Cortin P, Archer D. Maumenee IH, et al: Patterned macular dystrophy with yellow plaques and atrophic changes. *Br J Ophthalmol* 1980; 64:127–134.

Cotlier E, Maumenee IH, Berman ER: *Genetic Eye Diseases. Retinitis Pigmentosa and Other Inherited Eye Disorders.* New York, Alan R. Liss, 1982.

Deutman AF: Electro-oculography in families with vitelliform dystrophy of the fovea. *Arch Ophthalmol* 1969; 81:305–316.

Deutman AF, Jensen LM: Dominantly inherited drusen of Bruch's membrane. *Br J Ophthalmol* 1970; 54:373–381.

Eagle RC, Lucier AC, Bernardino V, Yanoff M: Retinal pigment epithelial abnormalities in fundus flavimaculatus. *Ophthalmology* 1980; 81:1189–1200.

Fetkenhour CL, Gurney N, Dobbie JG, Chromokos E: Central areolar pigment epithelial dystrophy. *Am J Ophthalmol* 1976; 81:745–753.

Fishman GA: Fundus flavimaculatus. *Arch Ophthalmol* 1976;94:2061–2067.

Fishman GA, Farber M, Patel BS, Derlacki DJ: Visual acuity loss in patients with Stargardt's macular dystrophy. *Ophthalmology* 1987;94:809–814.

Fishman GA, Rhee AJ, Blair NP: Blood-retinal barrier function in patients with cone or cone-rod dystrophy. *Arch Ophthalmol* 1986;104:545–548.

Fishman GA, Weinberg AB, McMahon TT: X-linked recessive retinitis pigmentosa. Clinical characteristics of carriers. *Arch Ophthalmol* 1986;104:1329–1335.

Foxman SG, Heckenlively JR, Bateman JB, Wirtshafter JD: Classification of congenital and early onset retinitis pigmentosa. *Arch Ophthalmol* 1985;103:1502–1506.

Franceschetti A, Francois J, Babel J: *Chorioretinal Heredodegenerations.* Springfield, Ill, Thomas, 1974.

Francois J, DeRouck A, Cambie E, DeLacy JJ: Visual functions in pericentral and central pigmentary retinopathies. *Ophthalmologica* 1972; 165:38–61.

Fraser HB, Wallace DC: Sorsby's familial pseudoinflammatory macular dystrophy. *Am J Ophthalmol* 1971;71:1216–1220.

Giuffrie G, Lodato G: Vitelliform dystrophy and pattern dystrophy of the retinal pigment epithelium. *Br J Ophthalmol* 1986;70:526–532.

Goldberg MF: *Genetic and Metabolic Eye Disease.* Boston, Little, Brown, 1974.

Gutman I, Walsh JB, Henkind P: Vitelliform macular dystrophy and butterfly-shaped epithelial dystrophy: A continuum? *Br J Ophthalmol* 1982;66:170–173.

Hadden OB, Gass JDM: Fundus flavimaculatus and Stargardt's disease. *Am J Ophthalmol* 1976;82:527–539.

Heckenlively JR, Weleber RG: X-linked recessive cone dystrophy with tapetal-like sheen. A newly recognized entity with Mizuo-Kurimoto phenomenon. *Arch Ophthalmol* 1986;104:1322–1328.

Hsieh RC, Fine BS, Lyons JS: Patterned dystrophies of the retinal pigment epithelium. *Arch Ophthalmol* 1977;95:429–435.

Kandori T, Tamia A, Watanabe T, Unilateral pigmentary degeneration of the retina. *Am J Ophthalmol* 1968;66:1091–1101.

Kinnear PE, Jay B, Witkop CJ: Albinism. *Surv Ophthalmol* 1985;30:75–98.

Krill AE: Retinitis pigmentosa: A review. *Sightsav Rev* 1972;42:21–28.

Krill AE: *Hereditary Retinal and Choroidal Diseases.* Hagerstown, Md, Harper and Row, 1972, vol. 1, p. 1.

Krill AE: *Hereditary Retinal and Choroidal Diseases.* Hagerstown, Md, Harper and Row, 1977, vol 2, p. 355.

Krill AE, Archer D, Marpin D: Sector retinitis pigmentosa. *Am J Ophthalmol* 1970;69:677–687.

Krill AE, Archer D: Classification of the choroidal atrophies. *Am J Ophthalmol* 1971;72:562–583.

Krill AE, Fold MR: Retinitis punctata albescens. *Am J Ophthalmol* 1962;53:450–454.

Krill AE, Deutman AF, Fishman M: The cone degenerations. *Docum Ophthalmol* 1973;35:1–80.

Kurstjens JH: Choroideremia and gyrate atrophy of the choroid and retina. *Doc Ophthalmol* 1965;19:1–122.

LaVail MM. Hollyfield JG, Anderson RE: *Retinal Degeneration. Experimental and Clinical Studies.* New York, Alan R. Liss, 1985.

Lesko JG, Lewis RA, Nussbaum RL: Multipoint linkage analysis of loci in the proximal long arm of the human x-chromosome: Application to mapping the choroideremia locus. *Am J Hum Genet* 1987;40:303–311.

Marmor MF: Vitelliform lesions in adults. *Ann Ophthalmol* 1979;11:1705–1712.

Marmor MF, Byers B: Pattern dystrophy of the pigment epithelium. *Am J Ophthalmol* 1977;84:32–44.

McDonnell PJ, Kivlin JD, Maumenee IH, Green WR: Fundus flavimaculatas without maculopathy. A clinicopathologic study. *Ophthalmology* 1986;93:116–119.

Newsome DA: Retinal fluorescein leakage in retinitis pigmentosa. *Am J Ophthalmol* 1986;101:354–360.

Newsome DA, Blacharski PA: Grid photocoagulation for macular edema in patients with retinitis pigmentosa. *Am J Ophthalmol* 1987;103:161–166.

Newsome DA, Stark WJ, Maumenee IH: Cataract extraction and intraocular lens implantation in patients with retinitis pigmentosa or Usher's syndrome. *Arch Ophthalmol* 1986;104:852–854.

Noble KC, Carr RE: Leber's congenital amaurosis. *Arch Ophthalmol* 1978;96:818–821.

Novack RL, Foos RY: Drusen of the optic disk in retinitis pigmentosa. *Am J Ophthalmol* 1987;103:44–47.

Patrinely JR, Lewis RA, Font RL: Foveomacular vitelliform dystrophy, adult type. A clinicopathologic study including electron microscopic observations. *Ophthalmology* 1985;92:1712–1718.

Piazza L, Fishman GA, Farber M, et al: Visual acuity loss in patients with Usher's syndrome. *Arch Ophthalmol* 1986;104:1336–1339.

Pinckers A, Craysberg JR: Pattern dystrophy of the retinal pigment epithelium. *Ophthalmic Paediatr Genet* 1986;7:35–43.

Prensky JG, Bresnick GH: Butterfly-shaped macular dystrophy in four generations. *Arch Ophthalmol* 1983;101:1198–1203.

Rabb MF, Tso MO, Fishman GA: Cone-rod dystrophy. A clinical and histopathologic report. *Ophthalmology* 1986;93:1443–1451.

Rabin J: Visual function in retinitis pigmentosa. *J Am Optom Assoc* 1986;57:840–842.

Rodrigues MM, Bardenstein D, Wiggert B, et al: Retinitis pigmentosa with segmental massive retinal gliosis. An immunohistochemical, biochemical, and ultrastructural study. *Ophthalmology* 1987;94:180–186.

Rodrigues MM, Wiggert B, Hackett J, et al: Dominantly inherited retinitis pigmentosa. Ultrastructure and biochemical analysis. *Ophthalmology* 1985;92:1165–1172.

Sheffield JB, Hilfer SR: *Hereditary and Visual Development.* New York, Springer-Verlag, 1985.

Takki K: Differential diagnosis between primary choroidal vascular atrophies. *Br J Ophthalmol* 1974;58:24–35.

Thompson JS, Thompson MW: *Genetics in Medicine,* ed 4. Philadelphia, WB Saunders, 1986.

Uliss AE, Gregor ZJ, Bird AC: Retinitis pigmentosa and retinal neovascularization. *Ophthalmology* 1986;93:1599–1603.

Vannas-Sulonen K, Sipila I, Vannas A, et al: Gyrate atrophy of the choroid and retina. A five year follow-up of creatine supplementation. *Ophthalmology* 1985;92:1719–1721.

Watzke RC, Folk JC, Lang RM: Pattern dystrophy of the retinal pigment epithelium. *Ophthalmology* 1982;89:1400–1406.

Appendix

ICD CODES

GLAUCOMA

Condition	ICD
Glaucoma—acute angle closure	365.22
Glaucoma—low tension	365.12
Glaucoma—pigmentary	365.13
Pigmentary dispension of iris	364.53
Glaucoma—primary open angle	365.11
Glaucoma—secondary to inflammation	365.62
File with anterior uveitis	364.00
Peripheral anterior synechiae	364.71
Peripheral posterior synechiae	364.71
Glaucoma—secondary to pseudoexfoliation	365.52
File with pseudoexfoliation	366.11
Glaucoma—steroid induced	365.31
Glaucoma—subacute angle closure	365.23
Glaucoma—suspect	365.00
Glaucoma—trauma	365.65
File with iridodialysis	364.76
File with hyphema	364.41
File with angle recession	364.77
File with contusion	921.30
Glaucoma—vascular	365.63
File with rubeosis	364.42
Glaucomatocyclitic crisis	364.22

MACULA

Condition	ICD
APMPPE	363.15
Age-related maculopathy—dry	362.51
Age-related maculopathy—wet	362.52
Angioid streaks	363.43
Choroidal rupture	363.63
Choroidal sclerosis	363.40
Cystoid macular edema	362.53
Degenerative myopia	360.21
Drusen—retinal degenerative	362.57
ICSC	362.41
Macular hole, lamellar hole	362.54
Toxic maculopathy	362.55

OPTIC NERVE

Condition	ICD
Autosomal dominant optic atrophy	377.15
Coloboma—optic nerve	
Acquired	377.23
Congenital	743.57
Compression—optic nerve	377.49
Demyelinizing optic neuropathy	377.32
Drusen—optic nerve	377.21
Inflammatory optic neuropathy	377.31
Ischemic optic neuropathy	377.41
Megalopapilla	377.20
Oblique (tilted) disc	377.90
Optic atrophy	377.10
Papilledema	377.00
Pigmentation	743.57
Pit—optic nerve	377.22
Pseudopapilledema	377.24
Toxic optic neuropathy	377.34

RETINA

Condition	ICD
Atrophic hole without detachment	361.31
Commotio retina	921.30
Detachment with dialysis	361.04
Detachment with giant tear	361.03
Detachment—old delimited	361.06
Detachment—rhegmatogenous with defect	361.00
Detachment of RPE	362.42
Detachment of RPE—hemorrhage	362.43
Detachment—serous without defect	361.20
Detachment—traction	361.81
Horseshoe tear without detachment	361.32
Lattice degeneration	362.63
Melanoma	
Choroid benign	224.6
Choroid malignant	190.6
Retina benign	224.5
Retina malignant	190.5
Multiple retinal defects without detachment	361.33
Pavingstone degeneration	362.61
Peripheral retinal degeneration	362.60
Posterior staphyloma	379.12
Reticular degeneration	362.64
Retinal break	361.30
Retinal coloboma	743.56
Retinal pigment acquired	362.74
Retinal pigment congenital	743.53
Retinoschisis	361.10
Retinoschisis—flat	361.11
Retinoschisis—bullous	361.12
Secondary vitreo retinal degeneration	362.66

RETINAL CHOROIDAL DYSTROPHIES

Condition	ICD
Achromatopsia	368.54
Albinism	270.20
Areolar choroidal dystrophy	363.53
Choroideremia	363.55
Dominant drusen	362.77
Fundus flavimaculatus	362.76
Geographic helicoid	363.52
Gyrate	363.54
Hereditary choroidal dystrophy unspecified	363.50
Hereditary retinal dystrophy unspecified	362.70
Juvenile (congenital) retinoschisis	362.73
Night blindness	368.60
Nystagmus unspecified	379.50
Oguchi's disease	368.61
Progressive cone-rod dystrophy	362.75
Retinitis pigmentosa	362.74
Stargardt's disease	362.75
Vitelliform	362.76

RETINAL INFLAMMATORY DISEASE

Condition	ICD
Chorioretinal scars	363.30
Chorioretinitis (disseminated)	363.10
Chorioretinitis (focal)	363.00
Chorioretinitis (unspecified)	363.20
Histoplasmosis	
Systemic	115.02
Choroidal neovascular net	362.16
Retinal pigment epithelial detachment	362.42
Serous retinal detachment	361.20
Pars planitis	363.21
Sarcoidosis	
Systemic	135.00
Chorioretinitis	363.00
Iritis	364.00
Periphlebitis	362.18
Toxocariasis	
Systemic	128.00
Ocular	363.03
Toxoplasmosis	
Systemic	130.20
Acquired	130.20
Chorioretinitis	363.00
Congenital	771.20
Iritis	364.00
Juxtapapillary	363.01
Optic nerve	377.30

RETINAL VASCULAR DISEASE

Condition	ICD
Angiomatosis retinae	362.17/759.60
Blind hypotensive eye	360.41
Blind hypertensive eye	360.42
Beçhet's disease	362.30
Branch retinal artery occlusion	362.32
Branch retinal vein occlusion	362.36
Cavernous hemangioma	228.03
Central retinal artery occlusion	362.31
Central retinal vein occlusion	362.35
Coat's disease	362.12
Diabetes	250.50
Background diabetic retinopathy	362.01
Proliferative diabetic retinopathy	362.02
Retinal hemorrhage	362.81
Retinal exudates	362.82
Retinal edema/cotton wool	362.83
Vascular tortuosity (acquired)	362.17
Retinal ischemia	362.84
Neovascularization retina/choroid	362.16
Eales' disease	362.18
Hollenhorst plaque	362.33
Hypertensive retinopathy	362.11
Incipient vascular occlusion	362.37
Neovascularization iris	364.42
Preretinal macular fibrosis	362.56
Proliferative retinopathy—other	362.20
Retinal periphlebitis	362.18
Retinopathy of prematurity	362.21
Telangiectasia	362.15
Vasculitis	362.18

VISUAL REHABILITATION

Condition	ICD
Abnormal ERG	794.12
Abnormal VER	794.13
Consultation complex	906.30
Hysterical blindness	300.11
Profound impairment, both eyes	369.00
Better eye: total impairment; lesser eye: total impairment	369.01
Better eye: near total impairment; lesser eye: total impairment	369.03
Better eye: near total impairment; lesser eye: near total impairment	369.04
Better eye: profound impairment; lesser eye: total impairment	369.06
Better eye: profound impairment; lesser eye: near total impairment	369.07
Better eye: profound impairment; lesser eye: profound impairment	369.08

Condition	ICD
Moderate or severe impairment; better eye, profound impairment lesser Eye	369.1
Better eye: severe impairment; lesser eye: total impairment	369.12
Better eye: severe impairment; lesser eye: near total impairment	369.13
Better eye: severe impairment; lesser eye: profound impairment	369.14
Better eye: moderate impairment; lesser eye: total impairment	369.16
Better eye: moderate impairment; lesser eye: near total impairment	369.17
Better eye: moderate impairment; lesser eye: profound impairment	369.18
Moderate or severe impairment, both eyes	369.2
Better eye: severe impairment; lesser eye: severe impairment	369.22
Better eye: moderate impairment; lesser eye: severe impairment	369.24
Better eye: moderate impairment; lesser eye: moderate impairment	369.25
Legal blindness as defined in United States	369.40
Profound impairment, one eye	369.60
Moderate or severe impairment, one eye	369.70

VISUAL FIELDS

Condition	ICD
Arcuate scotoma	368.43
Binasal hemianopsia	368.47
Bitemporal hemianopsia	368.47
Central scotoma	368.41
Chiasmal disorders	377.50
Conversion reaction	300.11
Defect—unspecified	368.40
Diplopia	368.20
Homonymous hemianopsia	368.46
Metamorphopsia	368.14
Paracentral scotoma	368.42
Stroke	
Unspecified	437.90
Aphasia	784.30
Agnosia	368.16
Dysphasia	784.50
Hemiplegia	342.90
Paralysis	344.90
Transient monocular blindness	368.12
Vision loss sudden	368.11
Visual cortex disorders	377.70
Visual pathway disorders	377.60

VITREOUS

Condition	ICD
Anomalies—vitreous congenital	743.57
Asteroid hyalosis	379.22
Degeneration/detachment	379.21
Floaters	379.24
Hemorrhage	379.23
Membranes	379.25
PHPV	379.29
Prolapse	379.26

Index